magic, myths and medicine

magic, myths and medicine

Richard Hunderfund
San Francisco State University

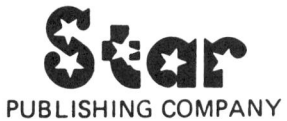
PUBLISHING COMPANY

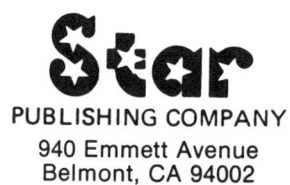

PUBLISHING COMPANY
940 Emmett Avenue
Belmont, CA 94002

Copyright © 1974 by Richard C. Hunderfund

Copyright © 1980, 1987 by Star Publishing Company

All rights reserved. No part of this publication may be reproduced, stored in an information storage and retrieval system, or transmitted, in any form or by any means, electronic, mechanical, photocopying, recording, or otherwise, without the prior written permission of the copyright owner.

Printed in the United States of America

Revised edition, 1987

ISBN: 0-89863-115-7

Contents

Pre-Historical Beliefs and Legends 1

Ancient Egypt – Kheme 7

The Hebrews and the Old Testament 35

Mesopotamia – The Land Between the Rivers 61

Ancient India 81

Ancient China 107

Crete – Mycenae – Greece – Rome 131

The New World 155

1500–Present. Explorations and Discoveries 195

New Diseases and Those Which Have Vanished 231

Index 235

pRE-hISTORICAL bELIEfS AnD LEGEnDS

The history of medicine begins somewhere in the past, beyond the written history of man, beyond even man himself. It has been postulated that the earth was formed approximately five billion years ago and that microoganisms were present more than three and one-half billion years ago. Amphibians developed about two hundred and fifty millions of years ago and man-like creatures, about three and one–half millions of years ago. Present man, *Homo sapiens,* appeared recently, about 100,000 years ago. Information concerning diseases can be found in the fossils, bones and the mummified remains of plants, animals and man. Paleopathologists can examine these remains from the past and frequently obtain information concerning diseases in antiquity. Fossil remains from the Age of the Amphibians are said to show lesions such as dental caries, bone fractures and evidences of parasitism. Evidences of diseases are lacking beyond this period.

The first attempts by animals to heal wounds or infections; the nonuse of an injured part of the body; the eating of certain vegetation; resting in the heat of the sun or the coolness of the shade; the special care (or destruction) of sick or injured offspring; these acts might all be thought of as the first attempts at the practice of medicine. These medicinal treatments can still be observed in our animal population and in primitive human cultures throughout the world.

The practice of medicine, for convenience, can be divided into several areas: infectious diseases; physiological diseases; treatment; prevention; and injuries.

Infectious diseases are those which are caused by parasites such as viruses, rickettsiae, bacteria, yeasts, molds, protozoans and worms. Examples are: influenza; Rocky Mountain spotted fever; typhoid fever; thrush; cryptococcosis; malaria and tapeworms. The infectious diseases may be passed directly from host to host, via fomites or may be transmitted by vectors such as mosquitos and flies. Physiological diseases are those malfunctions of the organisms which are not caused by infectious agents. Examples are hemophilia, diabetes, gout and arthritis. Injuries to organisms occur all the time; cuts, wounds and broken bones may lead to infection with an infectious agent which may cause death. In primitive cultures, diseases and injuries were prevented by the use of amulets, charms and spells. Today, they are prevented by Public Health methods and safety devices such as pedestrian crosswalks and automobile seat belts. The treatment of the sick or injured person has changed dramatically only in about the last one hundred years of man's history. The discovery of asepsis, microorganisms and "miracle drugs" has allowed the recovery of patients who, without treatment, would have normally died. These treatments were not available to primitive man. He had to rely mainly on his own body defence mechanisms to overcome the infection.

Primitive man must have observed that hitting, stabbing or choking another man or animal brought about either injury or death, depending on the location of the attack and the physical effort involved. There was no mystery about hitting something on the head with a club, or being hit oneself. However, this same primitive man might suddenly become hot (fever), become delirious and die. He might have strange fits periodically. He might suddenly fall to the ground, gasp for air and then die. What caused these strange events to occur? There were no wounds or broken bones.

Fortunately, there was someone around who could explain all these strange events. The interpreter might be given several different names such as seer, shaman, sorcerer, witch-doctor, witch, and medicine man. In advanced cultures, these persons have evolved into physicians, dentists, psychiatrists, members of various religious groups, faith-healers, chiropractors and others. These interpreters were certain skilled men and women who could treat cuts, wounds and broken bones and, when it came to an unknown condition, used magical powers to aid the afflicted. In general, primitive man (and modern man until the late 1800s) believed that sickness was caused by an evil spirit which had entered the body and, in order to bring about a cure, the evil spirit must be induced to leave. Various methods were used to bring this about which, in the majority, were not pleasant. Fire, water and obnoxious "medicines" were usually included in the treatment process or purification rite. However, the early physicians did have the following with which to treat their patients: amulets; charms; spells; herbs; amputations; fire (cauterization); opening the skull (trepanning); bleeding (phlebotomy); suction (cupping); leeches; fright and sewerage pharmacology.

The early history of man is shrouded by myths, legends and religious beliefs which were passed from person to person, and from generation to generation, orally, in story and song. Many tribes had a special person or persons who were responsible for remembering and retelling the history of the tribe. Eventually, with the discovery of writing, this information was recorded. Fortunately, some of these early records have survived, and it is from them that

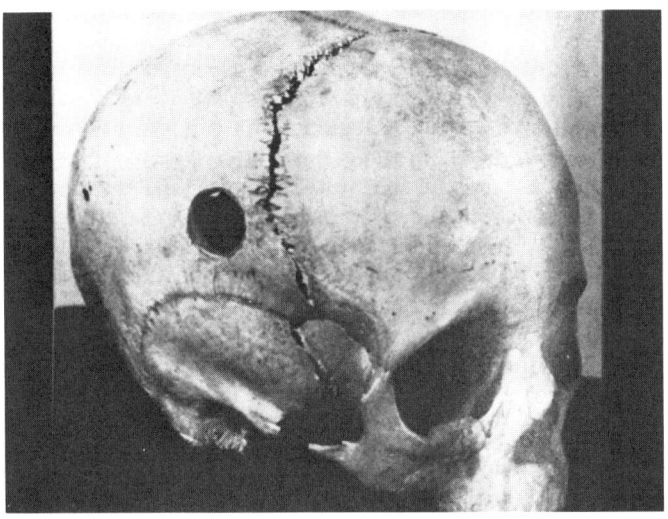

Trepanning was carried out in many ancient cultures to relieve pressure on the brain or to allow evil spirits to escape from the afflicted person. (Photograph courtesy of the National Museum of Anthropology and Archeology, Lima, Peru)

we can obtain knowledge concerning the practice of medicine in the early civilizations of the world: Ancient Egypt; Mesopotamia; India; China and later, Greece; Europe and North and South America.

Where did civilization, the act of living together in a community, develop? Many historians and archeologists believe that civilization began in the region of, what is today called, northern Iraq. One site investigated is believed to date back to 8000 B.C. By about 5000 B.C., agriculture had become widespread and some animals had been domesticated. Writing was developed by many cultures by about 3000 B.C. It would be very nice to say that from this region, civilization spread through the world. However, the subject is much too controversial to be handled in one small paragraph. How did the great civilizations of Ancient Egypt, India, China, Mexico and South America arise? More recently, in 1979, Fred Wendorf, U.S. Chief of a team that included scientists from Egypt and Poland, reported the discovery of grains of barley at a 17,000 year old Egyptian campsite near Aswan, U.A.R., which suggested that humans began practicing agriculture much earlier than had been thought. It is believed that these, and related discoveries, may place the origins of food production approximately 10,000 years earlier than previously thought.

There are legends and myths, both old and new, which tell of older civilizations. Churchward has popularized the legendary Pacific Ocean civilization in his books concerning the lost continent of Mu. He obtained his theory from translations of secret Naacal tablets which were hidden in a temple in India. Apparently, Mu had attained a very high state of civilization when it was suddenly destroyed by earthquakes and volcanic eruptions, and sunk beneath the waters of the Pacific Ocean. Scattered outposts of Mu survived, one of which was Atlantis. The legends concerning Atlantis are numerous and articles are still being published regularly, locating Atlantis off the Bahama Islands, off the Azores, off Spain and in the Mediterranean Sea. Wherever it was, the Ancient Egyptians knew about it because the Greek historian Solon obtained the information from them. This information was later popularized by Plato. Today, archeologists and historians believe that the Egyptian priests were actually relating the destruction of the Minoan Civilization which was brought about by the explosion of the volcanic island of Thera (Santorini) in the Mediterranean Sea. This had occurred about one thousand years earlier, in about 1500 B.C., but an extra zero had been included by the storyteller which caused the destruction to have occurred ten thousand years ago rather than one thousand years. However, there still are many people who do not believe this version of the story. In 1973, a large expedition from a University in the United States began explorations off the coast of Spain and Ireland for remnants of Atlantis, and recently, the Director of the Soviet Oceanology Institute reported finding, in the Atlantic Ocean, off Gibraltar, "ruins and a group of flat top mountains about 300 to 600 feet below the surface of the ocean."[1]

According to another legend, when Atlantis was destroyed, some of the inhabitants survived and traveled to other parts of the world. One of these survivors traveled to Ancient Egypt (Kheme), bringing knowledge and wisdom to the people. This man was Thoth. In the religion of Ancient Egypt, Thoth was one of the major Gods, the God of writing and science. According to legend, he composed 42 secret, sacred books which contained sections dealing with human anatomy, physiology, surgery and female ailments. He was also credited with many magical spells and charms and for the procedures used in the mummification of the dead.

The Ancient Egyptians also worshipped a God of Medicine, Imhotep. The Greeks later identified him with their God of Medicine, Aesculapuis. When dealing with myths and legends, one often wonders when the legend ends and truth begins. In this case, it was discovered that Imhotep, the God of Medicine, had been an actual person. He had been the Physician and Architect of King Djoser (Zoser) who had ruled Ancient Egypt in about 2780 B.C. He was responsible for the design and construction of the first large stone structure made by man, the famous step-pyramid of Djoser. He apparently was also very adept in medicine for he was so revered by the people of Ancient Egypt that he was eventually worshipped as a God. Thus we have Imhotep, the man, physician, architect and God, rescued by archeologists, historians and scholars, from myths and legends, to become the first well-known physician in the history of the world.

What occurred in the history of the development of medicine between the time of primitive man and the physician, Imhotep, in 2780 B.C., is difficult to ascertain. Imhotep was certainly not the first physician. He must have been

---

1. San Francisco Chronicle, April 4, 1979.

taught by someone. Records are very scarce for this period of time so it will not be until later, around 1500 B.C., when more detailed information is available. The careful work of scholars, translating the ancient texts, reveals much to us concerning ancient religious and medical works.

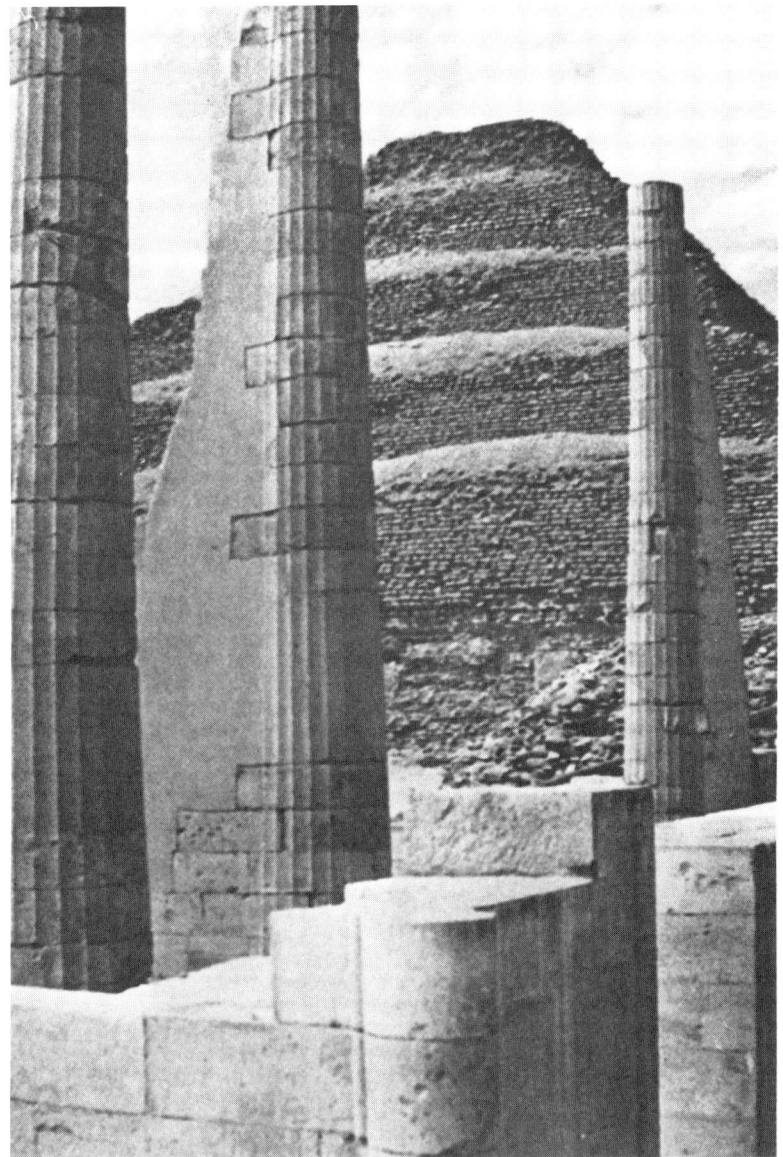

The step-pyramid of the pharaoh Djoser was designed by Imhotep, who later was worshipped as the Egyptian God of Medicine.

ancient egypt
kheme

When traveling through Egypt today, one is surrounded by the remains of a civilization that flourished thousands of years ago. Scholars are still unraveling the mysteries that surround this ancient culture. The Ancient Egyptians believed that, in the beginning, the universe was a primordial ocean called Nun. Eventually, a primeval hill appeared, rising from the waters. Atum, the God of Heliopolis, had created himself in Nun through his own efforts and, finding nowhere to stand, had created this piece of land. This first piece of land was later to become the site of the Temple of Heliopolis. Atum, since he was alone in the world, had to produce off-spring without a mate. He masturbated, swallowed the semen, and produced a son and daughter by spitting and vomiting them out, Shu and Tefnut. Shu and Tefnut produced Geb, the earth, and Nut, the sky. Geb and Nut were the parents of Osiris, Isis, Set and Nephtys. Horus, the Son of Osiris and Isis, was the predecessor of the future kings or pharoahs who were to rule Ancient Egypt. This age, in which the gods lived on the earth, was regarded as a golden age, in which the principles of justice ruled over the land, and were guarded by the goddess, Maat. This simplified version of the creation myth (there are several others) can be related to the annual inundation of the land by the Nile River; the rejuvenation of the land; and the production of vegetation. The tears of Atum fell to the earth and produced man.

By about 2600 B.C., Atum had become identified with the sun god, Ra. Ra, the sun, was frequently portrayed as the phoenix, or Bennu bird, perched on the pyramidial top of a obelisk. This obelisk, or Benben stone, symbolized a ray of the sun, and the primordial hill.

There are many myths surrounding these ancient gods, some of which indicate why and how certain customs originated. Within the stories are examples of the uses of charms and spells to ward off evil spirits and death. The following stories are, of course, extremely abbreviated.

In the beginning, Ra ruled the Earth but, as he grew older, his power weakened. Mankind became aware of Ra's weakness and plotted against him. Ra became enraged and sent his daughter Sekhmet, goddess of war and destruction, to subdue mankind. Sekhmet carried out her task so well that Ra feared all mankind would be destroyed, so he devised a plan to stop her slaughtering spree. Ra ordered large quantities of beer to be made and had the beer colored red with clay from Aswan. This was spread over the land. When Sekhmet discovered it, she thought that the colored beer was blood; consumed vast quantities of it; became drunk; and forgot about her mission and went to sleep. Thus, mankind was saved from destruction by the use of alcohol. Wines and beers were probably the most widespread medicines made by man and were used throughout the ancient civilizations of the world. The story also indicates that the flooding of the land saved mankind, which, of course, happened every year in Ancient Egypt.

Isis, the great-granddaughter of Atum-Ra, also recognized his weakened state and plotted to steal his power. Isis, great in spells and enchantments, collected the saliva that dribbled from Ra's lips, mixed it with dirt, and fashioned a serpent which she placed in Ra's path. He was bitten and suffered great pain. He could not cure himself and summoned help. Isis agreed to undertake his cure provided that he would tell her his secret name. In many ancient cultures (and in primitive cultures today) it was believed that if one could learn the secret name of another, one would then have power over that person. Do you willingly tell your name to strangers? Ra resisted, but Isis persisted and eventually learned his secret name. Ra, wearied of the earth, withdrew into the heavens. Horus, the son of Isis and Osiris, ruled on the Earth. The future pharaohs were the descendants of Horus.

The following is an Ancient Egyptian spell based on the previous story and was used in cases of snakebite. It was to be recited over images of Atum, Horus and Isis. It could be written and placed on the wound area, or swallowed, or mixed with wine or beer and be drunk by the patient:

> "Spew forth poison. Go from Ra. Eye of Horus, go from the God who created by his words. I am working this spell. I send out the powerful poison to fall on the ground. Behold, the great God has revealed his name. Ra lives, the poison dies. The poison dies, Ra lives."[1]

Isis is also one of the main characters in the drama concerned with the throne of Egypt; Osiris, Set and Horus; the mummification ritual and procedures; and the belief in life after death.

---

1. Author's arrangement from: "Wings of the Falcon," edited by Joseph Koster, Holt, Rinehart & Winston, N.Y., 1968, pg. 65.

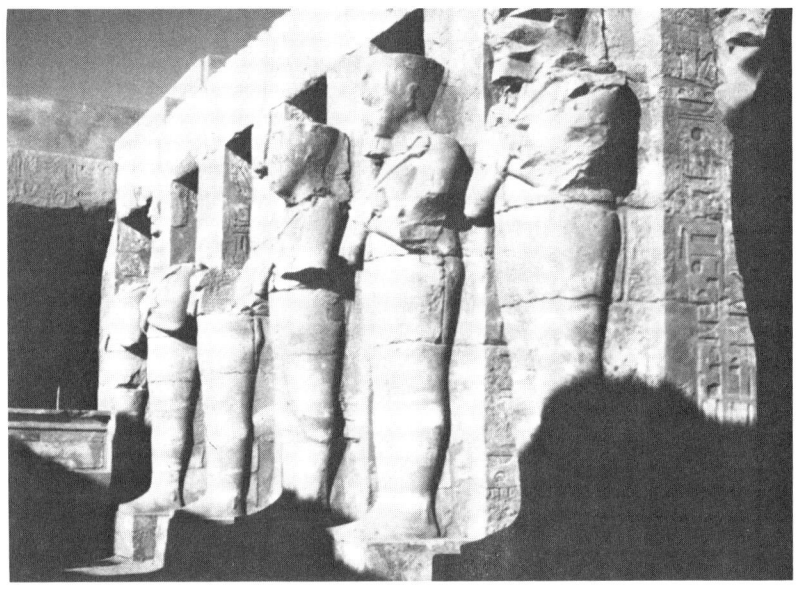
Colossal statues of Ramses III as Osiris at Midinet Habu, Thebes.

Osiris, the oldest son of Geb, the earth-god, had inherited the throne of Egypt, and was assisted by his sister-wife, Isis. Their brother, Set, was jealous of Osiris and plotted to steal the throne for himself. He had fashioned a beautiful humanoid-sarcophagus, built to the exact dimensions of Osiris, and then gave a party, at which the sarcophagus was offered as a prize to whomever it fitted. When Osiris lay down in the sarcophagus, Set slammed down the lid, fastened it, and had it thrown into the Nile River. Another version has Osiris thrown into the Nile where he is attacked and killed by "water-fleas." Many medical historians believe that this version indicates that Osiris died of Schistosomiasis, a disease which shall be discussed later. Isis, learning what had happened, set out in search of her husband's body and eventually went to Byblos, Phoenicia, where her magic powers told her that the sarcophagus had landed. The sarcophagus had washed ashore at the foot of a tamarisk tree which had, in the elapsed time, grown completely around it. The King of Byblos, noted the great tree, and had it cut down and used as a pillar in the palace. Isis became friendly with several of the maids of the palace and eventually was appointed the nurse of the King's son. Isis attempted to use her powers to make the child immortal, but the Queen surprised her and broke the spell. Isis revealed her identity and the King of Byblos gave her the pillar. On her return to Egypt, she hid in the marshes of the Delta and there, with the aid of Thoth and her magic spells, she assumed the form of a bird, fanned the breath of life into Osiris, and conceived a child. Set, hunting in the marshes, accidently discovered the body of Osiris. He tore the body into pieces which were scattered throughout Egypt except for the penis, which he threw into the Nile River where it was eaten by a crab. Isis searched throughout the land and found all the parts of his body, except the penis.

With the aid of Thoth, Isis attempted to revive Osiris, but since his body was incomplete, this could not be accomplished. Thoth instructed Isis in the embalming ritual which was accomplished with the aid of Anubis, who is thereafter the god of embalming and guardian of the cemeteries. Isis therefore, performed the first embalment ritual and provided the spells and charms for eternal life in the Land of the West (Dead).

Isis, fearing the power of Set, fled again into the deep marshes where she gave birth to her son, Horus. Set, entering the swamps in the form of a scorpion, found the infant Horus and stung him. Isis returned home to find him dying and enlisted the help of Thoth and the scorpion goddess, Serquet (Selket), to formulate a cure. The following spell was the result of their consultation:

> "Flow forth, scorpion, being of long back and many joints. Come here at my call as I utter it. I am the God who came into being by my own hand. Come, flow out at the command of Horus's wives. I am Horus, the *physician,* soothing the God. Flow out of the limbs. Etc. [2]

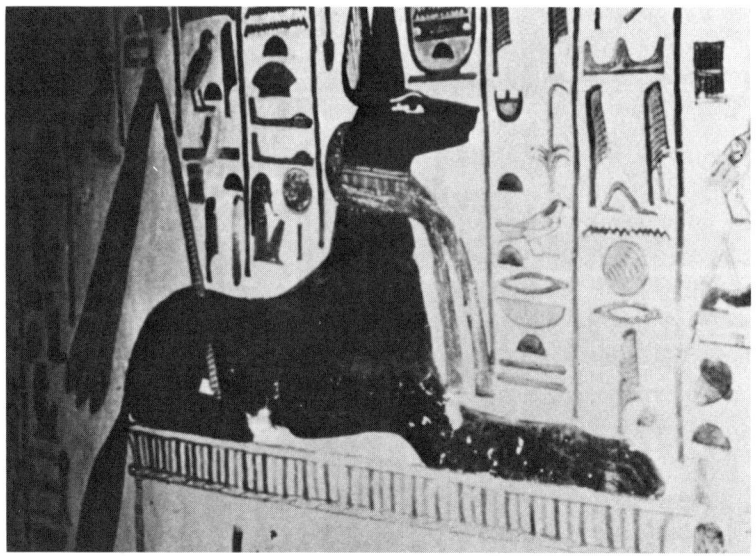

Anubis, God of Embalming and Burial Rituals, as portrayed in the tomb of Queen Nefertari.

---

2. Author's arrangement from: "Wings of the Falcon," edited by Joseph Koster, Holt, Rinehart & Winston, N.Y., 1968, pgs. 148-149.

Ancient Egypt – Kheme 11

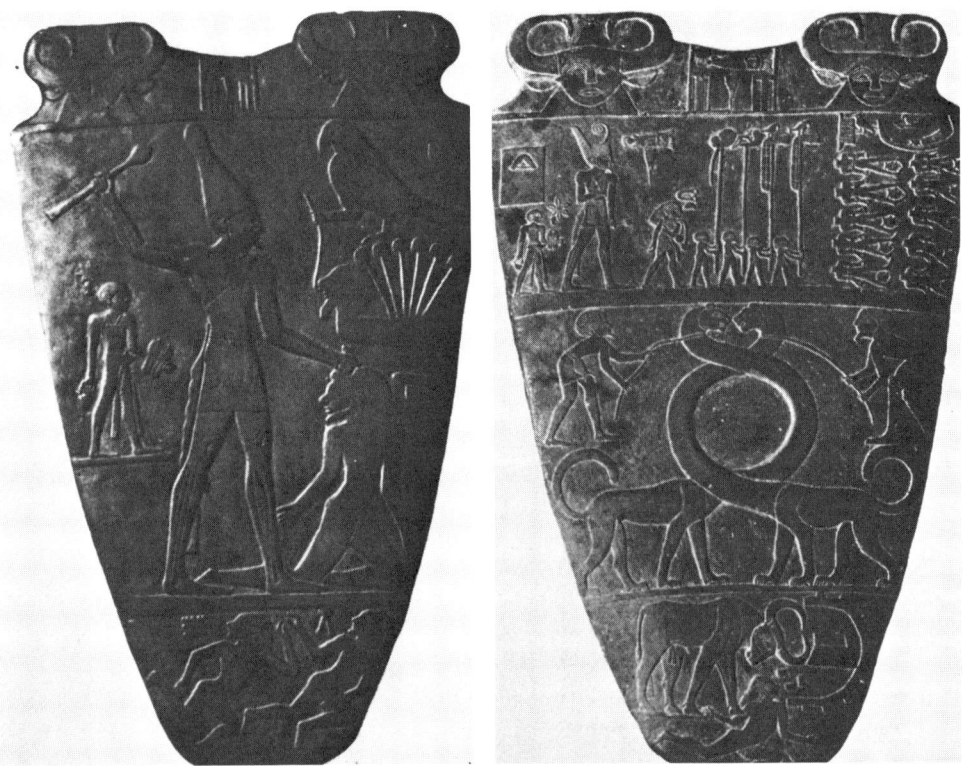

The palette of Narmer (Menes) which depicts the unification of Upper and Lower Egypt in about 3200 B.C. (Photographs courtesy the Egyptian Museum, Cairo)

The spell was successful, Horus recovered, attained manhood, and challenged Set for the throne. Horus, after numerous battles, defeated Set and placed him in chains. Isis, feeling sorrow for her captive brother, released him. Horus, enraged, severed the head from the body of Isis. Thoth, observing his favored Isis without a head, replaced it with the nearest at hand which, unfortunately, was that of a cow. (Ancient example of zenograft transplantation.) Horus finally defeated Set, who was sent to rule the deserts, while Horus and his descendents ruled the fertile lands along the Nile River. Historically, Upper and Lower Egypt were believed to have been united in 3200 B.C. by Menes-Narner, Little is known about the rulers of Upper Egypt and Lower Egypt prior to this time.

Some of the earliest artifacts of man have been found in the Nile Valley but little is known of the history of ancient Egypt prior to its unification by Menes-Narmer in approximately 3200 B.C. It is known that there were two kingdoms, Upper and Lower Egypt, and the rulers of the land stressed this in their claim to the throne as "Ruler of Upper and Lower Egypt." The unification is believed to be depicted in the "palette of Narmer," discovered by Sir

Flinders Petrie, which depicts the king wearing the white crown of Upper Egypt and the red crown of Lower Egypt and the killing and capturing of people of the marshes of Lower Egypt. The mace-head of an earlier king, Scorpion, has been found, who may have begun the unification plan. Sources do not agree on the chronology of the Egyptian Dynasties, some varying up to one thousand years. The following dates are from an official publication of the UAR and the information was collated from several books by authorities on Egyptian history.

Archaic Period: 3200-2680 B.C.

Dynasty I–Menes-Narmer united Upper and Lower Egypt. Other kings were Horaha, Zer (Athothis), Uadjii, Udimu, Enezib, Semerkhet, Ka'a.

Dynasty II–Khasekhemuwy and others.

Dynasty III–Djoser and Imhotep built step pyramid. Capital at Memphis.

Old Kingdom: 2680-2200 B.C.

Dynasty IV–Snefru and Queen Hetepheres; Cheops (Khufu); Cephren (Khafre); Mycerinus (Menkaure); true pyramids built at Dashur, Giza.

Dynasty V–Unas and others. Ra became the supreme god; Huge sun temples built.

Dynasty VI–Teti; Pepi I; Mernera; Pepi II. Pepi II and the Nubian dwarf. Nobles began construction of their own tombs.

Dynasty VII–At the death of Pepi II the kingdom collapsed and anarchy ensued,
  to Dynasty **X**

Middle Kingdom: 2150-1580 B.C.

Dynasty XI–Thebean Prince Intef reunited Egypt and established capital at Thebes.

Dynasty XII–Amenemhet and others. Capital moved to the north, near Fayum.

Dynasty XIII
  to
Dynasty XVII–The Aamu (Hyksos, Asiatics) invaded Egypt and introduced the horse and chariot and the compound bow. Aamu-king Aphophis in Avaris challenged by Sekenenre and Kamose of Thebes.

New Kingdom: 1580-1340 B.C.

Dynasty XVIII–Ahmose I, brother of Kamose, defeated the Aamu. This Dynasty established an Egyptian Kingdom extending from the Euphrates River in Mesopotamia to the Nile and extending southward into Nubia. Period of great trade.

Ahmose I; Amenhotep I; Thutmosis I; Thutmosis II; Hatshepsut; Thutmosis III; Amenhotep II; Thutmosis IV; Amenhotep III; Amenhotep IV-Akhenaton; Smenkhkare; Tutankhamon.

Dynasty XIX–General Horamhab became Pharaoh, followed by General Ramses I; Seti I; Ramses II; Merneptah. Legendary time of Hebrew Exodus.

Dynasty XX–Setinekht; Ramses III.

Late Period: 1165-332 B.C.

Dynasty XXI—Tanite Rule.

Dynasty XXII—Libyan Dynasty in Delta; Priest Kings in Thebes.

Dynasty XXIII

Dynasty XXIV—Saitic Rule.

Dynasty XXV—Nubian Rule. Egypt invaded by Mesopotamia under Esarhaddon and Ashurbanipol about 663 B.C.

Dynasty XXVI—Saitic rule. Necho sends expedition around Africa. Nebuchadrezzar in Babylon.

Dynasty XXVII
    to

Dynasty XXXI—Last of the Egyptian Kings and Persian Rule in 332 B.C.

Ptolemaic Dynasty—Alexander the Great; Ptolemy I-VIII; Cleopatra. 332-30 B.C.

Roman Rule—30 B.C. to 324 A.D.

Coptic Rule—324 to 640 A.D.

Arab Conquest—640 to 969 A.D.

Middle Ages—969 to 1517 A.D. Fatimids; Ayyubids; Mameluks.

Ottoman Empire—1517 to 1798 A.D.

Modern Period—Napoleon-1798; Mohammad Ali-1805; Arabi Revolt-1881; British Occupation-1882; Republic of Egypt-1953.

    The legends and spells utilized by the Ancient Egyptians could be said to be representative of any spell used by any primitive culture. From the texts of the spells, it can be seen that religion was closely involved with medicine. In Egypt, the physicians actually had to become priests in order to be qualified. Many of their treatments involved oral and manual rites; that is, they gave the treatment to the patient and also a spell to help the treatment work.

    The religion supplied the spells but where did the actual medical knowledge come from? Apparently from trial and error. According to legend, the god, Thoth, had compiled 42 books in antiquity, some of which dealt with medicine. Legends also mention other ancient books. In about 3100 B.C., the King Athothis (Zer) was credited with a book on anatomy. In 3050 B.C. King Usaphais was said to have produced a book concerned with the vessels of the body. The names of some well-known physicians of Egypt have also survived. The famous Imhotep, physician to the King Djoser, who was later worshipped as a god. The royal physician Iry, who lived about 2600 B.C., was a specialist concerned with the eyes of the king. One of his titles was "Guardian of the royal bowel movement." This title may seem strange to us but, since the King was responsible for the annual inundation of the Nile River, any malfunction of the body, such as constipation, might affect the flooding of the land. This could not be allowed to happen so the health of the King was carefully guarded.

In the Old Kingdom, the last king of the 6th Dynasty, Pepi II, ruled Egypt for approximately 100 years. He was crowned at the age of six and three years later, had the following letter sent to the leader of an expedition, Harkhuf, who was in "Yam," somewhere south of Aswan.

> "Come, then, when you come down the Nile, come straight to my palace. Make haste. Bring me this dwarf whom you are bringing back from the land of the Akhetiu; bring him back alive, well and healthy to dance like a god, to rejoice and delight King Neferkare. When he comes down the Nile with you, put vigilant men around him on both sides of the boat. Take care that he does not fall into the water. When he sleeps at night, send guards to sleep round him in his cabin, which guards must be changed ten times a night. My Majesty wants to see this dwarf more than the marvellous products of Punt. If you reach the palace and this dwarf is with you, alive, well, and healthy, My Majesty will do great things for you, more than was done for the divine sealer, Bawerded, in the time of Izozi, according to the delight which My Majesty will feel to see this dwarf."[3]

Dwarfs were brought to the Royal Court as entertainers and several statues and carvings have survived which depict dwarfs who were attached to the Courts of Egypt. Later, many of the Courts of Europe and the Aztecs in Mexico, kept large numbers of deformed people as entertainers.

Basically, there are two types of dwarfism; one in which the individual is not deformed but is merely small in stature and the other in which some portions of the body are normal in size while others are abnormal in size. The dwarf of Pepi II was an achondroplastic dwarf with short extremities, a trunk of normal size, a large globular head, stumpy nose and trident hands. This condition is usually caused by a defect in the formation of cartilage at the epiphyses of the long bones. The former type of dwarfism, without deforming characteristics, might best be represented by the famous "Tom Thumb" who was associated with a circus in the United States in the late 1800s. In 1979, the University of California announced that its scientists had found a new way to make human growth hormone, a promising aid for dwarfed children. It was estimated that one in 5000 to 7000 children of Western countries may have a growth hormone deficiency. A genetic research team succeeded in causing bacteria to synthesize relatively large amounts of the important but scarce enzyme.

Iry was not the only physician to specialize. Later, in 2550 B.C., there lived Sekhet-n-ankh, nose-doctor of the King Sahure. Apparently, the physicians had specialized in the treatment of various parts of the body for a very long time, just as physicians do today. Even evidence of dentistry appeared about 2500 B.C. Herodotus, a Greek traveler and historian, visited Egypt around 450 B.C. In his writings he stated that Egyptian medicine was practiced on a plan of separation, each physician specializing in a specific disorder and that because of this, there were a great number of medical practitioners in the country. The physicians studied their art in schools which were called "houses

---

3. "Lives of the Pharaohs," Pierre Montet, World Publishing Co., 1968, pg. 41.

Ancient Egypt – Kheme 15

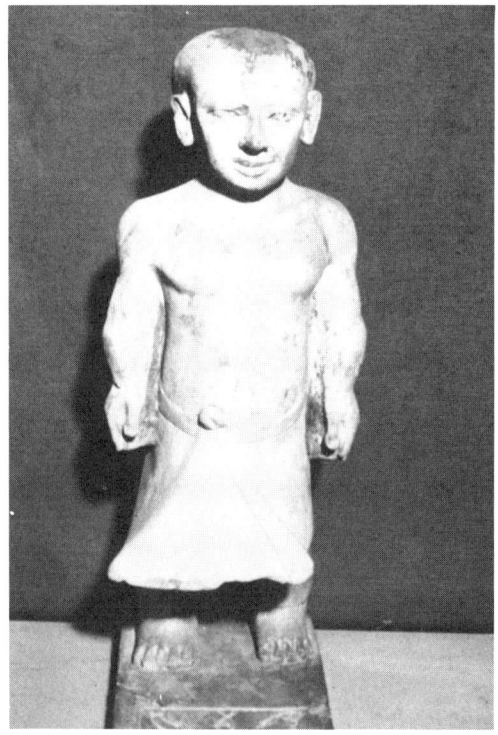

The statue of an achondrophlastic dwarf, Knum-Hotep, who lived during the Old Kingdom period. (Photo-graph courtesy the Egyptian Museum, Cairo)

of life." In about 500 B.C., Egypt was defeated by the Persians. The King of Persia, Darius (Daraya-vaush), ordered the Chief Physician, Usser-hor-resenet, to restore the houses of life which had fallen into disrepair. The order was carried out, and students from noble families were installed under the charge of wise men. The students were also equipped with all that they needed, including instruments.

Did the books of Thoth and those of the Kings Athothis and Usaphais actually exist? Some people think that they did, especially when certain ancient papyri were discovered in Egypt, some of which were concerned with medicine. Due to the Egyptian belief in life after death, valuable possessions were frequently buried with the mummy. Apparently, in some cases, medical papyri were buried with the deceased, who may have been physicians, and have been recovered and studied by scholars.

Copies and translations of Egyptian medical papyri can be found in most major libraries. The two best known medical papyri are the Edwin Smith papyrus and the Ebers papyrus. Both have been dated to the early part of the 18th Dynasty, about 1500 B.C., but archaic terminology found in certain portions of the papyri indicate that they were copied, in part, from sources of greater antiquity.

The Edwin Smith Papyrus is the most scientific of all the papyri and is devoted to the treatment of wounds, abscesses, bone dislocations and fractures.

It makes note of the brain, the pulse, and various organs and parts of the body. It contains 48 sections, each dealing with a specific problem in a specific area of the body. The wound or disorder is described and is followed by a discussion and treatment procedures. There are also 13 magical-medicinal incantations and prescriptions. The papyrus was not found intact. Approximately one-half is missing. In 1930, Breasted published a facsimile and translation of the papyrus, a portion of which follows:

> "One in whom an ailment is counted, like measuring the ailment of a man; in order to know the action of the heart. There are canals (or vessels) in it to every member. Now, if the priests of Sekhmet or any physician put his hands or fingers upon the head, upon the back of the head, upon the two hands, upon the pulse, upon the two feet, he measures to the heart, because its vessels are in the back of the head and in the pulse; and because its pulsation is in every vessel of every member."

> "If thou examinest a man having a gaping wound in his head, penetrating to the bone, smashing his skull, and rending open the brain of his skull, thou shouldst palpate his wound. Shouldst thou find that smash which is in his skull, like corrugations which form in molten copper, and something therein fluttering and throbbing under thy fingers, like the weak place of an infant's crown before it becomes whole, when it has happened there is no throbbing and fluttering under thy fingers until the brain of his skull is rent open and he discharges blood from both his nostrils, and he suffers with a stiffness in his neck. (Diagnosis) Thou shouldst say concerning him, an ailment not to be treated. (Treatment) Thou shouldst anoint that wound with grease. Thou shalt not bind it; thou shalt not apply two strips upon it; until thou knowest that he has reached a decisive point."

> "If thou examinest a man having a dislocation on his mandible (jaw) and shouldst thou find his mouth open and his mouth cannot close for him, thou shouldst put thy thumbs upon the ends of the two rami (bones) of the mandible in the inside of his mouth, and thy two claws (fingers) under his chin, and thou shouldst cause them to fall back so that they rest in their places. Thou shouldst say concerning him: One having a dislocation in his mandible, an ailment which I will treat."

> "If thou examinest a man having tumors with prominent head in his breast, (and) thou findest that the swellings have spread with pus over his breast, (and) have produced redness, while it is very hot therein, when thy hand touches him, (Diagnosis) Thou shouldst say concerning him: 'One having tumors with prominent head in his breast, (and) they produce (cysts) of pus. An ailment which I will treat with the fire-drill.' (Treatment) Thou shouldst burn for him over his breast (and) over those tumors which are on his breast. Thou shouldst treat him with wound treatment. Thou shouldst not prevent its opening of itself, that there may be no 'mnhy·w' in his wound (sore?). Every wound (sore?) that arises in his breast dries up as soon as it opens of itself."

> "If thou examinest a man having a diseased wound in his breast, while that wound is inflamed and a whirl of inflammation continually issues from the mouth of that wound at thy touch; the two lips of that wound are ruddy, while that man continues to be feverish from it; his flesh cannot receive a bandage, that wound cannot take a margin of skin; the granulation which is in the mouth

of that wound is watery, their surface is hot and secretions drop therefrom in an oily state, (Diagnosis) Thou shouldst say concerning him: 'One having a diseased wound in (his) breast, it being inflamed, (and) he continues to have fever from it. An ailment which I will treat. (Treatment) Thou shalt make for him cool applications for drawing out the inflammation from the mouth of the wound:

A. Leaves of willow (salicyn)
    nbs-tree
    ksnty
    Apply to it.

B. Leaves of ym'-tree
    dung
    hny-t'
    ksnty
    Apply to it.

Thou shalt make for him applications for drying up the wound:

A. Powder of green pigment (copper)
    wsb·t
    thn·t
    grease
    Triturate; bind upon it.

B. Northern salt
    ibex grease
    Triturate; bind upon it.

Thou shalt make for him poultices:
   Red spnn (poppy?)
   garden tongue
   d'r·t
   sycamore leaves
   Bind upon it.

If the like befalls in any member, thou shalt treat him according to these instructions."[4]

The Ebers Papyrus[5] is the longest (65 feet) and the most complete of all the medical papyri. It is believed that the scribe copied the magical-medicinal prescriptions and incantations from a variety of available sources, since portions of the Ebers papyrus can be found in other papyri (Smith, Kahun). In the Ebers papyrus, ailments are named and the treatment specified, along with the drugs to be used, the amounts to be used, a description of their preparation and how they are to be administered to the patient. Spells, charms and incantations are present in greater numbers than in the Smith papyrus.

---

4. "The Edwin Smith Surgical Papyrus," transliteration, translation and commentary by James H. Breasted, © The University of Chicago Press, Chicago, Illinois, 1930, Vol I.
5. "The Papyrus Ebers," translated by B. Ebbel, Levin & Munksgaard, Copenhagen, Denmark, 1937, pgs. 59, 69, 70, 97, 100, 101, 103, 108.

The following diseases were recognized and treated in the Ebers papyrus:

headache	tumors, innocent and malignant
migraine	baldness
giddiness	alopecia
constipation	scurf
diarrhea	eczema
indigestion	impetago
colic	scabies
dysentery	stings of wasps and tarantula
melaena	crocodile bite
piles	burns
inflammation of the anus	wounds
tumors and inflammations of the abdomen	abscesses
	gangrene
tapeworms and roundworms	pustules
guinea worms	menstrual irregularities
hookworms	aids to delivery, abortion and lactation
polyuria	
frequency of micturition	diseases of the breasts
accumulation and obstruction of urine	amenorrhea
	leucorrhea
cystitis	falling of the womb
chalazion	diseases of the female genitalia
enlarged prostate	
strictures	irregularities of the teeth
stones	coryza
cardiac pain and weakness	boils and abscesses
palpitation	catarrah
disorderly action of the heart	diseases of the tongue
atheroma	deafness
debility	diseases of the ear
diseases of the liver	diseases of the eyes
glandular swellings	blindness
cancer	blepharitis
chemosis	granulations
cataract	hemmorrhages
hydrothalmus	ophthalmoplegia
inflammations	trichiasis
iritis	pinguecula
leucoma	pterygium

The following plants were utilized in treatment of the patient:

acanthus	corn	garlic	pomegranate
aloes	crocus	grapes	poppy
arabian wood	cucumber	juniper berry	reeds
balsam	cyperus	lettuce	saffron
barley	dates	linseed	sycamore
beans	ebony	mint	willow tree

caraway	edelkraut	mulberry	wonderfruit
cedar tree	elderberry	nasturtium	lotus
cereals	fennel	onions	wheat
chaff	figs	palm tree	watermelon
coriander	flax	peppermint	turpentine

The following mineral and other remedies were used:

alabaster	lead
antimony	leather
an old book boiled in oil	myrrh
bread	natron—sodium carbonate
cake	plant and mineral oils
calamine	opal resin
clay	salt
collyrium-eye salve	saltpetre
copper	statue scrapings
dough	dust from a statue
slime from ships	soot
granite	various stones
gum	sulphur
haematite—iron ore	verdigris-copper compounds
honey	wax
indigo	writing fluids
lapis lazuli	yeasts
various animals	excretia

The following prescription from the Ebers papyrus was for the treatment of a headache and "When this remedy is used by him against all illnesses in the head and all sufferings and evils of any sort, he will instantly become well":

"Another remedy which the Goddess Isis prepared for the God Ra, to drive the pains that are in his head":

Berry of the coriander	1	stimulant
Berry of the poppy plant	1	narcotic, soporific
wormwood	1	stimulant, antihelminthic
Berry of the sames plant	1	
Berry of the juniper	1	stimulant, diuretic
honey		

It should be noted, that in this astounding list of ingredients used by the ancient Egyptian physicians, many are still in use today. Copper and antimony compounds are poisonous, but if taken in the correct dosages, can be used to combat various infectious diseases. In 1909, Paul Ehrlich developed Salvarsan, compounds of copper and arsenic, which was called the "Silver bullet," and was used to treat syphilis and protozoan infections. The Egyptians were using copper and antimony compounds prior to 1500 B.C., in medicinal treatments. Antimony compounds are useful in the treatment of Leishmaniasis, Schistsomiasis, Filariasis, Trypanosomiasis, ulcerating granulomas, *Etc.*

Some other selected excerpts from the Ebers Papyrus follow:

There are many formulas for treating a variety of eye infections and diseases. The majority of these utilize, among the various ingredients, stibium, or antimony, a metallic element, which was, and still is, used in the effective treatment of many infective diseases.

"Another to improve the sight by means of applying something to the eyelids: "tntj" fruit, the interior of "wdjt," stibium, water; these are finely ground, mixed together, and are applied to the eyelids."

"Another to expell trachoma in the eyes: stibium, red ochre, yellow ochre, red natron; are applied to the eyelids."

"Another for night-blindness: the liver of an ox is roasted and crushed out and given to the patient. Really excellent." (Vitamin A deficiency is the usual cause of night-blindness and it is stored in the liver!)

The following is a remedy for impotency, which is usually of a psychosomatic origin, and here, is treated with, among other drugs, hyoscyamus, commonly known as henbane, which is sedative and anti-spasmodic, in its effects, relaxing the patient.

"Another for weakness of the male member: hyoscyamus, beans, bran, sawdust of pine, "d3rt," sawdust of "mrj," sawdust of willow (aspirin), sawdust of zizyphus (pectoral), sawdust of sycamore, *Etc.*"

"Another to expell wrinkles of the face: gum of frankincense; wax; fresh balanites-oil; rush-nut; all are finely ground, put in a viscous fluid, and applied to the face every day. Make it and thou shalt see!"

"The beginnings of remedies to expel gonorrhea that constricts a man's or a woman's flesh: northern salt, 1 ro; frankincense, 8 ro; viscous fluid, 10 ro; are injected in the anus. It is also used without adding frankincense."

"Another: viscous fluid, 15 ro; balanites-oil, 2−1/2 ro; hammer-flakes from copper, 2 ro; stibium (antimony), 2 ro; honey, 4 ro; likewise. It is excellent to expel purulency." (The absorption of copper and antimony might bring about a cure).

"The beginnings of remedies to fasten a tooth: powder of ammi; yellow ochre; honey; are mixed together and the tooth is filled therewith."

"Another: scrapings of a millstone; yellow ochre; honey; the tooth is filled therewith."

"Remedy to expel cry from a crying child: spnnw of spn; fly dirt that is on the wall; are mixed together, strained, and taken for four days. It ceases immediately." (Many scholars have translated "spnnw of spn" as a derivative of the oriental poppy plant. If so, the treatment would be very effective.)

The Ebers Papyrus also contains a section on anatomy and physiology:

"The beginning of the physician's secret: knowledge of the heart's movement and knowledge of the heart.

"There are vessels from it to every limb. As to this, when any physician, any surgeon (Sachmet-priest) or any exorcist applies the hands or his fingers to the head, to the back of the head, to the hands, to the place of the stomach, to the arms, or to the feet, then he examines the heart, because all his limbs possess its vessels, that is: it speaks out of the vessels of every limb. (Compare this paragraph with the one in the Smith Papyrus which describes the heart. They are almost identical, indicating a similar source.)

"There are four vessels in his nostrils, two give mucus and two give blood. There are four vessels in the interior of his temples which then give blood to the eyes; all diseases of the eyes arise through them, because there is an opening to the eyes. As to the water that comes down from them: it is the pupils of the eyes that produce it; another lection: it is the sleep in the eyes which makes it. There are four vessels dispersing to the head which effuse in the back of the head and which produce (htp) a bald spot and loss of hair; this is their production upwards.

"As to the breath which enter the nose: it enters into the heart and the lung; these give to the whole belly.

"As to that through which the ears become deaf: there are two vessels that effect it, the ones leading to the root of the eye; another lection: to the whole eye. When he is deaf, his mouth cannot be opened (he cannot speak).

"As to inundation of the stomach: it is due to fluid of the mouth; all his limbs become faint.

"There are four vessels to his two ears together with the ear canal, two on his right side and two on his left side. The breath of life enters into the right ear and the breath of death enters into the left ear.

"There are six vessels that lead to the arms, three to the right and three to the left; they lead to his fingers.

"There are six vessels that lead to the feet, three to the right foot and three to the left foot, until they reach the sole of the foot.

"There are two vessels to his testicles; it is they which give semen.

"There are two vessels to the buttocks, one to the right buttock and the other to the left buttock.

"There are four vessels to the liver; it is they which give rise to it, humour and air, which afterwards cause all diseases to arise in it by overfilling with blood.

"There are four vessels to the lung and to the spleen; it is they which give humour and air to it likewise.

"There are two vessels to the bladder; it is they which give urine.

"There are four vessels that open to the anus; it is they which cause humour and air to be produced for it. Now the anus opens to every vessel to the right side and the left side in arms and legs, when it is overfilled with excrements.

"As to faintness: it is due to the fact that the heart does not speak or that the vessels of the heart are dumb, there being no perception of them under thy fingers; it arises through the air which fills them.

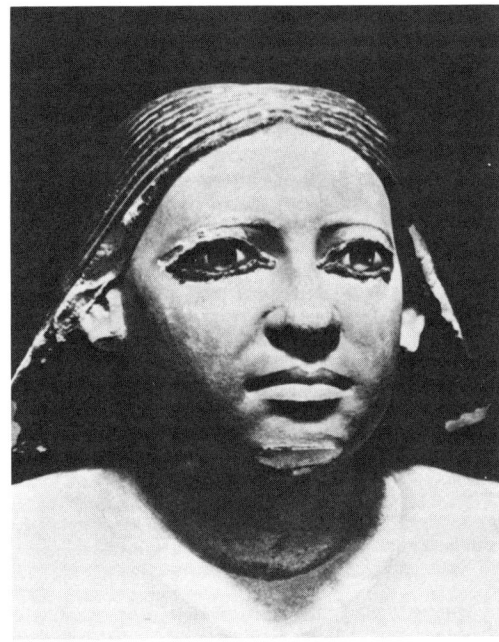

The portrait statue of a scribe from the 5th Dynasty which shows the use of heavy eye-makeup. (Photograph courtesy the Egyptian Museum, Cairo.)

"As to the feeling of sickness: it is due to debility of the heart through heat from the anus; if thou findest it great, something rotates in his cardia, likewise in the eye.

"As to his mind (consciousness) passes away: it is due to the fact that all the vessels of the heart are carrying feces."

Eye diseases were, and still are, prevalent in Africa and the Middle East. Described in the papyri are such eye ailments as conjunctivitis, cataracts, leucoma, glaucoma and tracoma. Tracoma is a disease of the conjunctiva which is attended by the formation of small elevations on the eyelids. Granulation and atrophy may occur. This painful, disfiguring, blinding disease is caused by a microorganism (Chlamydiae) of large particle size which is transmitted from person to person by means of the fingers, fomites and flies. Today, the disease is treated with sulfonamide and antibiotic therapy. Prior to their advent, copper, silver and sulfate compounds were used.

It is interesting that the Ancient Egyptians were very frequently portrayed with heavy make-up surrounding their eyes. The cosmetic was prepared by mixing powders of malachite (carbonate of copper), antimony, soot and goose grease. It is believed that the greasy cosmetic helped to ward off flies from the eyes, reduced the possibility of eye infection and helped to reduce the glare of the sun. The author has observed the use of a similar eye cosmetic on infants and children in the Middle East and you may have noticed people engaged in sports with a glare-reducing black material smeared under their eyes.

Papyri also indicate an area of dental specialization which included extractions, surgery and therapy. In 1976, University of Michigan researchers reported the discovery of three teeth found linked together by gold wire in an Egyptian tomb that was approximately 4500 years old. The three teeth were apparently part of a four-unit dental bridge. The gold wire was wrapped around two of the teeth and passed through a hole drilled in the third. However, the recent X-raying of royal mummies has revealed no evidence of dental treatments except extractions. There was excessive wear of teeth, exposure of pulp, peridontal disease, abscess, malocclusion and crowding of the teeth.

Trepanning is a very ancient surgical procedure which has been found to have been used by primitive man in many parts of the world. The procedure involved the removal of a piece of the skull in an apparent attempt to allow an evil spirit to leave the body of the patient. Some trepanned skulls which have been found exhibit the regrowth of bone, so the operation must have occasionally been successful. Amulets, found in burial sites, indicate that tribal members used the trepanned skulls of their associates as charms to ward off a similar affliction. Today, this operation can easily be performed by surgeons with modern equipment and aseptic techniques. Ancient man had stone tools and later, in Egypt, copper and bronze were in use. Recently, scientists from Thailand and the University of Pennsylvania announced the discovery of an ancient Bronze Age culture site at Ban Chiang in northeast Thailand which shows evidence of uses of metal alloys as early as 3600 B.C.. The discovery "challenges all the assumptions that have long been held about the development of our modern cultures." The use of iron was discovered about 1300 B.C., in the form of weapons which aided in the defeat of Babylon. The Egyptians observed many types of skull injuries and fractures and attempted to aid the afflicted. One treatment involved the covering of the injured skull area with a piece of ostrich eggshell.

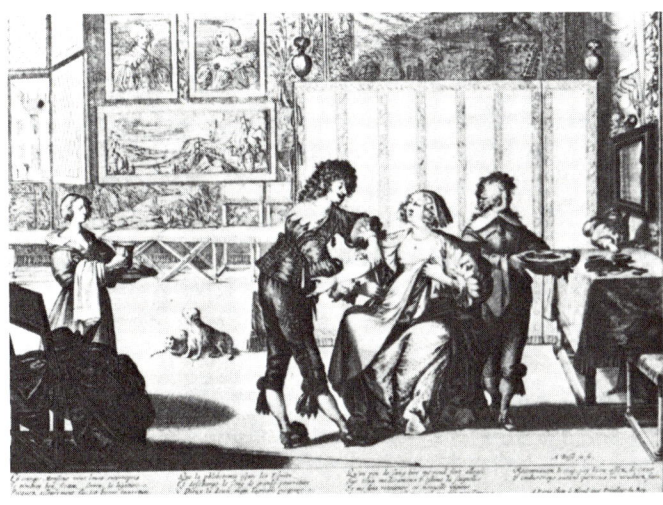

Phlebotomy. An etching by A. Bosse, Paris, 1635. From *Medicine and the Artist* by Carl Zigrosser, Dover Publications, Inc., New York, 1970. Reprinted through the permission of the publisher and the Philadelphia Museum of Art.

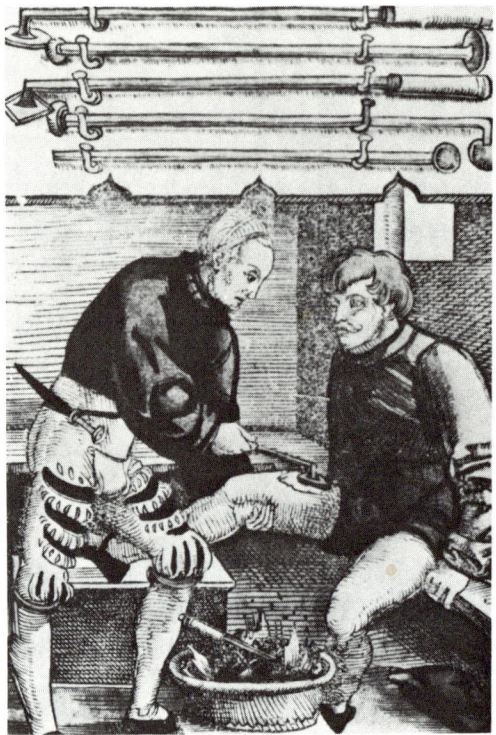

Cautery. Colored woodcut by J. Wechtlin from H. von Gersdorff's "Feldtbuch der Wundartzney," Strassburg, 1540. From *Medicine and the Artist* by Carl Zigrosser, Dover Publications, Inc., New York, 1970. Reprinted through the permission of the publisher and the Philadelphia Museum of Art.

Other procedures utilized by the physicians were phlebotomies (bleedings), enemas, leeching and cauterization. These were the mainstay of physicians until about 100 years ago and may still be found in use in primitive parts of the world. Cauterization has survived in modern medicine, but rather than using fire, our present physicians use electricity.

The Egyptian medical papyri and historical data indicate, until other evidence is uncovered, that Ancient Egypt can be credited with the earliest medical texts, containing anatomical and medical vocabulary, which were concerned with anatomy, surgery, pharmacology, diseases, injuries, and treatment procedures. Many of the rational treatments and procedures are accompanied by magical spells, incantations and sewage pharmacology. However, it should be remembered that the practice of medicine was actually to change very little from this period of time until the late 1800s, the time of Pasteur, Koch, Lister and others. Spells and incantations were altered to the forms of pilgrimages and prayers, and are still in use today.

We are fortunate that the medical and other papyri have survived from antiquity. It was due to the dry climate of Egypt and their religious beliefs that required the preservation of the bodies of the dead, and burial with prized possessions. How many people today are buried with books? Our writings are preserved in libraries. Unfortunately, the writings of the Egyptians that were preserved in the temples and the schools in Alexandria were partially destroyed by the Romans and later, were burned at the order of the Caliph Omar.

The preservation of the bodies of the dead was a religious rite based upon the Osirian beliefs of the people. The embalming procedures were necessary so that the deceased could have eternal life. If the body were destroyed, the spirit could not return to it in order to be nourished by offerings and religious ceremonies. Just when the embalming procedure began is unknown, but when one examines the mummies of the time of the 18th Dynasty, one finds that the preservation procedures were highly developed. The high temperatures, dry weather and burials in the desert sands probably brought about the first mummifications naturally, by dessication. Later, methods were developed for better preservation and the more lifelike appearance of the corpse. However, some of the later mummies were found to have deteriorated due to the excessive use of fats, oils and resins.

Herodotus, the Greek historian, gave a detailed account of the mummification procedures which he observed in ancient Egypt and stated that there were three procedures; one cheap, one expensive, and one very expensive. However, all were basically the same in that the soft tissues of the body were removed, either surgically or by dissolution, and the body was dessicated in natron, sodium carbonate, for approximately two months. The soft tissues might be embalmed and placed in canopic jars or wrapped and returned to the body cavity. Since this was a religious procedure, it must have involved priests. Priests were also involved with the medical schools and physicians were required to be priests, so there must have been some exchange of information concerning human anatomy, since many of the parts of the human body were mentioned in religious and medical papyri. The opening of the body of the deceased was only, to our knowledge, practiced by the ancient Egyptians. Other cultures buried or burned the dead intact. Later, Greek physicians and anatomists were to come to Egypt to study the human body, externally and internally, a practice which religious and popular custom forbade in their own country. Unfortunately, many of the observations were made incorrectly, so we find that the writings and observations of Galen (Greece-150 A.D.) were still in use until the work of Vesalius, in the 16th century, placed the study of human anatomy on a firmer foundation.

Another contribution from Ancient Egypt that involved mummification is that the preserved bodies can be studied and may reveal the diseases that could be found in antiquity. Pioneers in this area of paleopathology in Egypt were Armand Ruffer and Elliot Smith. Some diseases that have been identified or suggested are: smallpox–Ramses V; anthracosis and pneumonia–Horemhab; clubfoot–Siptah; excess weight–Thuthmosis II, Amenhotep III, Ramses III;

arterial disorders—Amenhotep III, Ramses II, Ramses III; schistosomiasis; tuberculosis; gall bladder and liver disorders; bone diseases, dental caries and sarcomas.

Schistosomiasis, a disease characterized by the infection of the body with blood flukes which generally localize in vesical or intestinal veins, was known in Egypt as early as 1250 B.C. In 1851, Bilharz found *Schistosoma haematobium* in the veins of an Egyptian. Since then, it has been found in many tropical and subtropical areas of the world. At the present time, about 200 million people are infected with schistosomiasis. The distribution of the disease is based upon the presence of their molluscan hosts, particularly snails. In Africa, the *Bulinus* and *Planorbarius* snails are involved. The life cycle of the parasite is unusual. Man and certain animals are infected by cercariae, which are microscopic, free-swimming forms found in infected waters, and which penetrate the skin and migrate to the vesical or intestinal veins where they mature. Copulation occurs and the female produces ova. The ova work their way through the venules and walls of the bladder and intestine, into the urine and feces. If the urine or feces are deposited in fresh water, the contained ova usually hatch within eight hours, releasing a free-swimming, microscopic, ciliated form called the miracidium. The miracidia die unless they penetrate a suitable snail within about eight hours. Within the snail, the miracidia form sporocysts which eventually each produce 200-400 daughter sporocysts. These, in turn, mature into cercariae which leave the snail and seek a human or animal host. The infective cercariae must find a suitable host within about 48 hours. The parasite may be found in the skin, heart, liver, spleen, bladder, genitalia, intestine and central nervous system. The chief complaints are abdominal enlargement and diarrhea. Death usually occurs from exhaustion, pneumonia or superimposed infections. Potassium and sodium *antimony* tartrate are effective in the treatment if the infection is in the early stages, but may be dangerous if administered in the advanced cirrhotic stage. Other drugs, such as Miracil D and Fuadin, are also in use today. Strangely, the building of the new Aswan Dam in Egypt, which supplies increased amount of power and water for the cultivation of more land, has also introduced Schistosomiasis into new areas where it was unknown, due to the lack of water.

Investigations into Egyptian history by scholars has resulted in a great controversy which is centered about the Pharaoh Amenhotep IV, who is better known as Ikhnaton (Akhenaton), one of the last Pharaohs of the 18th Dynasty. A tomb was found in the Valley of the Kings which contained a mummy, sarcophagus and other tomb furnishings and which had been burglarized in antiquity. Some of the furnishings had belonged to Ikhnaton and some to other members of the Royal Family. Statues and other art works produced during the reign of Ikhnaton had frequently portrayed him as having a rather large head with heavy, elongated features; a thin neck, arms and legs; a protruding abdomen; and heavy hips and thighs. Many scholars suggested that he had suffered from a glandular disorder, Frohlich's Syndrome, caused by a malfunction of the pituitary gland which results in adiposity, genital atrophies, changes in secondary sexual characters and development of the feminine type. Upon examination of the mummy, some investigators stated that the body was abnormal while others said that it was the normal body of a male of about twenty-eight years of age. Others have suggested that Ikhnaton was not afflicted with the disease and that the exaggeration of the body of Ikhnaton in the art works was merely a new innovation in the art forms of Ancient Egypt. This could be true because if Ikhnaton had been afflicted he would have been sterile; if he were sterile, then who was the father of the six daughters of his wife, Nefertiti? It is now generally accepted that the tomb contained the mummy of Smenkhkare, who was probably a half-brother to Ikhnaton, and who married the daughter of Ikhnaton and Nefertiti, Meritaton. Ikhnaton and Smenkhkare had ruled jointly for a time in the capital, Akhetaton (now called Tell el Amarna) and many have suggested a homosexual relationship between the two Kings which therefore would give credence to the theorized glandular disorder. Eventually, Smenkhkare was sent to rule in Thebes where he died and was replaced by Tutankhamon, who was later to become famous when his tomb was discovered, virtually intact, by Howard Carter. Recently, the mummy of Tutankhamon was x-rayed and it was discovered that the skull had been fractured. Tutankhamon and his wife, Ankhesenpaamon ruled at Thebes for about nine years. After the death of Tutankhamon, the Queen, Ankhhesenpaamon, wrote to the King of the Hittites requesting that he send one of his sons to Egypt to become her husband and Pharaoh. The Hittite Prince was murdered on his way to Egypt. The mummies of Ikhnaton, Nefertiti, Meritaton and Ankhesenpaamon have not, to the knowledge of the author, been identified. It is rather apparent, from all the rapid deaths in the Royal Family at the end of the 18th Dynasty, that something unusual was happening and that a reevaluation of that period is in order. Recently, the discovery of a large temple dedicated to Nefertiti indicates that she was not merely a beautiful woman but an important personage in her own right and, perhaps, the power behind the throne. It is also interesting that Amenhotep IV-Ikhnaton produced no male children and that apparently Smenkhare and Tutankhamon produced no children that survived infancy. This may have been due, in part, to the practice of incest by the royal family.

    Hormones are secreted by individual cells and glands and are chemical messengers that regulate body functions such as growth, metabolism, the utilization and storage of sugar and fats, the conversion of proteins to sugar, the elimination of body wastes, sexual development, emotions and body temperature. The deficiency or overproduction of a hormone can cause a disease, examples being Frohlich's Syndrome, just discussed, and diabetes. Many of these diseases are now being treated with synthesized hormones. the most widely used hormones today are estrogens and progesterones, found in the "pill," and used to suppress ovulation. The following list is of some of the major hormones and their effects on the body.

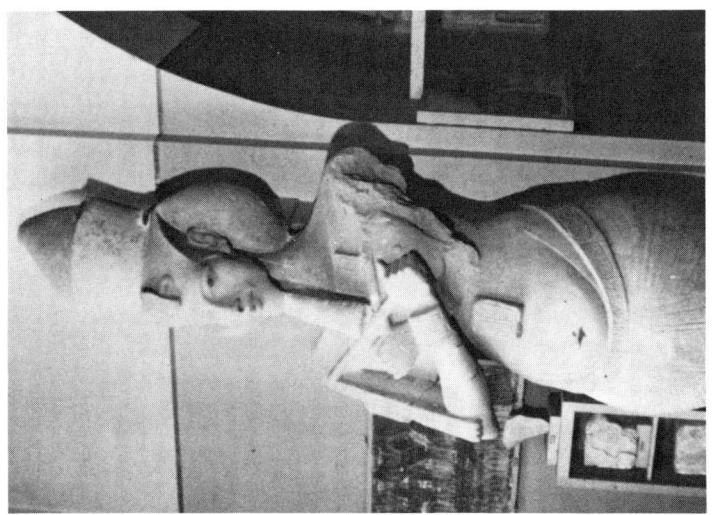

Two statues of Amenhotep III which originally were part of his mortuary temple, later used by others in building their temples. They were quarried near present day Cairo and brought to Thebes, approximately 450 miles to the south! Each is 64 feet in height. The statues are frequently called "The Colossi of Memnon" because the Romans claimed that the southern statue "spoke" at dawn and was therefore identified as Memnon, son of Aurora. Actually, the heat of the sun caused the rock to expand so that grating sounds were made by the cracked portions. Since the statues have been repaired, the sounds are no longer heard. In the background is the sacred pyramidal mountain which overlooks the Valley of the Kings. Tombs of the nobles and other important persons were cut into the cliffs facing the Nile River.

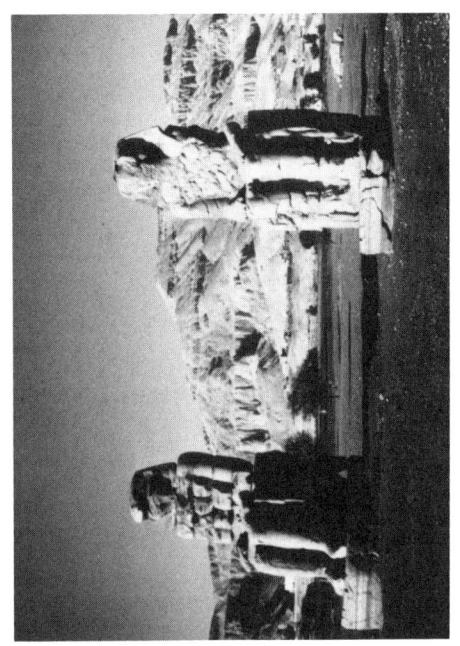

A statue of Amenhotep IV (Ikhnaton) reveals an unusual physique which may be a new art form of his period or the result of a disorder of the pituitary gland. (Photograph courtesy the Egyptian Museum, Cairo)

The Eighteenth Dynasty[1]

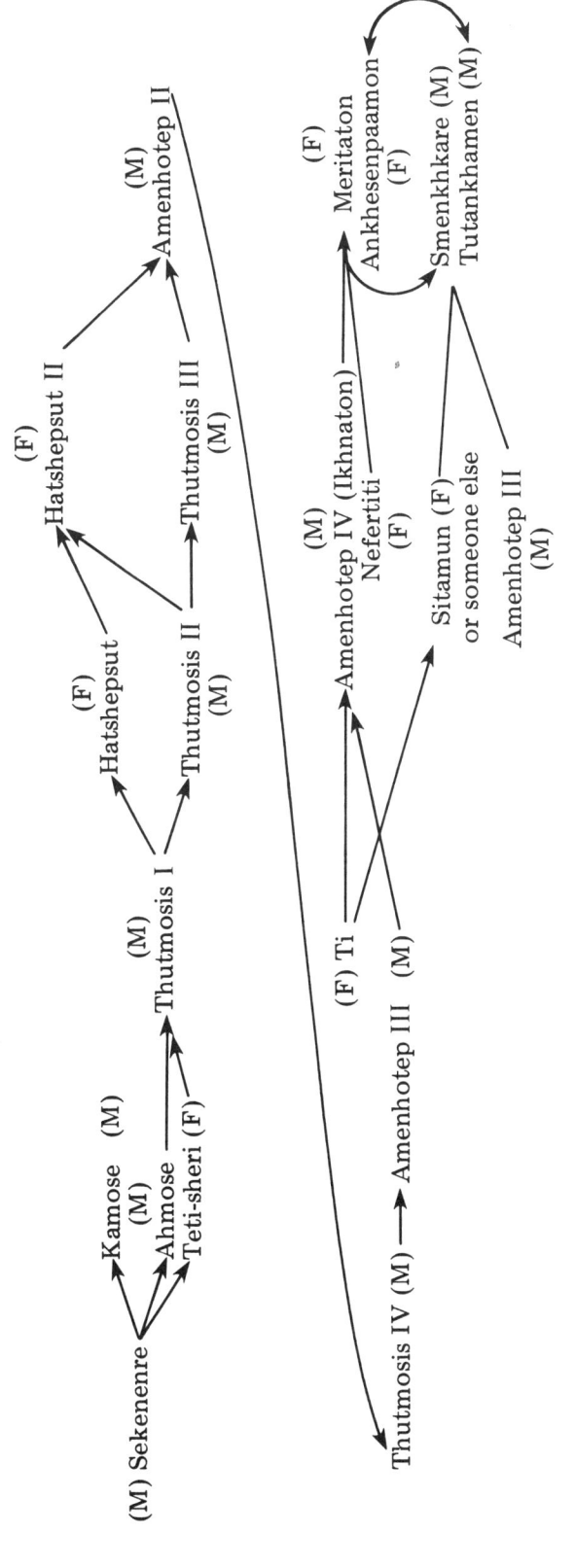

Ay (M)

Ay was a Vizier, high priest and, many believe, the brother of Queen Ti(Ty). He became pharaoh after the death of Tutankhamen. It is also believed by some that he fathered Nefertiti's children and that he later married Ankhesenpaamon.

1. Author's version.

Pituitary Gland

ACTH—adrenocorticotropic hormone—stimulates the adrenal cortex.
ADH—antidiuretichormone or vasopressin—regulates water absorption in the kidneys.
FSH—follicle stimulating hormone—stimulates egg or spermatozoa production.
Growth hormone—controls normal growth and regulates metabolism.
LH—luteinizing hormone—stimulates growth of egg follicles and the production of testosterone.
Oxytocin—stimulates the secretion of milk and the uterine muscles during parturition; aids sperm movement in Fallopian tubes.
Prolactin—regulates breast development and the production of milk.
TSH—thyrotropin—stimulates the thyroid gland.

Adrenal Cortex or Medulla

Adrenalin—stimulates heart rate, the brain, mobilizes fat and sugar.
Aldosterone and desoxycorticosterone—regulation of sodium, potassium and other minerals by the kidneys.
Cortisol and related hormones—regulates the metabolism of fat, minerals, protein, sugar and water.
Noradrenalin—constricts arterioles and increases heart contractions.

Thyroid Gland

Thyrocalcitonin—regulates calcium metabolism.
Thyroid hormones—regulates the overall body rate of metabolism.

Parathyroid Glands

Parathyroid hormone—regulates calcium metabolism.

Pancreas

Glucagon—regulates the utilization of sugar; antagonizes insulin.
Insulin—regulates the use of fats, protein and sugar.

Ovaries and Testes

Estrogen—regulates feminine characteristics and the ovulation cycle.
Progesterone—regulates the ovulation cycle and pregnancy.
Testosterone—regulates male characteristics and the reproductive tract.

Hypothalmus—Releasing factors for ACTH, TSH, LH, FSH, prolactin and the Growth hormone.

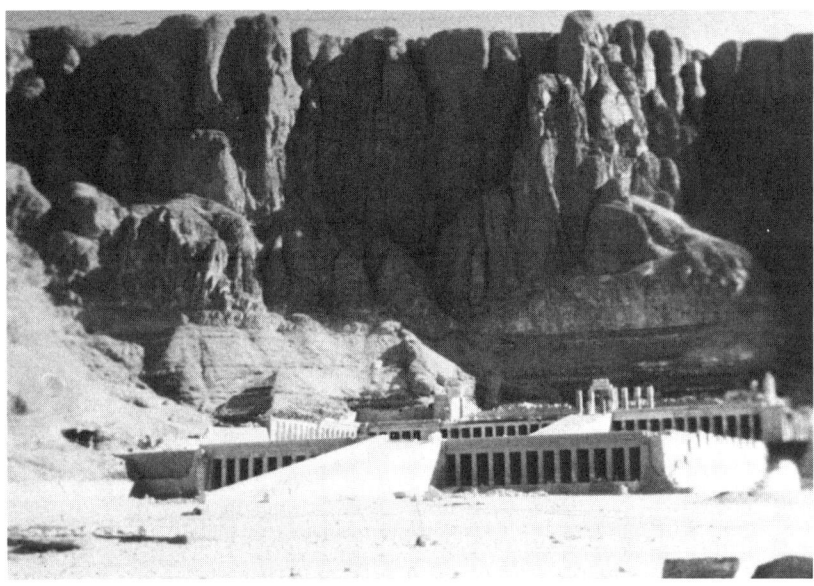

The mortuary temple of Hatshepsut (Ma'at-ka-re) at Der el-Bahri, on the western side of the Nile River, opposite the Temple of Amun at Karnak. Much of the temple was destroyed by Thutmosis III and others, and is still under reconstruction. Among the inscriptions found here are those concerning a voyage to the land of Punt, from which were brought, among other things, a collection of animals and plants, including incense-trees. The trees were planted in front of the temple where their locations can still be seen today. On the other side of the cliffs lies the famous Valley of the Kings.

Another very famous ruler of ancient Egypt was a woman named Hatshepsut (Makare). She was married to her half-brother, Thutmosis II. This union produced two daughters, Nefrure and Hatshepsut II. Thutmosis II produced a son, through a concubine, named Menkephrere who later became Thutmosis III. At the death of Thutmosis II, Thutmosis III was only a child. Hatshepsut was named regent to rule until he came of age, and the boy was married to her two daughters. However, Hatshepsut apparently planned to keep the throne for herself by declaring that she was none other than the daughter of the god Amon-Ra who had visited her Mother one night for the purpose of producing a child to rule Egypt. Hatshepsut assumed the role of Pharaoh; dressed in pharonic clothes; wore the double-crown of Egypt; and even wore the false-beard of the kings. She managed to hold the throne for about twenty years, then disappeared and Thutmosis III took his rightful place as the Pharaoh. During the reign of Hatshepsut, an expedition was sent to the east to a land called Punt, which is believed to have been at the southern end of the Red Sea. The expedition returned with gold, animals, plants and incenses. A botanical collection was established by Hatshepsut which was later added to by Thutmosis III, with plants that he brought back from expeditions into the region of Mesopotamia and from Nubia. Hatshepsut had a large funerary temple constructed at Dier el Bahri upon whose walls she had recorded the expedition to Punt. Among the many carvings is one of an overweight, misshaped woman who, many investigators believe, represented a person who was suffering from Elephantiasis.

Elephantiasis occurs in certain persons after long exposure to repeated filarial worm infections and recurrent attacks of lymphangitis. Elephantiasis usually affects the genitalia, legs, arms and breasts. It is a fibromyositis or collagenous hypertrophy of subcutaneous connective tissue with redundant skin and pockets of lymph. The skin becomes rough and nodular.

The filarial or thread worms are parasites of the circulatory and lymphatic systems, connective tissues and muscles of many vertebrates. The principal parasites in man are: *Wuchereria bancrofti; W. malayi; Onchocerca volvulus; Loa loa; Acanthocheilonema perstans;* and *Mansonella ozzardi*. The adult worms are found in the lymph vessels, subcutaneous nodules, tissues, and body cavities of man. Copulation occurs and the female produces microscopic microfilariae at the rate of about 12,000 per day. The microfilariae migrate into the circulatory system and can be found in the peripheral blood. The microfilariae are removed by bloodsucking insects in which they develop into infectious filariform larvae. The infective larvae are transmitted to the skin of a new host by the proboscis of the biting insect. The larvae enter the body of the new host through the bite wound and develop into mature filarial worms at its selected site. Obstructive inflammation of the lymphatic system may lead to Elephantiasis. There is no effective chemotherapeutic agent for destroying both adult worms and microfilariae but complete cures have been reported after treatment with arsenical compounds and hetrazan, a piperazin derivative.

Infection with *Wuchereria bancrofti* and *W. malayi* may result in damage to the lymphatic system and Elephantiasis; *O. volvulus* infections usually produce lesions of the arms, nodules or calabar swellings and blindness. *Loa loa* infections are generally not serious except when there is eye involvement during which the worm may actually pass in front of the eyeball or across the bridge of the nose. *A. perstans* causes little tissue reaction but has been associated with enlarged, painful livers. The same applies to *M. ozzardi*. These parasitic worms disfigure or blind about 300 million people today.

When reading about Ancient Egypt, one cannot ignore the pyramids, mainly because some are of the largest man-made structures on the Earth. From the beginning of the 4th Dynasty to the collapse of the Old Kingdom, about three hundred years later, every Pharaoh, except one, had a pyramid constructed, presumably as a tomb. The largest pyramind, that of Cheops (Khufu), was originally about 490 feet high and its base covers an area of approximately thirty-one acres: an area in which could be fitted Westminster, St. Paul's and the cathedrals of Milan, Florence and St. Peter's. It has been estimated that

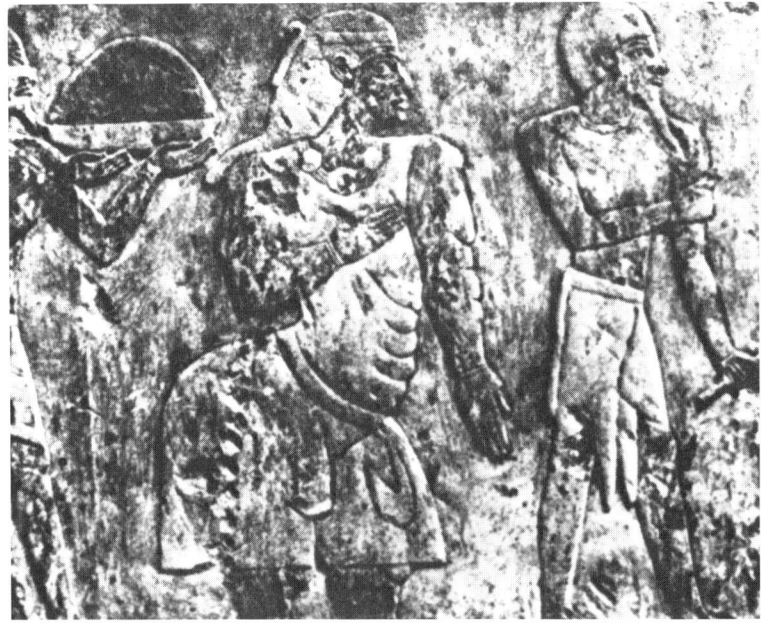

A portion of the Punt inscriptions on the walls of the mortuary temple of Hatshepsut which depicts the wife of the ruler of Punt. The woman may merely be obese or she may have had repeated filarial worm infections which led to elephantiasis.

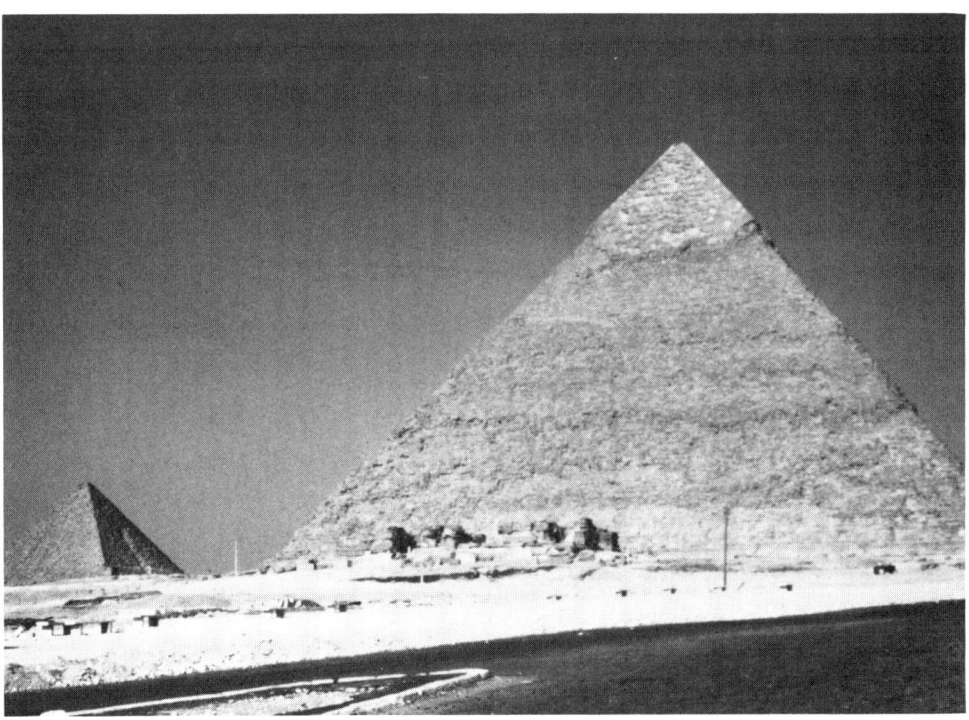

The great Pyramids of Chephren and Mycerinus at Giza.

there are 2,300,000 blocks of stone contained in the pyramid, some weighing as much as 30 tons.

Reasons other than the building of a royal tomb have been postulated by scholars for the construction of the pyramids. The most recent being that their construction was a huge public works project used to keep the population under control during the flood season and to bring about a more stable unification of Upper and Lower Egypt.

It has also been proposed that the form of the pyramid, when aligned in an East-West, North-South axis, in some manner, prevents decomposition of materials and allows mummification or dessication of once living material to occur. Razor blades and knives are said to remain sharp for long periods of time if stored in this manner. For the interested reader, the directions for construction of such an object follow.

The construction of the pyramid requires four identical isosceles triangles measuring 14.94 × 14.94 × 15.7 units. These are joined together to form a pyramid which is exactly 10.0 units in height. A shelf to hold objects is constructed exactly 3.33 units from the base of the pyramid. Orient the pyramid precisely so that the base lines face magnetic north-south and east-west.

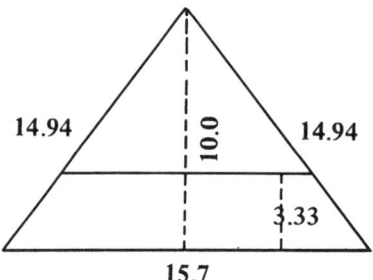

Tombs, pyramids, catacombs and caves are actually dangerous places to enter, not because of the supposed curses that were placed on the burial places, but because of the possible presence of rabid bats and the accumulated fecal material of birds and bats which might contain pathogenic fungi such as *Histoplasma capsulatum* or *Cryptococcus neoformans*. The inhalation of the organisms or spores may result in a tuberculosis-like infection in the lungs or the infection may become disseminated throughout the body. *C. neoformans* has a predilection for the central nervous system. Once dissemination of the infection occurs, death may occur rapidly. Today, the infections are treated, with some success, with the antifungal drug Fungizone (Amphotericin B). It is interesting to note that many of the Egyptian tomb robbers were said to watch the cliffs in the burial areas on the west bank of the Nile River, at dawn and at dusk, to discover where the bats and birds flew to and from, since frequently they found hidden tombs in which to roost undisturbed.

the hebrews and the old testament

It is believed that the Hebrews were a group of nomads who migrated from the Arabian Peninsula, through Mesopotamia, into Lower Egypt, and then returned to the area of the Middle East surrounding present day Jerusalem. Their legends and history are preserved in the Old Testament and other works. It is believed that the early Books of the Old Testament were organized by scribes under the direction of Ezekial, in about 550 B.C., during the Babylonian Captivity of some of the Hebrews by Nebuchadrezzar. It is interesting to note that in the first Book of the Old Testament, Genesis, Abram, from whom all Hebrews claim descent, arrived with his family at Harran, from Ur of the Chaldees. The Chaldeans ruled Ur at the time of the Babylonian captivity, but not 1500 years earlier during the time of Abram. In 1976, a treasure trove of clay tablets was discovered at Ebla, in northern Syria, which provides evidence of a kingdom that existed in the area between about 2400 and 2250 B.C., and numerous biblical connections. The tablets contain accounts of the creation and flood which are very similar to those in Mesopotamian literature and the Old Testament. The tablets mention a place called "Urusalina" (Jerusalem?) and Ebrium (Eber), who is identified in the Old Testament as the great-great-great-great grandfather of Abraham (Abram). The quotations used in the discussion of the Hebrews are from "The Holy Scriptures of the Old Testament."[1]

The Creation:
Genesis I: 1,2,6,9,11,16,24,26,27,48,31

"In the beginning God created the heaven and the earth. And the earth was without form, and void; and darkness was upon the face of the deep. And the Spirit of God moved upon the face of the waters. And God said, Let there be a firmament in the midst of the waters, and let it divide the water from the

---

1. "Extracts from the authorized version of the Holy Bible (King James Version), which is Crown copyright in England, are included with permission."

waters. And God said, Let the waters under the heaven be gathered together unto one place, and let the dry land appear: and it was so. And God said, Let the Earth bring forth grass, the herb yielding seed, and the fruit tree yielding fruit after his kind, whose seed is in itself, upon the earth: and it was so. And God made two great lights; the greater light to rule the day, and the lesser light to rule the night: he made the stars also. And God said, Let the earth bring forth the living creature after his kind, cattle and creeping thing, and beast of the earth after his kind: and it was so. And God said, Let us make man in our image, after our likeness: and let them have dominion over the fish of the sea, and over the fowl of the air, and over the cattle, and over all the earth, and over every creeping thing that creepeth upon the earth. So God created man in his own image, in the image of God created he him; male and female created he them. And God blessed them, and God said unto them, Be fruitful, and multiply; and replenish the earth, and subdue it: and have dominion over the fish of the sea, and over the fowl of the air, and over every living thing that moveth upon the earth. And God saw everything that he had made, and, behold, it was very good. And the evening and the morning were the sixth day."

Genesis II: 5,6,7,8,16,17, 21, 22, 23

"And every plant of the field before it was in the earth, and every herb of the field before it grew: for the Lord God had not caused it to rain upon the earth, and there was not a man to till the ground. But there went up a mist from the earth, and watered the whole face of the ground. And the Lord God formed man of the dust of the ground, and breathed into his nostrils the breath of life; and man became a living soul. And the Lord God planted a garden eastward in Eden; and there he put the man whom he had formed. And the Lord God commanded the man, saying, Of every tree of the garden thou mayest freely eat: But of the tree of the knowledge of good and evil, thou shalt not eat of it; for in the day that thou eatest thereof thou shalt surely die. And the Lord God caused a deep sleep to fall upon Adam, and he slept; and he took one of his ribs, and closed up the flesh instead thereof; and the rib, which the Lord God had taken from man, made he a woman, and brought her unto the man. And Adam said, This is now bone of my bones, and flesh of my flesh: she shall be called Woman, because she was taken out of Man."

It should be noted that in the above, there were apparently two sources for the creation of man. According to legend, the first woman created was Lilith, who was an equal of Adam. The second woman, Eve, was created from Adam's rib, and was therefore subserviant. The Hebrew Creation should be compared with the Egyptian and Mesopotamian Creation legends for similarities.

Genesis VI: 1,2,3,4,5,7,8,13,14,15,17,18,19,21,22

"And it came to pass, when men began to multiply on the face of the earth, and daughters were born unto them, that the sons of God saw the daughters of men that they were fair; and they took them wives of all which they choose. And the Lord said, My spirit shall not always strive with man, for that he also is flesh: yet his days shall be a hundred and twenty years. There were giants in the earth in those days; and also after that, when the sons of God came in unto the daughters of men, and they bare children to them, the same became mighty men which were of old, men of renown. And God saw that the wickedness of man was great in the earth, and that every imagination of the thoughts of his heart was only evil continually. And the Lord said, I will destroy man whom I have created from the face of the earth; both man, and beast, and the creeping thing, and the fowls of the air; for it repenteth me that I have made them. But Noah found grace in the eyes of the Lord. And God said unto Noah, the end of all flesh is come before me; for the earth is filled with violence through them; and, behold, I will destroy them with the earth. Make thee an ark of gopher wood; rooms shalt thou make in the ark, and thou shalt pitch it within and without with pitch. And this is the fashion which thou shalt make it of: The length of the arc shall be three hundred cubits (from elbow to end of middle finger), the breadth of it fifty cubits, and the height of it thirty cubits. And behold, I, even I, do bring a flood of waters upon the earth, to destroy all flesh, wherein is the breath of life, from under heaven; and everything that is in the earth shall die. But with thee will I establish my covenant; and thou shalt come into the ark, thou and thy sons, and thy wife, and thy son's wives with thee. And of every living thing of all flesh, two of every sort shalt thou bring into the ark, to keep them alive with thee; they shall be male and female. And take thou unto thee of all food that is eaten, and thou shalt gather it to thee; and it shall be food for thee and for them. Thus did Noah; according to all that God commanded him, so did he."

The beginning of Chapter VI, Genesis, has been taken by some authors to indicate that there were different types of people on the earth, including giants, who interbred to produce modern man. Some writers have postulated that the "sons of God" who bred with the "daughters of men" were travelers from outer space. Many cultures around the world have in their mythology, stories about giants, who are usually portrayed as being evil. It is entirely possible that isolated tribes, by inherited traits, were giants, when compared with other persons. Giantism may result from a disease of the anterior lobe of the hypophysis or hyperfunctioning of the pituitary gland. The body may be large, but normal in appearance, as observed in some present day basketball players; or the body may be enlarged in only specific areas, as in acromegaly.

The epic of the flood in the Old Testament, can be found in the Sumerian myth concerning a deluge and the Sumerian epic, Gilgamesh. The destruction of mankind is also found in Egyptian mythology but there, the land is flooded to save mankind. The Egyptians knew that the Nile River would flood at the heliacal rising of Sirius, the dog-star, and could plan accordingly. In other parts of the world, floods could occur at any time and could cause many deaths because there was no advance warning for the people.

Abram and the Covenant

Genesis XI: 31

"And Terah took Abram his son, and Lot, the son of Haran his son's son, and Sarai his daughter in law, his son Abram's wife; and they went forth with them from Ur of the Chaldees, to go into the land of Canaan; and they came unto Haran, and dwelt there.

Genesis XII: 10

"And there was a famine in the land: and Abram went down into Egypt to sojourn there; for the famine was grievous in the land."

Genesis XVII1,5,8,10,11

"And when Abram was ninety years old and nine, the Lord appeared to Abram, and said unto him, I am the Almighty God; walk before me, and be thou perfect. Neither shall thy name any more be called Abram, but thy name shall be Abraham; for a father of many nations have I made thee. And I will give unto thee, and to thy seed after thee, the land wherein thou art a stranger, all the land of Canaan, for an everlasting possession; and I will be their God. This is my covenant, which ye shall keep, between me and you and thy seed after thee; Every man child among you shall be circumcised. And ye shall circumcise the flesh of your foreskin; and it shall be a token of the covenant betwixt me and you."

The story of Abraham and the ritual of circumcision is not unique. Many primitive cultures utilize the ritual of circumcision during puberty rites. In some cultures, females are also circumcised. Circumcision was practiced in Ancient Egypt, and it may be that Abram learned of the practice there while waiting for the famine to subside. Just when the ritual of circumcision began is unknown but it was widespread in Ancient Egypt, among the Hebrews and other peoples in the Middle East and Africa. Today, many reports indicate that there is less cancer of the penis among circumcised males than uncircumcised males and that the wives of circumcised males have a lower incidence of cancer of the cervix than the wives of males who have not been circumcised. It is believed that the common Herpes virus can be harboured under the foreskin of males and transmitted to females during sexual intercourse. The Herpes virus, in some manner, is believed to stimulate the growth of another virus or viruses which cause the cancers of the penis and cervix. Circumcision also allows for the easier cleaning of the penis following intercourse and a lower incidence of venereal diseases.

Genital herpes simplex infection, a venereal disease, is caused by the herpes simplex virus, of which there are two types. Type I usually causes cold sores, fever blisters on the face, and eye infections. It also causes about 10 percent of genital herpes infections. Type II is usually acquired through sexual contact and is the predominant cause of genital herpes infections. Women with Type II herpes simplex are eight times more likely to get cervical cancer than are women who do not have the infection. An experimental drug, 2-deoxy-D-glucose, which interferes with the multiplication of the herpes virus, is being tested at the University of Pennsylvania.

The Book of Genesis concludes with the story of Joseph, who had served the Pharaoh, and the mummification of Joseph's father, Jacob, and later when Joseph died, the mummification of his body. It is unusual that mummification was utilized by the Hebrews in these two cases, since the process involved the use of Egyptian religious rites. The Book of Exodus starts with a new king ruling over Egypt who did not look with favor upon the Hebrews, and made them work for the use of his land.

Exodus I: 11

"Therefore they did set over them taskmasters to afflict them with their burdens. And they built for Pharaoh treasure cities. Pithom and Raamses."

Exodus I: 16

"And he (Pharaoh) said, When ye do the office of a midwife to the Hebrew women, and see them upon the stools; if it be a son, then ye shall kill him: but if it be a daughter, then she shall live."

The cities of Pithom and Ramses were located in the eastern Delta region (Goshen) and were probably fortified in order to protect the route from the Middle East into Egypt. The Hebrews were in this area with their grazing animals. Previously, Joseph had interpreted the Pharaoh's dreams and the Pharaoh had made him ruler over Egypt.

Genesis XLI: 40

"Thou shalt be over my house, and according unto thy word shall all my people be ruled: only in the throne will I be greater than thou."

This was very unusual, to place a foreigner to rule Egypt. Egyptian writings rarely mention the Hebrews and it is uncertain under which two Pharaohs Joseph, and later, Moses, served, since the Old Testament does not call them by name. Many scholars date the Exodus in the 13th century B.C.; about the time of Ramses II and his son, Merneptah. In 1250 B.C., Merneptah's records state that Israel was destroyed and had no seed; but how could Israel be destroyed if this was the time of the Exodus? One thing that is definitely known is that about 300 years later, in about 945 B.C., King Sheshonk (Shishank) of the Libyan Dynasty sacked Jerusalem during the reign of King Rehoboan.

Unfortunately, in Book I, Kings XI: 17,19, is the following:

"That Hadad fled, he and certain Edomites of his father's servants with him, to go into Egypt; Hadad being yet a little child. And Hadad found great favor in the sight of Pharaoh, so that he gave him to wife the sister of his own wife, the sister of Tahpenes the queen."

Hadad fled into Egypt during the reign of Solomon. Ahmose I, one of the founders of the 18th Dynasty, about 1580 B.C., had a queen named Tanethap (Tenthape). If this is the same Queen stated in the Old Testament and in Egyptian records, then the Exodus must have occurred prior to the time of David and Solomon and of Ahmose I of the 18th Dynasty.

An interesting inscription[2] was found at Tell el Arish, in the eastern Egyptian Delta, which has been assigned to the Pharaoh Taui Thom (Tau Timaeus) who ruled at the end of the Middle Kingdom, before the time of Ahmose I. Portions of the inscription follow:

"Now behold the majesty of Shu was in his palace in Memphis: his majesty said, Come now, let us proceed to my palace in At Nebes (locality in Goshen, Eastern Delta) and see our father, Ra-Harmakhis in the Eastern horizon: Then the children of the dragon, Apep, the evil-doers of Usheru and of the red country (desert), came upon the road of At Nebes; then the majesty of Shu caused to be fortified all the places around At Nebes; in At Nebes is a pool upon the east of Hat Nebes in which the majesty of Ra proceeded; Now it came to pass that the majesty of Shu obtained the whole land, none could stand before him, but sickness came upon him, confusion seized his eyes, he made his chapel, evil fell upon the land, a great disturbance in the palace; the palace was in great affliction; Shu had departed to heaven; there was no exit from the palace by the space of nine days; Now these nine days were in violence and tempest; none, whether god or man could see the face of his fellow. The majesty of Seb came forth appearing on the throne of his father Shu: every royal dwelling did him homage. Behold, he went to the East of Usher (desert) and entered the house of Aar at the eastern gate of At Nebes; he discussed the history of the city and they told him all that had happened when the majesty of Ra was at At Nebes, the conflicts of *King Tum* in this locality, and the valor of the majesty of Shu in this city: Now when the majesty of Ra-Harmachis fought with the evil-doers in this pool, the Place of the Whirlpool, the evil-doers prevailed not over his majesty; his majesty leaped into the so-called Place of the Whirlpool; he smote the evildoers in the Place of the Whirlpool: he slew the children of Apep."

Interesting points in the inscription concern a Pharaoh who fought and defeated some peoples from the Eastern deserts at the Place of the Whirlpool where he was wounded or became sick and died. His son, the next Pharaoh, after a period of nine days of violence and tempest, took the throne and then

---

2. "The Antiquities of Tell el Yahudiyeh," F.L. Griffith, The Egypt Exploration Fund, Memoir Seven, 1889. London, 1890, pg. 72.

returned to the East to learn what had happened there. Whether this refers to the time of the Exodus of the Hebrews is unknown, but there are many similarities.

Although it is, at this time, unfortunate that the time of the Exodus cannot be stated with certainty, it apparently did occur since the Hebraic observance of Passover is one of the great celebrations of that religion and must have had some foundation in the past. Within the story of the Exodus are included some great feats of magic which were caused to happen by the God of the Hebrews and the Egyptian magicians.

When Moses was born, his mother hid him for three months in order to escape the Pharonic order for the death of male infants, and then placed him in an ark of bulrushes. He was found by a daughter of Pharaoh, became her son, and she called him Moses. When Moses was grown, he killed an Egyptian who was "smiting an Hebrew, one of his brethren." When the Pharaoh heard of the murder, "he sought to slay Moses. But Moses fled from the face of Pharaoh and dwelt in the land of Midan." While there Moses married Zipporah. "And it came to pass in process of time, that the King of Egypt died: and the children of Israel sighed by reason of the bondage." God appeared to Moses saying "Come now therefore, and I will send thee unto Pharaoh, that thou mayest bring forth my people the children of Israel out of Egypt." "And I will stretch out my hand and smite Egypt with all my wonders which *I* will do in the midst thereof; and after that he will let you go." "But every woman shall borrow of her neighbor . . . jewels of silver and jewels of gold, and raiment: and ye shall spoil the Egyptians." Moses hesitated so God changed a staff which Moses held into a serpent; caused leprosy to appear and disappear from his hand and showed him how to change water into blood. Moses still hesitated because he did not speak well and he was allowed to take Aaron, his brother, along as his spokesman.

Exodus VII: 10, 11, 12

"And Moses and Aaron went in unto Pharaoh, and they did so as the Lord had commanded: and Aaron cast down his rod before Pharaoh, and before his servants, and it became a serpent. Then Pharaoh also called the wise men and the sorcerers; now the magicians of Egypt, they also did in like manner with their enchantments. For they caste down every man his rod and they became serpents: But Aaron's rod swallowed up their rods."

However, Pharaoh's heart was hardened and he refused to let the Hebrews leave Egypt. Therefore, ten plagues were put upon Egypt. The stories of the plagues are well-known, but if there are examined, the majority of them were things that happened frequently in Egypt. The Hebrews, being recent immigrants, were not aware that many of these so-called plagues had visited Egypt before. It has been reported that the Egyptian cobra can be induced, by pinching behind the head, to remain rigid for a period of time, and would thus resemble a stick or rod, if held in one's hand.

Plague I

Exodus VII: 20,21,22,23,24

"And Moses and Aaron did so, as the Lord commanded; and he lifted up the rod, and smote the waters that were in the river, in the sight of Pharaoh and in the sight of his servants; and all the waters that were in the river were turned to blood. And the fish that was in the river died; and the river stank, and the Egyptians could not drink of the water of the river; and there was blood throughout all the land of Egypt. And the magicians of Egypt did likewise with their enchantments: and Pharaoh's heart was hardened and Pharaoh turned and went into his house. And all the Egyptians digged around about the river for water to drink; for they could not drink of the water of the river."

Every summer, when the Nile River began to flood, the turbulence of the waters would dissolve the red clay of the Cataract region and color the waters red. In mythology, Ra had colored beer with this same clay so that it appeared to be blood, and stopped the Goddess Sekhmet from destroying mankind. The great amounts of decaying organic material carried by the flooding waters could utilize large amounts of oxygen during their decomposition, removing it from the water and killing the fish. The flooding Nile would be so dirty it would be unfit to drink. The Egyptians dug wells near the edge of the river which would provide clear, filtered water for drinking.

Plague II

Exodus VIII: 6,7,14

"And Aaron stretched out his hand over the waters of Egypt; and the frogs came up, and covered the land of Egypt. And the magicians did so with their enchantments, and brought up frogs upon the land of Egypt. And they gathered them together upon heaps: and the land stank." When the Nile River flooded inland, it drove the frogs from the edge of the river before flooding, to the new edge of the river after flooding. This new edge of the river was where the people were, so the frogs would be seen more easily. The Hebrews, being nomadic herders of arid regions, would not be accustomed to seeing frogs. An Egyptian fertility god was portrayed as a frog.

Plague III

Exodus VIII: 17,18

"And they did so: for Aaron stretched out his hand with his rod, and smote the dust of the earth, and it became lice in man, and in beast; all the dust of the land became lice throughout all the land of Egypt. And the magicians did so with their enchantments to bring forth lice, but they could not: so there were lice upon man, and upon beast."

Lice have been, and still are, common parasites of man and animals. They have been found on the mummified bodies of Ancient Egyptians and Nubians and, for some reason, are suddenly appearing in epidemic proportions in the populations of countries of the world today, such as the United States. They can be easily passed from person to person during sexual intercourse or through fomites such as clothing or haircombs. Associated with lice is typhus fever. Typhus fever is an acute infectious disease, with no characteristic lesions but with great prostration. It is accompanied by a possible softening of the spleen; darkness of the blood; and congestion of the lungs. It is caused by *Rickettsia prowazeki* and occurs in two forms. In the epidemic form, the organism is transmitted by lice; in the endemic or murine form, by the rat flea, *Xenopsylla cheopis.* The disease is usually accompanied by a high fever, headache and generalized rash. The case-fatality rate in epidemics is about twenty percent. The description by Fracastoro, in 1546, is the earliest medical record which is sufficiently clear to identify typhus fever as a separate entity. Typhus fever has always been associated with wars, famine, misfortunes and the crowding together of people. This crowding together of people occurred, naturally, when the Nile River flooded and therefore, facilitated the spreading of lice from person to person. Today, typhus fever can be prevented by immunization. Lice can be controlled with insecticides. The tetracyclines and chloramphenicol are highly effective in the treatment of typhus infections.

Plague IV

Exodus VIII: 24

"And the Lord did so; and there came a grievous swarm of flies into the house of Pharaoh, and into his servants' houses, and into all the land of Egypt: The land was corrupted by reason of the swarm of flies."

The flooding of the Nile River had resulted in the death of fish and later, the frogs died and "they gathered them together upon heaps: and the land stank." The bodies of the dead fish and frogs provided the environment for the production of swarms of flies. In Egypt and the Middle East, flies are involved in the transmission of tracoma and other diseases.

Plague V

Exodus IX: 3,6

"Behold, the hand of the Lord is upon thy cattle which is in the field, upon the horses, upon the asses, upon the camels, upon the oxen, upon the sheep: there shall be a very grievous murrain. And the Lord did that thing on the morrow, and all the cattle of Egypt died: but of the cattle of the children of Israel died not one."

Epidemic diseases can attack both people and cattle. Isolation is one method of combatting infectious diseases. In Plague IV, the Hebrews went three days journey into the wilderness in order to make a sacrifice to remove the plague of flies. Perhaps the cattle were also three days journey into the wilderness. Nevertheless, it can be assumed that the two groups of cattle were not mixed together. Viral diseases of animals, such as hoof and mouth disease and encephalitis, some of which are transmitted by arthropods, others by direct contact or fomites, could result in the deaths of large numbers of animals. The flooding environment would favor the reproduction of mosquitos. The flies have already been mentioned in great numbers. Encephalitis can also be transmitted from animals to humans by certain mosquitos. Several outbreaks have occurred in the United States which resulted in the deaths of many of those persons who were infected.

Plague VI

Exodus IX: 10,11

"And they took ashes of the furnace, and stood before Pharaoh; and Moses sprinkled it up toward heaven; and it became a boil breaking forth with blains upon man and upon beast. And the magicians could not stand before Moses because of the boils; for the boil was upon the magicians, and upon all the Egyptians."

Leishmaniasis or Egyptian ulcer, or Oriental sore, or Bagdad boil are the names given to a prevalent infection found in the Mediterranean regions. The infective agent, *Leishmania donovani,* and others, is a flagellate protozoan which is parasitic in man and certain animals, attacking various organs of the body, and causing lesions to appear on the skin. There is a general loss of weight and debility. Death may occur within weeks or years. Antimony compounds are used today in the treatment of this disease. It is transmitted among hosts by sand flies of the *Genus Phlebotomus.* The Ancient Egyptians, crowded together in the sandy regions at the edge of the flooding Nile, made easy targets for the blood-seeking sand flies. Sand flies may be controlled today by the destruction of their breeding grounds and the use of insecticides.

Plague VII

Exodus IX: 23,24,25,26

"And Moses stretched forth his rod toward heaven: and the Lord sent thunder and hail, and the fire ran along the ground; and the Lord rained hail upon the land of Egypt. So there was hail, and fire mingled with hail, very grievous, such as there was none like it in all the land of Egypt since it became a nation. And the hail smote throughout all the land of Egypt all that was in the field, both man and beast; and the hail smote every herb of the field, and brake every tree of the field. Only in the land of Goshen, where the children of Israel were, was there no hail."

It is believed by some scholars that the word which, in the above, is translated as "hail," should be written as "stone(s)"; the description would then fit that of a volcanic eruption. It is possible that the eruption and destruction of the volcanic island of Thera (Santorini), in about 1500 B.C., is described here by the falling of stones and fire.

Hail, or stones, and fire could certainly destroy man, beasts, herbs and trees. However, it should be pointed out that in Plague V, all the cattle of the Egyptians had died. Rain is very scarce in the Nile Valley. The plague described could also be a violent thunderstorm, with hail and lightning which would be something unusual for the Egyptians to experience, but not the well-traveled Hebrews.

Plague VIII

Exodus X: 13,15

"And Moses stretched forth his rod over the land of Egypt, and the Lord brought an East wind upon the land all that day, and all that night; and when it was morning, the east wind brought the locusts. For they covered the face of the whole earth, so that the land was darkened; and they did eat every herb of the land, and all the fruit of the trees which the hail had left: and there remained not a green thing in the trees, or in the herbs of the field, through all the land of Egypt."

This is not an unusual thing to happen in the Middle East or Africa where large swarms of locusts still occur today. When the Mormons settled in Salt Lake City, in the United States, they were visited by a swarm of locusts and, according to their writings, were saved by the arrival of a large flock of seagulls.

Plague IX

Exodus X: 22,23

"And Moses stretched forth his hand toward heaven; and there was a thick darkness in all the land of Egypt three days: And they saw not one another, neither rose any from his place for three days: but all the children of Israel had light in their dwellings."

An eclipse of the sun could cause a temporary darkness, but not for three days. The thick darkness could refer to ashes, powder and dirt in the air caused by a volcanic eruption as previously described. This could last three days or more. The Hebraic account is similar to the darkness described in the Tell el Arish inscription, of Egyptian origin.

Plague X

Exodus XII: 21,22,23,24,29,30,31,35,41

"Then Moses called for all the elder of Israel, and said unto them, Draw out and take you a lamb according to your families, and kill the passover. And ye shall take a bunch of *hyssop,* and dip it in the blood that is in the bason, and strike the lintel and the two side posts with the blood that is in the bason; and none of you shall go out at the door of his house until the morning. (The hyssop plant contains an anti-coagulant which prevents the clotting of blood.)

"For the Lord will pass through to smite the Egyptians; and when he seeth the blood upon the lintel, and on the two side posts, the Lord will *pass over* the door, and will not suffer the destroyer to come in unto your houses to smite you. And ye shall observe this thing for an ordinance to thee and to thy sons for ever. And it came to pass that at midnight the Lord smote all the firstborn in the land of Egypt, from the firstborn of Pharaoh that sat on his throne unto the firstborn of the captive that was in the dungeon; and all the firstborn of cattle. And Pharaoh rose up in the night he, and all his servants, and all the Egyptians; for there was not a house where there was not one dead. And he called for Moses and Aaron by night, and said, Rise up and get you forth from among my people. . . . And the children of Israel did according to the word of Moses; and they borrowed of the Egyptians, jewels of silver and jewels of gold, and raiment: And it came to pass at the end of four hundred and thirty years, even the selfsame day it came to pass, that all the hosts of the Lord went out from the land of Egypt."

There are some scholars who believe that the deaths of the Egyptians were caused by an earthquake. The Egyptians lived in houses of clay, supported by wood which, during the earthquake, fell upon them, killing many of them. The Hebrews, living in tents of hides with wooden supports, survived the earthquake and fled during the confusion that followed.

The Hebrews traveled "not through the way of the land of the Philistines, although that was near," but "through the way of the wilderness of the Red Sea." They were pursued by the Pharaoh who "made ready his chariot, and took his people with him: and he took six hundred chosen chariots, and all the chariots of Egypt." The Pharoah and his army overtook the Hebrews who were "encamping by the sea, beside Pi-hahiroth."

Exodus XIV: 21,22,27,28

"And Moses stretched out his hand over the sea; and the Lord caused the sea to go back by a strong east wind all that night, and made the sea dry land, and the waters were divided. And the children of Israel went into the midst of the sea upon the dry ground: and the waters were a wall unto them on their right hand, and on their left. And Moses stretched forth his hand over the sea, and the sea returned to his strength when the morning appeared; and the Egyptians fled against it; and the Lord overthrew the Egyptians in the midst of the sea. And the waters returned, and covered the chariots, and the horsemen, and all the host of Pharaoh that came into the sea after them; there remained not so much as one of them."

Many scholars believe that the escape by the Hebrews occurred, not in the Red Sea, but, in the "Sea of Reeds," a swampy area near the Red Sea, in which the chariots of the Egyptians became mired. The Hebrews, on foot with their herds, escaped.

An interesting story can be found in Egyptian literature which tells about the Pharaoh Seneferu, founder of the Fourth Dynasty, and father of the Pharaoh Cheops, who built the great pyramid. The Pharaoh was being rowed about a lake by a crew of beautiful girls when they stopped because one of the girls had dropped a new pendant into the water and refused to row until it was found. The Chief Lector-priest was sent for and when he arrived and heard what had happened, "He said words of magic, and he placed the one side of the water of the lake upon the other, and he found the fish pendant lying on a potsherd. Then he said what he said, words of magic, and he brought the waters of the lake back to their place."

Although the Hebrews had lived in Egypt for "Four hundred and thirty years," they failed to record any of the Egyptian medical lore in their writings in the Old Testament. However, they did establish certain dietary laws which, we know today, prevented the Hebrews from contracting certain diseases. They also established the custom of examination, isolation and expulsion of individuals who exhibited signs of certain infectious diseases. Hebraic medicine was, at this time, more preventative than curative.

Leviticus XI: 2,3,4,5,6,7,9,10,12,13,14,15,16,17,18,19,20,21,22,23,29,30

"Speak unto the children of Israel, saying, These are the beasts which ye shall eat among all the beasts that are on the earth. Whatsoever parteth the hoof, and is clovenfooted, and cheweth the cud, among the beasts that shall ye eat. Nevertheless these shall ye not eat of them that chew the cud, or of them that divide the hoof: as the camel, because he cheweth the cud, but divideth not the hoof; he is unclean to you. And the coney . . . And the hare . . . And the swine. . ."

Today, we know that the coney and the hare are associated with the bacterial disease, Tularemia; and swine with the nematode infection, Trichinosis, and others.

Tularemia derives its name from Tulare, California, the district in which the disease was first described. It is a disease of rodents, resembling plague, which may be transmitted to man. The causative agent is a bacterium, *Francisella tularensis* (formerly *Pasteurella*). In man the disease takes the form of an undulant fever, lasting several weeks, with much malaise and depression. The disease is transmitted by deer flies, stable flies, certain fleas and the bedbug. The Hebraic taboo against touching, eating or use of the skins of rodents for clothing, prevented the establishment of the infection in the community. Today, vaccination can prevent infection; if infected, the patient can be treated with Streptomycin, the drug of choice. The tetracyclines and chloramphenicol are also effective in the treatment of Tularemia.

Trichinosis is a worm infection of carnivorous and omnivorous animals, including man; the infective agent is the nematode, *Trichinella spiralis.* Infective larvae are found coiled in a cyst in the muscles of the host. When the infected tissue is eaten, the cyst dissolves and the parasite is liberated in the intestinal tract, where it matures. Copulation occurs, and the female deposits its larvae in the deep mucosa. The larvae are carried by the blood and lymphatics to all parts of the body, and again, encyst. Their effect on the host depends upon their numbers and location. In overwhelming infections, death may occur in two to three weeks. In 1947, it was estimated that there were approximately 28 millions of infected persons in the world and that 3/4 of them were in the United States. This high incidence was probably due to the custom of feeding garbage to hogs. The thorough cooking of all food given to hogs could eliminate the infection in the United States. The thorough cooking of all meats obtained from hogs, and all carnivorous and omnivorous animals, could prevent human infection. The holding of pork at $-15°C$. for 30 days will destroy the larvae, but thorough cooking is still recommended. Many chemotherapeutic agents have been tried against adult and larval worms without success. During the first few days of infection, the intestinal worms may be removed with purgatives or antihelminthics. Hetrazan, a piperazine derivative, may be effective in destroying the larvae.

"These shall ye eat of all that are in the waters: whatsoever has fins and scales in the waters, in the seas, and in the rivers, them shall ye eat. And all that have not fins and scales in the seas, and in the rivers, of all that move in the waters, and of any living thing which is in the waters, they shall be an abomination unto you. Whatsoever hath no fins nor scales in the waters, that shall be an abomination unto you."

This dietary law prohibits the eating of any thing found in the waters except animals with fins and scales, which is to say, fish. It is known today that shellfish, and other organisms taken from polluted waters, may be contaminated with a great number of diseases such as: hepatitis, typhoid fever, amoebic dysentery, bacillary dysentery, a variety of worm infections and, may also contain toxins from ingested marine organisms. If the shellfish are eaten raw, or if they are not properly cooked, the consumer may contract one of the previously mentioned diseases.

Whoever originated the dietary law was unaware that fish may also be capable of transmitting several diseases to man, including a tapeworm. The fish tapeworm, *Diphyllobothrium latum,* was recognized as a distinct species in 1602 and was differentiated from the pork tapeworm, *Taenia solium,* in 1777. The first cases in the United States were reported in 1906. The parasite is prevalent in temperate areas of the world where fresh-water fish are a part of the diet. The ova of tapeworms are taken into the alimentary canal of the host, from which they make their way into the tissues, where they form small, cystlike masses, called scolices or cysticerci. When the flesh of the original host is eaten, the scolices develop within the alimentary canal of the new host into a strobilis, or adult tapeworm. The adult worm is composed of a scolex (head), neck, and numerous hermaphroditic segments called proglottids. It may attain the length of ten meters. The proglottids produce the ova which, if they enter fresh water, as they must for the fish-tapeworm, release a free-swimming ciliated form called the coracidium. If it is ingested by certain copepods, such as *Diaptomus* or *Cyclops,* it develops into an elongated procercoid larva. When the infected copepod is ingested by a suitable fresh-water fish, such as carp, burbot or pike, the larva penetrates the intestinal wall and is transformed into the encysted form previously mentioned, the cysticerci. When the raw or improperly cooked fish is eaten, a tapeworm infection may result.

Unfortunately, one very well-known Hebraic fish preparation, gefilte fish, is prepared from fresh-water fish. During the preparation of the speciality, the cook tastes the mixture to be certain of the flavor prior to cooking. If the flesh of the fish were infective, the individual could contract the tapeworm infection. Until recently, women did most of the preparation of food for a family or group so, Hebrew women had a high incidence of fish tapeworm when compared with children or males. Infection may display no symptoms or the host may show nervous disturbances, digestive disorders, abdominal discomfort, pain, loss of weight, weakness, malnutrition and anemia. When the worm is attached to the jejunum, the vomiting of proglottids with severe abdominal pain is characteristic. Removal of the adult worms is brought about with the administration of purgatives and antihelmintic drugs. Atabrine, the drug that is also used against malaria, has a great affinity for the holdfast organs of the worms, and a single treatment may result in the expulsion of the entire worm. The scolex (head) must be identified to insure that the entire worm was eliminated. Other successful drugs have been Oleoresin of aspidium (shield ferns), hexylresorcinol, carbon tetrachloride, thymol and others. When traveling, one may be offered local food delicacies, especially in the Orient, where raw fish is frequently served. One should be cautious and inquire whether the fish is from fresh water or salt water if one wishes to avoid a fish-tapeworm.

"And these are they which ye shall have in abomination among the fowls; they shall not be eaten, they are an abomination: the eagle, the ossifrage, and the osprey, and the vulture, kite, raven, owl, night hawk, cuckow, hawk, owls, cormorant, swan, pelican, gier eagle, stork, heron, lapwing, bat and all fowls that creep, going upon all four, shall be an abomination unto you."

Most scavengers, carnivores and birds which ate various seafoods were forbidden. Because of their eating habits they were considered unclean. They also could be infected with many of the water-bourne diseases and parasitic worms. Most insects were forbidden except for the following:

"Even these of them ye may eat; the locust after his kind, and the bald locust after his kind, and the beetle after his kind, and the grasshopper after his kind."

Again, however, one should be cautious about eating beetles. There are two acanthocephalid worm infections which have as their intermediate hosts, larval or adult beetles. They are *Macracanthorhynchus hirudinaceus* and *Moniliformis moniliformis.* The definitive hosts are hogs, boars, rats, mice, dogs, cats and others. Man, the accidental host unless beetles are included in the diet, may suffer from abdominal pain, diarrhea and exhaustion. A violent ringing in the ears has also been reported. The life cycle and treatment of these infections is similar to that of the tapeworms.

"These also shall be unclean unto you among the creeping things that creep upon the earth; the weasel, the mouse, the tortoise, the ferret, the chameleon, the lizard, the snail and the mole."

All are possible carriers of diseases, either due to their diets or the body parasites such as fleas or ticks, which might act as vectors. Strangely, the rat is not mentioned here.

Women were considered to be unclean after childbirth for varying lengths of time. This time period would allow the woman to recover from possible trauma during delivery and prevented sexual intercourse for the prescribed time period.

Leviticus XII: 2,3,4,5

"Speak unto the children of Israel, saying, If a woman have conceived seed, and born a man child: then she shall be unclean seven days; according to the days of separation for her infirmity shall she be unclean. And in the eighth day the flesh of his foreskin shall be circumcised. And she shall then continue in the blood of her purifying three and thirty days; she shall touch no hallowed thing, nor come into the sanctuary, until the days of her purifying be fulfilled. But if she bear a maid child, then she shall be unclean two weeks, as in her separation: and she shall continue in the blood of her purifying three score and six days."

Skin diseases and leprosy were present in the Hebrews. A person with a disease of the skin was examined by the priest in order to determine whether the infection was leprosy. If it was determined that the infection was leprosy, the person was expelled from the village. His personal effects were burned and his house was dismantled and disposed of in an unclean place outside of the village. After seven days of isolation, the afflicted person was again examined by the priest. If he were found to be healed of the leprosy (or skin disease) the following purification ritual was performed. It is interesting because contained in it is the primitive method of the attempt to transfer the disease from the afflicted to an animal. (Leprosy is discussed in medicine of India)

Leviticus XIV: 3,4,5,6,7

"And the priest shall go forth out of the camp; and the priest shall look, and, behold, if the plague of the leprosy be healed in the leper; Then shall the priest command to take for him that is to be cleansed, two birds alive and clean, and cedar wood and scarlet, and hyssop: And the priest shall command that one of the birds be killed in an earthen vessel over running water: As for the living bird, he shall take it, and the cedar wood, and the scarlet, and the hyssop, and shall dip them and the living bird in the blood of the bird that was killed over the running water. And he shall sprinkle upon him that is to be cleansed from the leprosy seven times, and shall pronounce him clean, and shall let the living bird loose into the open field."

Most scholars present gonorrhea as an ancient disease but the descriptions referred to into ancient writings are very vague and do not necessarily indicate the specific infection. In 130 A.D., Galen first employed the term, "Gonorrhea," or flow of seed, which again does not specifically mean the bacterial infection caused by *Neisseria gonorrhoeae*. The microorganism was identified by Neisser, in 1879, as the agent causing the disease. Man is the only known host and the source of infection is the exudate from the mucous membranes of those who are infected. Transmission of the disease occurs during intimate contact. Asymptomatic carriers have been reported. An infected woman may pass the infection to her child during birth. Eye involvement, unless prevented with silver nitrate or antibiotics, frequently occurs and may result in blindness. Untreated infections may result in sterility. Spontaneous cures of anterior penile gonorrhea in males have been reported in the absence of sexual activity. Rest and sexual inactivity was one of the early methods of treatment along with various ineffective medicines. Sandalwood oil was a well-known agent until urethral irrigation with potassium permanganate was introduced in 1892. Sulfonimides later were found to be effective and may be administered today along with the drug of choice, Penicillin. Resistant strains of the organism may require the use of other antibiotics.

Leviticus XV: 2,16,17,18,19,24,32

"Speak unto the children of Israel, and say unto them, When any man hath a running issue out of his flesh, because of his issue he is unclean. And if any man's seed of copulation go out from him, then he shall wash all his flesh in water and be unclean until the even. And every garment and every skin, whereon is the seed of copulation, shall be washed with water, and be unclean until the even. The woman also with whom the man shall lie with seed of copulation, they shall both bathe themselves in water and be unclean until the even. And if a woman have an issue and her issue in her flesh be blood, she shall be put apart seven days: and whosoever toucheth her shall be unclean until the even. And if any man lie with her at all, and her flowers be upon him, he shall be unclean seven days; and all the bed whereon he lieth shall be unclean. This is the law of him that hath an issue, and of him whose seed goeth from him, and is defiled therewith."

While traveling through the arid regions around the Red Sea, the Hebrews had a strange encounter which was recorded:

Numbers XXI: 4,5,6,8,9

"And they journeyed from Mount Hor by the way of the Red Sea, to compass the land of Edom: and the soul of the people was much discouraged because of the way. And the people spake against God and against Moses. Wherefore have ye taken us out of Egypt to die in the wilderness? for there is no bread, neither is there any water; and our soul loatheth this light bread. And the Lord sent fiery serpents among the people, and they bit the people; and much people of Israel died. And the Lord said unto Moses, Make thee a fiery serpent, and set it upon a pole: and it shall come to pass, that everyone that is bitten, when he looketh upon it, shall live. And Moses made a serpent of brass, (Nehushtan) and put it upon a pole, and it came to pass, that if a serpent had bitten any man, when he beheld the serpent of brass, he lived."

It is believed that the "fiery serpents" which attacked the Hebrews were actually worms which today are called Guinea, Medina, serpent or dragon worms. The worm, *Dracunculus medinensis,* was first described, in 1863, by Bastian and the larval form by Fedtschenko, in 1870. The disease is found in Africa, the Middle East, Asia and North and South America. The threadlike worm, 20-30 inches in length, inhabits the subcutaneous and intermuscular tissues of man and several animals. The gravid female migrates to the tissues of the body which are likely to come in contact with water, such as the legs or arms. An ulcer forms over the cephalic (head) end of the worm which, when it contacts water, ruptures. Motile larvae are discharged into the water from a loop of the uterus which has prolapsed through a rupture in the anterior end of the worm. The larvae are ingested by small copepods named *Cyclops,* in which they develop into infective, tightly coiled, larvae. When man, or a susceptible animal, drinks the water containing the infected *Cyclops,* the larvae penetrate the wall of the digestive tract and migrate to other parts of the body. There may be allergic reactions to the worm but these usually occur just before the rupture of the ulcer, which is accompanied by local irritation, a severe inflammatory reaction, and perhaps, a secondary bacterial infection. Treatment involves the removal or destruction of the worm. The ancient method of rolling the worm very slowly, day by day, on a stick, is still used in many parts of the world today. Surgical removal is preferable but is not always available. Prior to removal, the worm may be killed by injections of bichloride of mercury or other compounds.

Intramuscular injections of phenothiazine in olive oil and the oral administration of the minced roots of the banyan tree, *Ficus bengalensis,* have been reported to cause a partial expulsion of the worm which permits an easier removal. The sap of other *Ficus* species is used to expell other intestinal worms. The fig tree is of this *Genus* and, of course, is common in the Middle East and Egypt, and is mentioned in several Egyptian medical papyri. The Hebrews, traveling through the arid regions, could find water only in stagnant pools in which the *Cyclops* thrives. Running water is relatively free from the infection.

Suspected waters should be boiled before drinking. It has been estimated that 50 million cases may exist today in Africa, the Middle East and India and Asia. In India, the native religious practice of ablution favors contamination of the waters and infection of the *Cyclops.* It is very possible that the act by Moses, that of placing a brass serpent on a pole, refers to the primitive method of removing the worm by twisting it on a stick, slowly, until it has been completely removed from the body.

Sorcery, witchcraft and allied practices have been in existence since before recorded history. A Hebraic interdict includes, apart from sorcery and witchcraft, the practices of divination, soothsaying, the consulting of auguries, magic spells and necromancy.

Deuteronomy XVIII: 10,11,12

"There shall not be found among you anyone that maketh his son or his daughter to pass through the fire, or that useth divination, or an observer of times, or an enchanter, or a witch, or a charmer, or a consulter with familiar spirits, or a wizard, or a necromancer. For all that do these things are an abomination unto the Lord: and because of these abominations the Lord thy God doth drive them out from before thee."

Possibly the most well-known witch in literature is the Witch of En-dor, who is consulted by Saul, in Samuel I: XXVIII: 3,5,7,8,9,10,11,12,13,14,15,19 and Samuel I: XXXI: 4,5.

"Now Samuel was dead, and all Israel had lamented him, and buried him in Ramah, even in his own city. And Saul had put away those that had familiar spirits, and the wizards, out of the land. And when Saul saw the host of the Philistines, he was afraid, and his heart greatly trembled. Then said Saul unto his servants, seek me a woman that hath a familiar spirt, that I may go to her, and inquire of her. And his servants said to him, Behold, there is a woman that hath a familiar spirit at En-dor. And Saul disguised himself and put on other raiment, and he went, and two men with him, and they came to the woman by night: and he said, I pray thee, divine unto me by the familiar spirit, and bring me him up, whom I shall name unto thee. And the woman said unto him, Behold, thou knowest what Saul hath done, how he hath cut off those that have familiar spirits, and the wizards out of the land: wherefore then layest thou a snare for my life, to cause me to die? And Saul sware to her by the Lord saying, As the Lord liveth, there shall be no punishment happen to thee for this thing. Then said the woman, Whom shall I bring up unto thee? And he said, Bring me up Samuel.

And when the woman saw Samuel, she cried with a loud voice: and the woman spake to Saul saying, Why hast thou deceived me? For thou art Saul. And the King said unto her, Be not afraid: for what sawest thou? And the woman said unto Saul, I saw gods ascending out of the earth. And he said unto her, What form is he of? And she said, An old man cometh up; and he is covered with a mantle. And Saul perceived that it was Samuel, and he stooped with his face to the ground, and bowed himself. And Samuel said to Saul, Why hast thou disquieted me, to bring me up? And Saul answered, I am sore distressed; for the Philistines make war against me, and God is departed from me, and answereth me no more, neither by prophets, nor by dreams: therefore I have called thee, that thou mayest make known unto me what I shall do. Samuel answered, Moreover the Lord will also deliver Israel with thee into the hand of the Philistines: and tomorrow shalt thou and thy sons be with me: the Lord also shall deliver the host of Israel into the hand of the Philistines. Then said Saul unto his armourbearer, Draw thy sword, and thrust me through therewith; lest these uncircumcised come and thrust me through and abuse me. But his armourbearer would not; for he was sore afraid; therefore Saul took a sword, and fell upon it. And when his armourbearer saw that Saul was dead, he fell like-wise upon his sword, and died with him."

Later, in Europe and the New England colonies of North America, the Hebraic interdict against witchcraft was revived, and many innocent people were accused of witchcraft, were tried, convicted and killed. However, the "Talmud," expressly excludes from the ban of superstitious practices, "anything done for the sake of healing." It permits the carrying, as an amulet, the egg of a locust to ward off an earache; the tooth of a fox to ward off insomnia or drowsiness; and the nail from a gallows to prevent swellings.

During the seige of Jerusalem by Nebuchadrezzar, in about 597 B.C., the people within the city were starving, due to a lack of food.

Lamentations IV: 4,5,7,8,9,10,12

"The tongue of the sucking child cleaveth to the roof of his mouth for thirst: the young children ask bread, and no man breaketh it unto them. They that did feed delicately are desolate in the streets: They that were brought up in scarlet embrace dunghills. Her Nazarites were purer than snow, they were whiter than milk, they were more ruddy in body than rubies, their polishing was of sapphire: Their visage is blacker than a coal; they are not known in the streets: their skin cleaveth to their bones; it is withered, it is become like a stick. They that be slain with the sword are better than they that be slain with hunger: for these pine away, stricken through for want of the fruits of the field. The hands of the pitiful woman have sodden (cooked) their own children: they were their meat in the destruction of the daughter of my people. The kings of the earth, and all the inhabitants of the world, would not have believed that the adversary and the enemy should have entered into the gates of Jerusalem."

This is a rather vivid account of what could happen when people are deprived of food, or have certain foods missing from their diet. Scurvy, Beriberi and pellagra are well-known diseases caused by deficiencies in the diet.

Scurvy is a deficiency disease caused by the lack of vitamin C in the diet. The afflicted is marked by weakness, anemia, spongy gums, a tendency to muco-cutaneous hemorrhages (Their visage is blacker than a coal), and induration of the muscles of the calves and legs. The use of fresh vegetables and citrus fruits are preventative and remedial measures. The Ancient Chinese and later, Captain Cook, on his long voyage, used freshly sprouted seeds in their diets, which prevented this disease.

The following list is of the vitamins required by man and the conditions which result from the deficiency of the vitamin or the ingestion of an excess amount of the substance.

Vitamin A: a deficiency causes poor fetal development, a variety of skin diseases and night blindness. An excess of the vitamin may cause deformities of the skin and bones, mental disturbances, nausea and vomiting. Found in eggs, liver, butter, cheese, carrots, tomatoes and others.

The B Vitamins

Vitamin B-1: Thiamine; a deficiency of this vitamin impairs the brain, heart and nerves; may lead to the disease, Beriberi. Found in eggs, liver, grains.

Vitamin B-2: Riboflavin; a deficiency impairs the functioning of the nervous system. Found in eggs, milk, meats, liver.

Vitamin B-6: Pyridoxine; a deficiency impairs the nervous system and may lead to convulsions. Found in various plants and animals.

Vitamin B-12: Cyanocobalamin; impairs the production of erythrocytes and blood platelets causing pernicious anemia, if deficient, and damages the CNS. Found in various plants and animals.

Niacin: a deficiency causes diarrhea, skin disorders, brain disorders and eventually Pellagra. Found in various plants and animals.

Vitamin C: Ascorbic acid; a deficiency causes the swelling and bleeding of the gums, and disorders of the joints and brain leading to Scurvy. Found in citrus fruits, tomatoes and other vegetables.

Vitamin D: a deficiency affects absorption of calcium and therefore causes bone disorders; Rickets. An excess of the vitamin causes high blood calcium levels, kidney damage and brain disorders. Found in eggs, milk, liver.

Vitamin E: a deficiency affects erythrocyte longevity, and some claim infertility. Found in grains and vegetables.

Vitamin K: a deficiency affects the clotting of blood. Found in vegetables.

Biotin: a deficiency causes skin disorders. Found in eggs, milk, liver.

Folic Acid: a deficiency causes anemia and poor growth and development. An excess of the vitamin may mask pernicious anemia. Found in green plants, fruits, meats.

Pantothenic Acid: a deficiency causes several nutritional disorders. Found in liver and other tissues.

During the reign of Hezekiah, the Assyrians attempted to conquer the Hebrews. In about 701 B.C., Sennacherib lay siege to Jerusalem but was forced to withdraw. The Old Testament, Herodotus and historians differ, as to the reason for the withdrawal.

II Kings XVIII: 1,4,13; XIX: 32,33,35,36

"Now it came to pass in the third year of Hoshea son of Elah king of Israel, that Hezekiah the son of Ahaz king of Judah began to reign. He removed the high places, and brake the images, cut down the groves, and brake in pieces the brasen serpent that Moses had made: for unto those days the children of Israel did burn incense to it: and he called it Nehushtan. Now in the fourteenth year of King Hezekiah did Sennacherib king of Assyria come up against all the fenced cities of Judah, and he took them. Therefore thus saith the Lord concerning the king of Assyria, He shall not come into this city, nor shoot an arrow there, nor come before it with shield, nor caste a bank against it. By the way that he came, by the same shall he return, and shall not come into this city, saith the Lord. And it came to pass that night, that the angel of the Lord went out and smote in the camp of the Assyrians an hundred fourscore and five thousand: and when they arose early in the morning, behold, they were all dead corpses. So Sennacherib king of Assyria departed and went and returned, and dwelt at Nineveh."

This account of the deaths of the Assyrians is similar to the account of the deaths of the Egyptians during the "Pass over." In about 450 B.C., Herodotus related that the Assyrians withdrew from Jerusalem because they had been visited by a plague of mice which ate away the strings of their bows. Historically, there was a revolt in Babylon and an Egyptian army marched to relieve Jerusalem, so apparently, Sennacherib withdrew for military reasons. However, the deaths of many of the Assyrians and the account by Herodotus of the plague of mice, have lead my writers to postulate that the Assyrians may have experienced an outbreak of bubonic plague.

Bubonic plague is an acute, febrile and exceedingly fatal epidemic disease produced by the bacterium, *Yersinia* (formerly *Pasteurella*) *pestis*. It begins with fever and chills, quickly followed by great prostration, and later by swelling of the lymphatic glands and the formation of buboes. It is frequently attended with delirium, headache, vomiting and diarrhea. The plague attacks rodents and various mammals, including man. The disease is almost always transmitted through the bites of fleas, such as *Xenopsylla cheopis*, which have become infected by feeding on an animal or person infected with the disease. Most generalized infections are fatal unless treatment is available. Historically, the disease can be traced, almost unbroken, to the Third century, B.C., when Dionysius mentioned it as a fatal disease occurring in Egypt, Syria and Libya. During the 1600s-1700s, epidemics occurred in Europe where the disease was called the Black Death or Black Plague. The bacterium was discovered in Hong

Kong, in 1894, by Alexander Yersin. Immunization against the disease was initiated in 1896 and Yersin developed an antiplague serum for use in therapy. The therapeutic value of sulfonamides and various antibiotics, such as streptomycin, was established by field tests in endemic areas. The disease can be controlled by vaccination, rodenticides and insecticides; however, recently, it has been reported that many rodents and arthropods are becoming highly resistant to the chemicals used for their destruction. It was recently estimated that the rat population of the United States is equal to the human population. This does not take into account other animals that could harbor the infection. It is entirely probable that, in the near future, an epidemic of Bubonic Plague could occur in the United States, as it has in the past.

Medical researchers believe that a very rare disease is described in Genesis XXV: 19,20,21,22,23,24,25,26,27 and XXVII: 11.

"And these are the generations of Isaac, Abraham's son: Abraham begat Isaac: And Isaac was forty years old when he took Rebekah to wife; And Isaac intreated the Lord for his wife was barren: and the Lord was intreated of him, and Rebekah his wife conceived. And the children struggled together within her; and she said, If it be so, why am I thus? And she went to inquire of the Lord. And the Lord said unto her, Two nations are in thy womb, and two manner of people shall be separated from thy bowels; and the one people shall be stronger than the other people; and the elder shall serve the younger. And when her days to be delivered were fulfilled, behold, there were twins in her womb. And the first came out, red all over like a hairy garment; and they called his name Esau. And after that came his brother out, and his hand took hold on Esau's heel; and his name was called Jacob: and Isaac was threescore years old when she bare them. And the boys grew: and Esau was a cunning hunter, a man of the field; and Jacob was a plain man, dwelling in tents. And Jacob said to Rebekah his mother, Behold, Esau my brother is a hairy man, and I am a smooth man."

Hypertrichosis, or excessive hair, is a rare disease which is estimated to occur in one per billion persons. At birth, the excessive hair is usually limited to the ears, but later, it becomes generalized. The hair is lanugo (fine and downy), up to ten inches in length, and varies in color from silvery gray to pale yellow. Hypertrichosis is transmitted as a dominant trait. Accompanying the excessive hair, usually, is the absence of teeth in the cuspid, bicuspid and molar areas. Due to the abnormalities of the hair and teeth, the disease is classified as a congenital ectodermal defect. The hair is found on all parts of the body except the palms, soles, lips, tips of the fingers and the glans penis. There are case studies concerning this disease which date to the 16th Century. Often, persons with this condition would be sent to a Royal court to entertain the nobility, and later, appeared in carnival exhibits. The author believes that this abnormality, excessive hair and an unusual teeth arrangement, may be the origin of the legends of the werewolf. It is interesting that in the Old Testament, "Esau was a cunning hunter, a man of the field."

58   *Magic, Myths and Medicine*

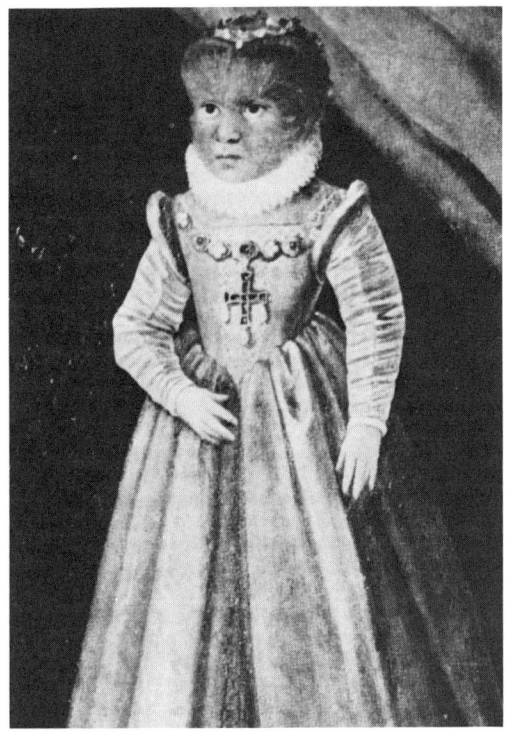

A portrait of a girl with hypertrichosis in the court of King Henry II, at Valois, France, in about 1585. The "Daughter of Gonzales" reproduced by courtesy of the Kunsthistorisches Museum, Vienna, and the Schloss Ambras, Innsbruck, Austria.

An early example of resuscitation is found in Kings I: XVII: 17,18,19,21,22,23. "And it came to pass after these things, that the son of the house, fell sick; and his sickness was so sore, that there was no breath left in him. And she said unto Elijah, What have I to with thee, O thou man of God? Art thou come unto me to call my sin to remembrance, and to slay my son? And he said unto her, Give me thy son. And he took him out of her bosom, and carried him up into a loft, where he abode, and laid him upon his own bed. And he stretched himself upon the child three times, and cried unto the Lord, and said, O Lord my God, I pray thee, let this child's soul come into him again. And the Lord heard the voice of Elijah; and the soul of the child came into him again, and he revived. And Elijah took the child, and brought him down out of the chamber into the house, and delivered him unto his mother: and Elijah said, See, thy son liveth."

The disposal of human wastes has been, and still is, a problem due to the possibility of the contamination of the earth and waters with disease producing microorganisms. The Hebrews disposed of human wastes in the following manner. Deuteronomy XXIII: 12,13. "Thou shalt have a place also without the camp, wither thou shalt go forth abroad: And thou shalt have a paddle upon thy weapon: and it shall be, when thou wilt ease thyself abroad, thou shalt dig therewith, and shalt turn back and cover that which cometh from thee."

These observations cited from the Old Testament of the Hebrews indicate that their concepts and traditions were absorbed into their moral and legislative system and that their diety was given the power of healing. Centuries later, Christianity will turn away from empirical medicine and return to the pure virtue of the healing power of faith, an initial Hebraic concept. The Hebrews fought contagious diseases and plagues by isolation and expulsion of the infected persons or by flight. These concepts were later adopted by many peoples who had incorporated the Old Testament teachings into their religions.

mesopotamia— the land between the rivers

The "fertile crescent" is the name given to the area of land that stretches from present-day Israel, around northern Arabia to the Persian Gulf. Much of the eastern half of the crescent which lies between the Tigris and Euphrates Rivers, falls within the territory of the country, today, called Iraq. It is in this area of the world that many scholars believe arose the world's earliest civilization. In 1948, the archeologist Braidwood excavated at Jarmo, in northern Iraq, and uncovered a town which had consisted of one to three hundred people and which was dated to approximately 8000 B.C. Stone implements were found for the cutting of wheat and barley; for the storage of foods, stone pots were utilized. Animals, such as the goat and dog, had been domesticated. By about 5000 B.C., agriculture had spread westward into the region of the Tigris and Euphrates Rivers where improved strains of cereals were cultivated, and cattle and sheep had been domesticated. Towns and cities, with age, came to stand on mounds, or "tells," which were the results of the accumulation of garbage, debris and ruined buildings. Most of the building was done with sun-dried bricks which softened and collapsed during heavy rains or floods. The tell, when it became high enough, protected the inhabitants against flooding and enemies. The people were forced to cooperate with one another in order to maintain the elaborate system of irrigation which was required to grow crops. Irrigation systems were developed in the north by about 5000 B.C., and within one thousand years, had spread to the south where large city-states developed, some having populations of perhaps ten thousand people. Little is known of these early cultures, such as the Ubaids, but the Directorate General of Antiquities of Iraq has extensive plans for archeological investigations funded by oil revenues. The main cereal crop of the area was barley which could withstand the high salt content of the soil, caused by the necessity of constant irrigation.

In approximately 4000 B.C., the Sumerians entered Mesopotamia from the northeast and conquered the lower Euphrates region, establishing a civilization which lasted until about 2800 B.C. Their country is called Sumer, the

Shinar mentioned in the Old Testament of the Hebrews. There were many Sumerian cities along the rivers such as Eridu, Lagash, Uruk, Nippur and Ur. Ur was the city where, according to the Old Testament, Abraham, the patriarch of the Hebrews, originated. The cities were built with a series of walls which surrounded the central temple or ziggurat. The ziggurats were built to great heights, and one, that of Babylon, was probably the "Tower of Babel" of the Old Testament.

Writing was developed, by about 3400 B.C., in order to keep records of crops and taxes required to maintain the city-states. It became fully developed by 3100 B.C. Also developed were astronomy, astrology, mathematics, the calendar, weights and measures, a postal system and wheeled vehicles.

In the early 1930s, Wooley excavated the Sumerian city of Ur and reported that he had found a layer of silt in the excavation which was eleven feet deep, and which contained no relics. He postulated that this was the sediment of a great flood which had covered the land to a depth of twenty-five feet, and had covered an area of land measuring 100 × 300 miles. This superflood is believed to have taken place in about 2800 B.C. and had destroyed all records that had been recorded on sun-baked clay.

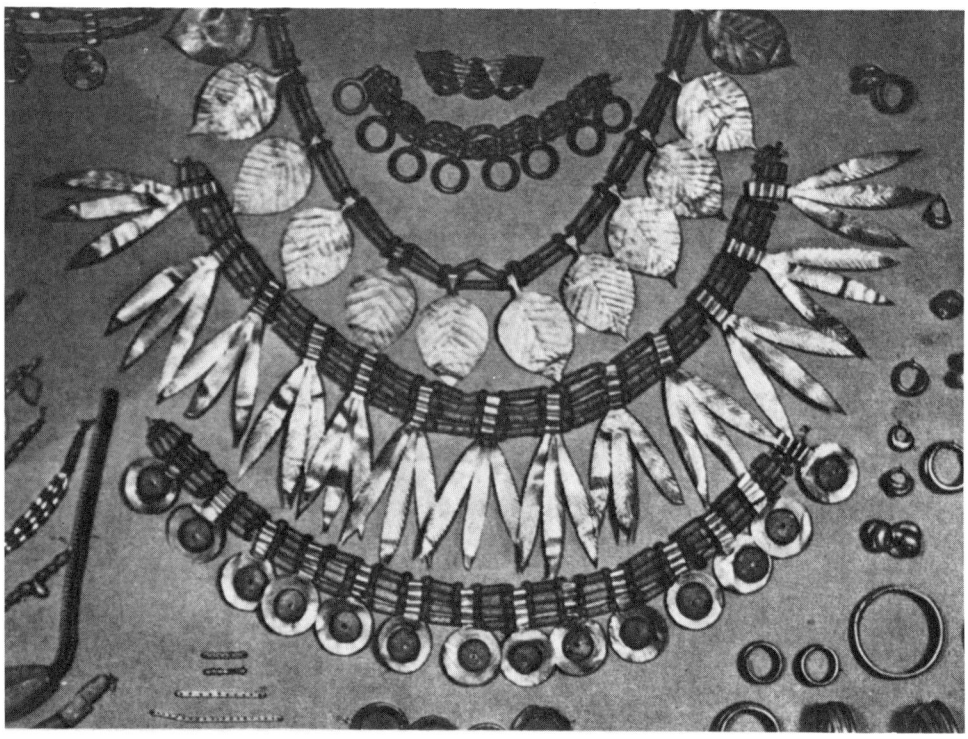

The golden ornaments of Queen Shub-ad from the royal graves of Ur discovered by Leonard Wooley. (Photograph by courtesy of the Trustees of the British Museum)

Mesopotamia – The Land Between the Rivers 63

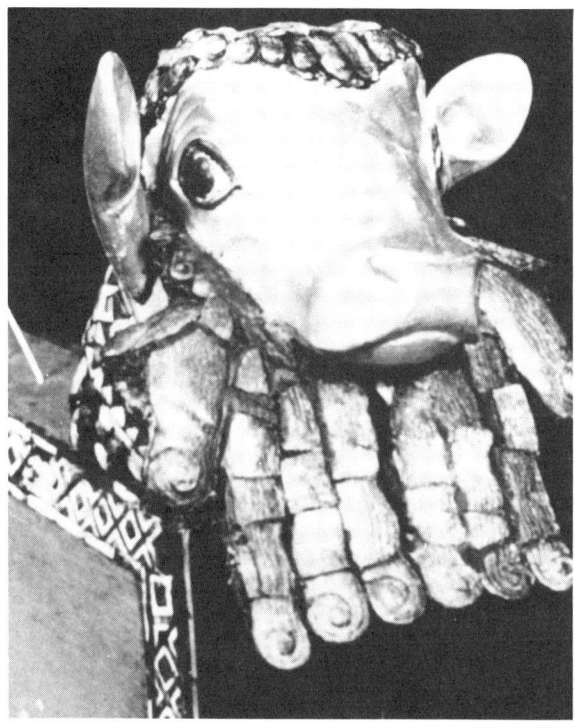

A bull's head of gold and lapis lazuli decorated a harp found in the pit-tombs of Ur by Leonard Wooley. (Photograph by courtesy of the Trustees of the British Museum.)

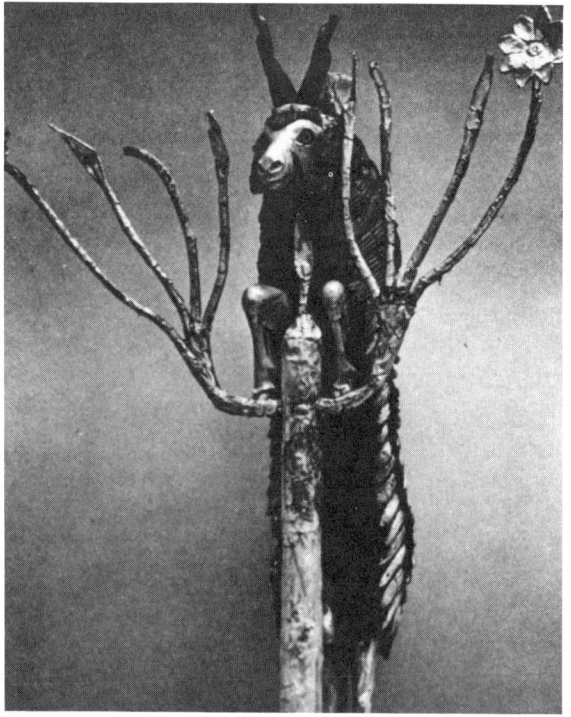

The tree of life is being mounted by a goat in a beautiful work of ancient sculpture (2500 B.C.) discovered in the ruins of Ur. (Photograph by courtesy of the Trustees of the British Museum.)

Prior to the flood mentioned in the Sumerian writings, in about 2800 B.C., a group of people, the Akkadians, attempted to enter Mesopotamia, but were turned northward by the powerful Sumerians. The language of the Akkadians was polysyllabic and structured similar to ancient Hebrew or modern Arabic. The Old Testament describes these people as having descended from Shem, a son of Noah, from which is derived the term "semetic language." These invaders eventually conquered much of Mesopotamia. One of the invaders, Sargon, had a new city constructed which he called Agade. He was called Sargon of Agade from which was derived the name Akkad or Akkadians. Connected with Sargon is the earliest of the caste-away legends which precedes that of Moses, Oedipus, Perseus, and Romulus and Remus.

According to the legend, Sargon was the illegitimate son of a woman of high birth who, in order to avoid a scandal, decided to dispose of her son. She made a small boat of reeds; smeared it with pitch; and placed it in the river. The boat and child drifted away and were later found by a poor gardener who raised the child. When grown, the child took service with the king and eventually secured the throne for himself.

A creation myth of the Akkadians has survived which is much more violent than those of the Egyptians, Hebrews and Sumerians and which represents a struggle between cosmic order and chaos. Selected portions of the myth to follow which was translated by E.A. Speiser.*

"O Marduk, thou art indeed our avenger. We have granted thee kingship over the universe entire. Thy weapons shall not fail; they shall smash thy foes. Go and cut off the life of Tiamat (chaos). Then he sent forth the winds he had brought forth, the seven of them. To stir up the inside of Tiamat they rose up behind him. Then the Lord raised up the flood-storm, his mighty weapon. He mounted the storm-chariot, irrestible and terrifying. He harnessed and yoked to it a team-of-four; sharp were their teeth with poison. For a cloak, he was wrapped in an armor of terror; with his fearsome halo his head was turbaned. Towards the raging Tiamat he set his face. In his lips he held a spell.

"Tiamat emitted a cry, without turning her neck, framing savage defiance in her lips. She was like one possessed; she took leave of her senses. In fury Tiamat cried out aloud. To the roots her legs shook both together. She recites a charm, keeps casting her spell while the gods of battle sharpened their weapons. Then joined issue, Tiamat and Marduk. They strove in single combat, locked in battle. When Tiamat opened her mouth to consume him, he drove in the Evil Wind that she close not her lips. As the fierce winds charged her belly, her body

---

Selections from "Akkadian Myths and Epics," transl. E.A. Speiser, "Myths and Epics from Mesopotamia," transl. S.N. Kramer, "Collection of Laws from Mesopotamia," transl. Albrecht Goetze, and "The Code of Hammurabi," transl. Theophile J. Meek in James B. Pritchard, *The Ancient Near East: An Anthology of Texts and Pictures,* (copyright © 1958 by Princeton University Press) pgs. 32-36, 28-30, 137-138, and 139-167. Reprinted by permission of Princeton University Press.

was distended and her mouth was wide open. He released the arrow, it tore her belly, it cut through her insides, splitting the heart. Having thus subdued her, he extinguished her life. He caste down her carcass to stand upon it. The lord trod on the legs of Tiamat; with his unsparing mace he crushed her skull. When the arteries of her blood he had severed, the North Wind bore it to places undisclosed. He split her like a shellfish into two parts: half of her he set up and ceiled it as sky, pulled down the bar and posted guards. He bade them to allow not her waters to escape. He constructed stations for the great gods, fixing their astral likenesses as constellations."

"Blood I will mass and cause bones to be. I will establish a savage, man shall be his name. Verily, savage man will I create. He shall be charged with the service of the gods, that they might be at ease."

Sargon and his armies overran the Sumerian city-states to the south and he established himself as "King of Sumer and Akkad," establishing an empire which lasted almost 150 years. The Akkadians were defeated by the Guti, from the Zagros mountains to the east, who ruled for about 100 years until the local ruler of several of the city-states defeated them. In about 2112 B.C., Ur Nammu, king of Ur, united all of Mesopotamia and had the laws written down. The laws of Ur-Nammu are the oldest written laws that are known and stressed monetary payments rather than punishments for the offences. The following excerpts are from the "Laws of Eshunna," translated by Albrecht Goetze, and which are dated to about 2000 B.C.[1]

"If a man bites the nose of another man and severs it, he shall pay 1 mina of silver. For an eye he shall pay 1 mina of silver; for a tooth 1/2 mina; for an ear 1/2 mina; for a slap in the face 10 shekels of silver."

"If a man severs another man's finger, he shall pay 2/3 of a mina of silver."

"If a man throws another man to the floor in an altercation and breaks his hand, he shall pay 1/2 mina of silver. If he breaks his foot, he shall pay 1/2 mina of silver."

"If a man hits another man accidentally, he shall pay 10 shekels of silver. And in addition, in cases involving penalties from 2/3 of a mina to 1 mina, they shall formally try the man. A capital offence comes before the king.

"If an ox is known to gore habitually, and the authorities have brought the fact to the knowledge of its owner, but he does not have his ox dehorned, it gores a man and causes his death, then the owner of the ox shall pay 2/3 of a mina of silver. If it gores a slave and causes his death, he shall pay 15 shekels of silver."

1. The Ancient Near East, edited by James B. Pritchard, Princeton University Press, 1958, pgs. 137, 138.

"If a dog is vicious, and the authorities have brought the fact to the knowledge of its owner, if nevertheless he does not keep it in, it bites a man and causes his death, then the owner of the dog shall pay 2/3 of a mina of silver. If it bites a slave and causes its death, he shall pay 15 shekels of silver."

The previous paragraph is one of the oldest references that we have to rabies. The history of the disease has been primarily associated with the domesticated dog but now, due to immunization procedures, wild animals living close to man, such as bats, skunks, and raccoons, are becoming more involved in the transmission of the disease in the human population, especially in the United States.

Rabies is a type of encephalitis, caused by a virus, that is communicated from animal to animal, and from animal to man, usually by the bite of the infected animal. After an incubation period of from one to six months, the disease begins with malaise, depression and a swelling of the lymphatics in the wound area. There are choking and spasmodic catchings of the breath and tetanic-type spasms, especially of those muscles utilized in respiration and swallowing. The spasms are increased at the attempts to drink water and later, at the sight or sound of water. Fever, vomiting, mental derangement and profuse salivation may occur. The disease is generally fatal, death occurring in from two to five days. Characteristic and diagnostic cytoplasmic inclusion bodies, called Negri bodies, are found in the brain. Pasteur and his associates, in 1884, modified the pathogenicity of the virus by drying the spinal cords of infected rabbits. In 1885, Pasteur saved the life of a boy who had been bitten by a rabid dog by inoculation of the attenuated virus into his body. The boy survived and the vaccine treatment for rabies was soon adopted in medical centers throughout the world. Once the symptoms of the disease are evident, it is usually too late to attempt the Pasteur treatment, and the patient dies. Recently, in the United States, a boy developed the symptoms of rabies and was put under intensive care by his physicians with a total life support system. The boy survived, with no apparent damage, and is now fully recovered. The disease may be prevented by the control and vaccination of animals in close contact with man. Many countries have very rigid laws which govern the importation of wild and domestic animals and which require isolation of the animals for periods of 30 days to six months. Rabies may be treated with hyperimmune serum, vaccine, barbiturates for relieving anxiety, anesthesia for the control of spasms and intravenous injections of liquids for combatting dehydration and lack of nourishment.

Later king-lists record that ten kings had ruled for 10,000 years prior to the flood. The Old Testament lists ten patriarchs, from Adam to Noah, as having lived prior to the flood. The patriarchs lived for very long periods of time, but less than 1000 years, although Methusaleh lived for 969 years. The

Sumerian flood-legend has survived and, as do the Ebla tablets, offers a striking parallel to Hebraic material. The legend is also encountered in the "Epic of Gilgamesh," who, according to king-lists, was the 5th King of the 1st Dynasty of Uruk, of about 2700 B.C. Much of the Sumerian myth is incomplete, but the introductory passages include statements concerning the creation of man, the origin of kingship and the existence of several antediluvian cities.

The Deluge; translator: S.N. Kramer[2]

"On the earth he . . . d, placed the . . . there. After Anu, Enlil, Enki, and Ninhursag had fashioned the black-headed people (mankind), vegetation luxuriated from the earth; Animals, four-legged creatures of the plain, were artfully brought into existence. (thirty-seven lines destroyed) After the exalted tiara and the throne of kingship had been lowered from heaven, He perfected the rites and the exalted, divine ordinances . . .; founded the five cities in the pure places; called their names; apportioned them as cult centers. The first of these cities, Eridu, he gave to Nudimmud (water-god); the second, Badtibira, he gave to . . .; the third, Larak, he gave to Endurbilhursag; the fourth, Sippar, he gave to the hero, Utu (sun-god); the fifth, Shuruppak, he gave to Sud (wife of Enlil). When he had called the names of these cities, apportioned them as cult-centers, he brought . . . (probably water); established the cleaning of the small rivers as . . . (37 lines destroyed)

"Then did Ziusudra, the king, the pasisu of . . . Build giant . . . Humbly obedient, reverently he . . . Attending daily, constantly he . . . Bringing forth all kinds of dreams, he . . . Uttering the name of heaven and earth he . . . the gods a wall . . . Ziusudra, standing at its side, listened. 'Stand by the wall at my left side . . . by the wall I will say a word to thee, Give ear to my instruction.

" 'By our . . . a flood will sweep over the cult-centers; To destroy the seed of mankind . . ., is the decision, the word of the assembly of the gods. By the word commanded by Anu and Enlil . . ., its kingship, its rule, will be put to an end. (forty lines destroyed)

"All the windstorms, exceedingly powerful, attacked as one. At the same time, the flood sweeps over the cult-centers. After, for seven days and seven nights, the flood had swept over the land, and the huge boat had been tossed about by the windstorms on the great waters. Utu (sun) came forth, who sheds light on heaven and earth. Zuisudra opened a window of the huge boat. The hero Utu brought his rays into the giant boat. Zuisudra, the king, prostrated himself before Utu. . . . Zuisudra the king, prostrated himself before Anu and

---

2. The Ancient Near East, edited by James B. Pritchard, Princeton University Press, 1958, pgs. 29, 30.

Enlil. Anu and Enlil cherished Zuisudra; Life, like that of a god they gave him; breath eternal, like that of a god they gave him. Then, Zuisudra the king, the preserver of the name of vegetation and of the seed of mankind; in the land of crossing (east), the land of Dilmun, the place where the sun rises, they caused him to dwell. (remainder, 39 lines destroyed)

The "Epic of Gilgamesh" was found inscribed on clay tablets excavated from the ruins of Nineveh, Nimrud, Uruk, Nippur and others. The cuneiform writing was first deciphered by Rawlinson, who used as the "key," the inscription of Darius, on the Behistun Rock, in Persia. Publication was begun in 1855. In this legend, Zuisudra of the flood epic is called Utnapishtim. The story of Gilgamesh is extremely long so it cannot be reproduced here. A synopsis by the author follows.

Gilgamesh, tyrannical ruler of Uruk, was superior to all other men in beauty and strength and was wearing out his subjects with the games of love and war. The gods heard the laments of the people and caused the goddess Aruru to create a man from clay, which she dropped in the wilderness. Enkidu, was a wild man, whose body was "covered with matted hair, like Samuqan's, the god of cattle." (hypertrichosis?) He was reared with the wild animals and was as swift as a gazelle. In time, Enkidu was seduced by a harlot from the temple of Uruk, at the order of Gilgamesh, and lost his innocence; whereupon, the animals then rejected him and he eventually arrived in Uruk and became the companion of Gilgamesh. After many adventures, Enkidu died and Gilgamesh mourned him. Gilgamesh, fearing death, set out to find Utnapishtim (Zuisudra) to whom the gods had given eternal life. After many adventures, he arrived at the sun's garden by the shores of the Ocean. This was an earthly paradise similar to the "Garden of Eden" in the Old Testament. An old woman told him to find the boatman to carry him over the waters of death to the land of Dilmun where lived Utnapishtim. Gilgamesh arrived in Dilmun and found Utnapishtim who then related to him the story of the flood. Gilgamesh learned that the plant which confers everlasting life grew at the bottom of the sea, so he tied two rocks to his ankles and plunged to the bottom, where he found the plant. He did not eat it, and began his journey homeward, planning to share the plant with his people. On the way, he saw a pool of water and went to bathe, leaving the plant nearby. However, deep in the pool was lying a serpent and, sensing the sweetness of the plant, the serpent snatched it away and immediately shed its skin and returned to the pool. Gilgamesh wept; then he returned to Uruk, where later he died and was lamented by his people.

Gilgamesh named the miraculous plant "The Old Men are Young Again." The search for a method with which to regain lost youth has apparently inspired mankind for thousands of years. Later, the search for the Philosopher's

Stone and the Fountain of Youth would occupy the time of many researchers and explorers. Scientists are still interested in the unraveling of the process of ageing. Recent investigations indicate that heredity and diet play an important role in the life span of the individual.

In about 2000 B.C., invaders entered Mesopotamia from the south and west who settled in Akkad, their most populous city being Babilum. In 1850 B.C., they established a dynasty that was to last about 1000 years and set the foundations of the future state of Assyria. The Hebrews called these people the Amalikites and their city, Babylon. These are also the people who invaded Egypt prior to the 18th Dynasty and were called the Amu or Hyksos. In 1792 B.C., the sixth Amurru (Amorite) ruler, Hammurabi, conquered much of Mesopotamia and established a new empire, called Babylonia. Hammurabi is remembered for his code of laws which were carved into a stele of dorite for everyone to see. The stele was later carried away by the Elamites, in 1174 B.C., to Susa, where it was found by Morgan, in 1901. Today the stele is located in the Louvre Museum, Paris. Portions of the "Code of Hammurabi" follow which were translated by Theophile J. Meek.[3]

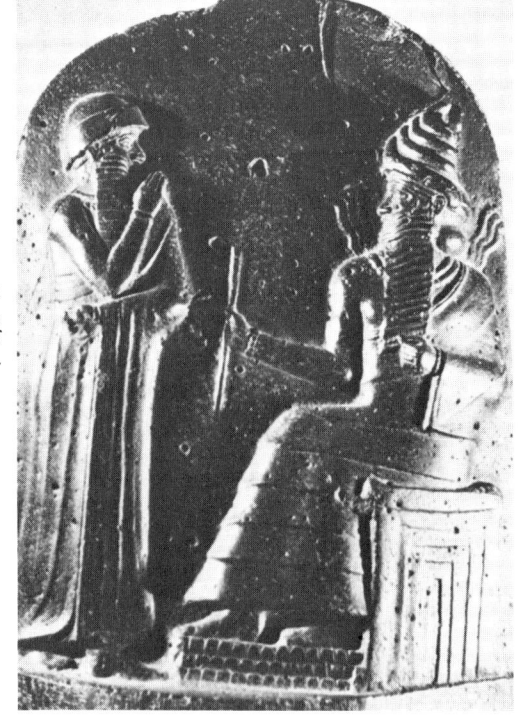

A portion of the stele of Hammurabi which depicts Hammurabi and the God of the Sun, Shamash, on a mountain top where the code of laws, which is below, is being formulated. (Photograph courtesy the Louvre, Paris)

3. The Ancient Near East, edited by James B. Pritchard, Princeton University Press, 1958, pgs. 139, 161, 162, 163, 167.

"If a seignor accused another seignor and brought a charge of murder against him, but has not proved it, his accuser shall be put to death."

"If a seignor brought a charge of sorcery against another seignor, but has not proved it, the one against whom the charge of sorcery was brought, upon going to the river (Euphrates), shall throw himself into the river, and if the river has then overpowered him, his accuser shall take over his estate; if the river has shown that seignor to be innocent, and he has accordingly come forth safe, the one who brought the charge of sorcery against him shall be put to death, while the one who threw himself into the river shall take over the estate of the accuser."

"When a seignor gave his son to a nurse and that son has died in the care of the nurse, if that nurse has then made a contract for another son without the knowledge of his father and mother, they shall prove it against her and they shall cut off her breast, because she made a contract for another son without the knowledge of his father and mother."

"If a son has struck his father they shall cut off his hand."

"If a seignor has destroyed the eye of a member of the aristocracy, they shall destroy his eye. If he has broken another man's bone, they shall break his bone. If he has destroyed the eye of a commoner or broken the bone of a commoner, he shall pay one mina of silver. If he has destroyed the eye of a seignor's slave or broken the bone of a seignor's slave, he shall pay one-half of his value."

"If a seignor has knocked out a tooth of a seignor of his own rank, they shall knock out his tooth. If he has knocked out a commoner's tooth, he shall pay one-third mina of silver."

"If a seignor has struck the cheek of a seignor who is superior to him, he shall be beaten sixty times with an oxtail whip in the assembly."

"If a seignor has struck another seignor in a brawl and has afflicted an injury on him, that seignor shall swear, "I did not strike him deliberately," and he shall pay for the *physician*."

"If a seignor struck another seignor's daughter and has caused her to have a miscarriage, he shall pay ten shekels of silver for her fetus. If that woman has died, they shall put his daughter to death. If by a blow he has caused a commoner's daughter to have a miscarriage, he shall pay five shekels of silver. If that woman has died, he shall pay one-half mina of silver. If he struck a seignor's female slave and has caused her to have a miscarriage, he shall pay two shekels of silver. If that female slave has died, he shall pay one-third mina of silver."

"If a *physician* performed a major operation on a seignor with a bronze lancet, and has saved the seignor's life; or he opened up the eye-socket of a seignor with a bronze lancet and has saved the seignor's eye, he shall receive ten shekels of silver. If it was a member of the commonalty, he shall receive five shekels. If it was a seignor's slave, the owner of the slave shall give two shekels of silver to the physician."

"If a *physician* performed a major operation on a seignor with a bronze lancet and has caused the seignor's death, or he opened up the eye-socket of a seignor and has destroyed the seignor's eye, they shall cut off his hand. If a physician performed a major operation on a commoner's slave with a bronze lancet and has caused his death, he shall make good, slave for slave. If he opened up his eye-socket with a bronze lancet and has destroyed his eye, he shall pay one-half his value in silver."

"If a *physician* has set a seignor's broken bone, or has healed a sprained tendon, the patient shall give five shekels of silver to the physician. If it was a member of the commonalty, he shall give three shekels of silver. If it was a seignor's slave, the owner of the slave shall give two shekels of silver to the physician."

"If a *veterinary surgeon* performed a major operation on either an ox or an ass, and he has saved it life, the owner of the ox or ass shall give to the surgeon one-sixth shekel of silver as his fee. If he performed a major operation on an ox or an ass and has caused its death, he shall give to the owner of the ox or ass, one-fourth its value."

"If a seignor purchased a male or female slave and when his month was not yet complete, epilepsy (or heart trouble) attacked him, he shall return him to his seller and the purchaser shall get back the money which he paid out."

The laws of Hammurabi clearly indicate that there were physicians and surgeons who treated the people and animals for set fees and who were punished or fined if their performance was in error. It therefore, is unusual to find that in about 450 B.C., the Greek historian Herodotus made the following observation. "They have no doctors, but bring their invalids out into the street, where anyone who comes along offers the sufferer advice on his complaint, either from personal experience, or observation of a similiar complaint in others."

After the death of Hammurabi, the semites of Assyria began expanding and eventually conquered Mesopotamia, the Hebrews and Egypt, thus establishing the great Assyrian Empire. Well-known rulers of the Assyrians were the Sargons, Sennacherib and Ashurbanipol. Ashurbanipol, ruling from Nineveh, had collected for his library, a copy of every worthwhile cuneiform tablet in Babylonia. When Nineveh was excavated, these tablets were found and yielded a new light on the literature of ancient Mesopotamia. The "Epic of Gilgamesh" and the "Flood legend" were found in this collection as well as other tablets, some of which deal with sickness. Excerpts from these tablets were obtained from "Sacred Books and Early Literature of the East," edited by C.F. Horne.[4]

"I removed the bodies of those who had been struck down by the pestilence, and whose carcases, devoured by dogs and pigs, were blocking the streets and open places of Babylon. Even those who had lost their lives in the terrible famine."

---

4. Sacred Books and Early Literature of the East, edited by C.F. Horne, Vol. I, 1917, Parke, Austin, and Lipscomb, Inc., N.Y. and London, pgs. 71, 72, 73, 255-259, 428-430.

"The noxious god, the noxious spirit of the neck, the neck-spirit of the desert, the neck-spirit of the mountains, the neck-spirit of the sea, the neck-spirit of the morass, the noxious cherub of the city, this noxious wind which seizes the body and the health of the body. Spirit of heaven remember, spirit of earth remember."

"The burning spirit of the neck which seizes the man, the spirit of the neck which works evil, the creation of an evil spirit. Spirit of heaven remember, spirit of earth remember."

"Wasting, want of health, the evil spirit of the ulcer, spreading quinsy of the gullet (acute tonsillitis), the violent ulcer, the noxious ulcer. Spirit of heaven remember, spirit of earth remember."

"Sickness of the entrails, sickness of the heart, the palpitation of a sick heart, sickness of bile, sickness of the head, noxious colic, the agitation of terror, flatulency of the entrails, noxious illness, lingering sickness, nightmare. Spirit of heaven remember, spirit of earth remember."

"He who makes an image which injures the man, an evil face, an evil eye, an evil mouth, an evil tongue, evil lips, an evil poison, spirit of heaven remember, spirit of earth remember." (This is, perhaps, one of the oldest references to the making of images which are used in witchcraft. Similar images were later used by the Romans and are well-documented during the Middle Ages).

"The cruel spirit, the strong spirit of the head, the head-spirit that departs not, the head-spirit that goes not forth, the head-spirit that will not go, the noxious head-spirit. Spirit of heaven remember, spirit of earth remember."

"The poisonous spittle of the mouth (tuberculosis?) which is noxious to the voice, the phlegm which is destructive to the . . . , the pustules of the lungs, the pustule of the body, the loss of the nails, the removal and dissolving of old excrement, the skin which is stripped off, the recurrent ague of the body, the food which hardens in a man's body, the food which returns after being eaten, the drink which distends after drinking, death by poison, from the swallowing of the mouth which distends, the unreturning wind from the desert. Spirit of heaven remember, spirit of earth remember."

"May Nin-cigal (Queen of the Underworld), the wife of Nin-a'su, turn her face toward another place; may the noxious spirit go forth and seize another; may the propitious cherub and the propitious genie settle upon his body. Spirit of heaven remember, spirit of earth remember."

"May Nebo, the great steward, the recliner supreme among the gods, like thy god who has begotten him, seize upon his head; against his life may he not break forth. Spirit of heaven remember, spirit of earth remember."

"On the sick man by the sacrifice of mercy may perfect health shine like bronze; may the Sun-god give this man life; may Marduk, the eldest son of the deep, give him strength, prosperity, and health. Spirit of heaven remember, spirit of earth remember."

The Lament of the Pious Ruler: "An evil demon has come out of its lair; from yellowish, the sickness became white. It struck my neck and crushed my back, it bent my high stature like a popular; like a plant of the marsh, I was uprooted and thrown on my back. Food became bitter and putrid, the malady dragged on its course. Though without food, hunger diminished; the sap of my blood he drained. In my stall I passed the night like an ox, I was saturated like a sheep in my excrements; the disease of my joints baffles the chief exorcizer, and my omens were obscure to the diviner, the exorcizer could not interpret the character of my disease, and the limit of my malady the diviner could not fix. He (Marduk) drove back the evil demon into the abyss. My entire body he restored, he wiped away the blemish, making it resplendent, the oppressed stature regained its splendor, on the banks of the stream where judgement is held over men the brand of slavery was removed, the fetters taken off. Into the jaw of the lion, about to devour me, Marduk inserted a bit. Marduk has seized the snare of my pursuer, has encompassed his lair."

"O Marduk, lord of the lands, the mighty. . . . O lord, at this time stand beside me and harken to my cries, give judgement, make my decision. The sickness . . . do thou destroy, and take thou away the disease of my body. O my god and goddess, judge ye mankind, and possess me. By the command of thy mouth may there never approach anything evil, the magic of the sorcerer and the sorceress. May there never approach me the poisons of the evil of men. May there never approach the evil of dreams, of powers and portents of heaven and of earth."

Fourteen years after the reign of Ashurbanipol, the empire collapsed under a siege by the Medes and the Babylonians, under Nebuchadrezzar. Thus commences the New Babylonian or Chaldean Empire. Nebuchadrezzar is noted further for ending the Davidic Dynasty of the Hebrews and carrying the leaders off to Babylon. He beautified Babylon with "hanging gardens" in order to please his mountain-borne Median wife and made the city the center of trade, science and technology. Many early Greek philosophers, such as Thales and Pythagoras, traveled to Babylon for their education. Nebuchadrezzar died in about 562 B.C.

About twenty years later, in 539 B.C., Cyrus of Persia conquered Babylonia and his son, Cambyses conquered into Egypt. There, he and most of his army disappeared. Recently, in Egypt, near the Siwa Oasis, about 350 miles west of Cairo, an Egyptian archeological mission discovered the remains of the Persian Army, tens of thousands strong, which had apparently been overwhelmed by a sandstorm. A cousin, Darius, came to the throne and organized the Persian Empire. The priests of the Persians were called Magi, and were believed to have occult powers. It was Darius who had his accomplishments carved into the Behistun Rock in Old Persian, Elamite and Akkadian, the discovery of which led to the decipherment of cuneiform writing. He also established a new capital, Parsa, known today as Persepolis.

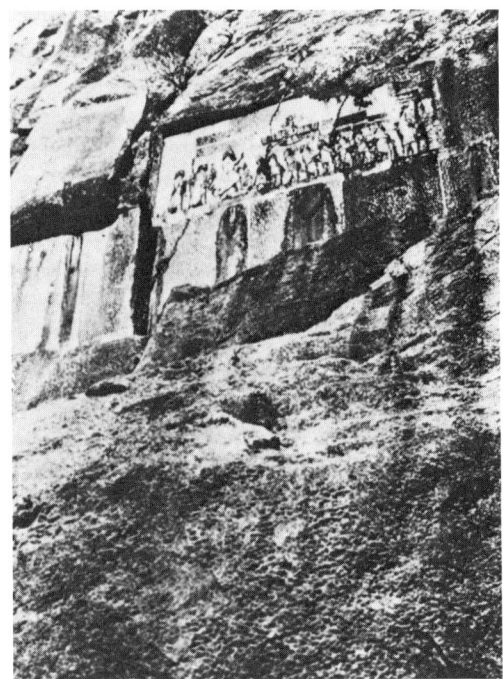

Into this two thousand foot cliff, the Behistun Rock, Darius, King of Persia had chiseled inscriptions which Henry Rawlinson observed in 1837 and published in 1846 as "The Persian Cuneiform Inscriptions at Behistun," which led to the deciphering of the ancient scripts. (Photograph courtesy Phototeque Musee de l'Homme, Paris)

In 480 B.C., the son of Darius, Xerxes, marched against the Greeks, but was defeated. In 338 B.C., Philip of Macedon succeeded in uniting the Greek city-states and in 331 B.C., his son, Alexander, defeated the Persians near the ruins of ancient Nineveh. Recently, Professor Andronikos, at Salonica University, Greece, announced the discovery of the tomb of King Philip under a forty foot mound, in the village of Vergina, in northern Greece.

Alexander conquered the land around the Mediterranean Sea from Greece to Egypt; and from Mesopotamia to the Indus River in India. He destroyed Persepolis, in revenge for the Persian burning of Athens, and made Babylon his capital. According to legend, his magicians warned him that if he entered Babylon, he would die. Alexander died in Babylon, in 323 B.C., reportedly of the effects of repeated infections with malaria. The Empire then split into the Ptolemy Empire of Egypt and Judea; and the Seleucid Empire which consisted of Asia Minor, Syria and Mesopotamia. During this period, Greek language, customs and writing were introduced into the Near East and Africa, and much of the history of these areas was written in Greek, by Greek historians. The knowledge of the various countries was assimilated by the Greeks, including the practices of medicine. Later, when only the Greek language could be read by scholars, it was believed that the Greeks were the "fathers of medicine."

Malaria is a febrile disease, formerly supposed to be due to poisonous emanations from damp ground and marshes, but now known to be caused by protozoal blood parasites of the *Genus Plasmodium*. Early Chinese physicians, and later, Hippocrates, divided fevers into four groupings: continuous; quotidian; tertian; and quartan; with the latter three being identified with malaria. Of the malarial parasites of man, *Plasmodium malariae* was described in 1880 by Lavaran. *Plasmodium vivax, P. falciparum* and *P. ovale,* other species parasitic in man, were described shortly after by other investigators.

The life history of the plasmodia occurs in two hosts: a mosquito, in which the sporulating sexual cycle (sporogony) occurs; and a vertebrate, in which takes place the asexual cycle (schizogony). Infective sporozoites from the salivary glands of infected mosquitos enter the vertebrate host through the bite of the insect, and are carried to the liver and other tissues of the body. In these tissue cells, the sporozoite develops into a schizont which contains several thousand merozoites. The merozoites are released and attack erythrocytes, in which further asexual multiplication occurs which results in the formation of additional merozoites. The erythrocytic merozoites, in turn, are released from the red blood cells and infect other erythrocytes. In some erythrocytes, sexual malarial gametocytes develop: the macrogametocyte, or female cell; and the microgametocyte, or male cell. The gametocytes are ingested by the mosquito when taking a blood meal and fertilization occurs in the stomach of the insect. Within 24 hours, the fertilized zygote develops into the wormlike form, the ookinete, which penetrates the gut wall and develops into a spherical oocyst. Within the oocyst, thousands of sporozoites may develop which, after liberation, may penetrate the salivary glands and infect the next vertebrate host bitten by the mosquito.

The clinical manifestations of the disease are caused by the destruction of the erythrocytes and the resultant disruption of metabolism. The infection is characterized by intermittent febrile attacks, secondary anemia and enlargement of the spleen. When both the circulatory and nervous systems are affected, the disease may result in a rapid loss of strength, cardiac weakness, coma and death. A frequent complication with falciparum malaria is "Blackwater fever," in which there is an enormous hemolysis of erythrocytes and necrosis of the liver, spleen and kidneys, with a fatality rate of approximately 25 per cent.

Protection against infection is passively transferred from infected mothers to their children. An acquired, active infection during childhood results in an acquired immunity for life, against superinfection with the antigenically-similar parasite. It is believed that the continued presence of the specific strain of the parasite is necessary within the body to prevent superinfection with that specific strain of malaria. A host may be infected with more than one species of the malarial parasite. It infects about 150 million people each year and kills more than one million children in Africa alone.

Malaria can be controlled by the elimination of mosquitos and carriers, and the protection of noninfected persons. Human infections are treated with a variety of drugs which usually attack the asexual, erythrocytic forms of the parasite and suppress the infection: they are Quinine; Atabrine; Chloroquine;

Primaquine; and others. Casual prophylactic and suppressive treatments of malaria have resulted in the appearance of resistant strains of the parasite.

Drugs were not readily available for the treatment of malaria until about 1820, when two Frenchmen, Pelletier and Caventou, isolated the antimalarial substance from the bark of the Chinchona tree and it appeared on the world markets as quinine-sulfate. The effectiveness of the powdered bark of the Chinchona tree, in treating fevers, was noted by Father Calancha, in Peru, in 1633. Unfortunately, not all the bark which was sent to Europe was from the correct tree, so the acceptance of quinine took approximately 200 years. In Ancient China, according to legend, the Emperor Shen Nung, who lived about 2700 B.C., composed a herbal which described the drug "Ch'ang Shan" which was used in the treatment of malaria. This plant is *Dichroa fibrifuga*. During World War II, when the forces of Japan threatened to cut off the world's major source of Chinchona bark, which was plantation-grown in southeast Asia by the Dutch colonies, cultivation of this plant was begun in the United States. Synthetic quinine was chemically prepared in the laboratory which ended dependence on the growth of the Chinchona tree and *Dichroa fibrifuga*.

The physicians of ancient Mesopotamia were, as in ancient Egypt, a part of the priesthood. Associated with the practice of medicine were also independent exorcists, bleeders, cuppers and layers-on of plasters. Diseases were thought to have been introduced into the body from without and, most frequently, were thought to have been caused by evil spirits, the expulsion of which brought about the recovery of the patient. In the treatment of various diseases, the procedures and medicinal treatments are usually accompanied or obscured by prayers, rituals, exorcisms, magic formulas and amulets. The use of astrology and divination through hepatoscopy were also utilized in medicinal predictions and therapy. The interest of the priesthood in the so-called demonical diseases, gave impetus to the collection of observations of various diseases, thus developing a clinical history of certain diseases. At first, the clinical history was used to make prophecies, but later, it was used to predict the fate of the patient. The separation of the religious beliefs from the actual medicinal beliefs could only occur when the divorce between the priests and the physicians was accomplished. The Greeks, perhaps, were the first people to bring about this separation of religion and medicine.

Cuneiform tablets, unearthed from the sites of the early cities of Mesopotamia, reveal a variety of diseases that were recognized, treatments that could be utilized, predictions as to the recovery of the patient, and omens related to incurable diseases and congenital deformities. The oldest pharmaceutical prescriptions of man have been found on Babylonian cuneiform tablets which are approximately 4000 years old. Unfortunately, the tablets seldom describe the disorders for which the prescriptions were compounded.

Eye diseases were, and still are, a problem in the Middle East. Cuneiform tablets describe such conditions as: night blindness, which we now know is caused by a vitamin A deficiency; xerophthalmia, a drying of the eyes due to an improper diet and which was treated by the application of an onion; nystagmus, the rapid movement of the eyes from side to side; ophthalmoplegia, the paralysis of the eyes in a fixed position; trachoma (previously described); trichiasis, an ingrowing of the eyelashes; entropion, the inturning of the eyelid; dacrocystitis, an abscess of the lacrymal sac; and others. The "Code of Hammurabi" refers to physicians who "opened up the eye-socket" with a bronze lancet and either saved or destroyed the eye of the patient. It is highly unlikely that in 1790 B.C., physicians were cutting into the eye of a patient with a lancet in order to remove cataracts or tumors. Until discoveries prove otherwise, it would be more reasonable to assume that the surgery was for the removal or lancing of cysts or abcesses of the eye region. Since the punishment for the physician who destroyed the eye of his patient could be the cutting off of the hand of the physician, it would seem unlikely that a physician would perform an operation, such as that of cataract removal, which could so easily result in the destruction of the eye of the patient. That the law concerning the eye-operation is included in the "Code" indicates that it was performed quite frequently and therefore required regulation. Perhaps paramedical personnel had been attempting to perform the operation along with their phlebotomies and cuppings.

Other noninfectious diseases that were observed are: general paralysis; paresis, a partial paralysis, edema, the accumulation of body fluids in the tissues, scurvy; lung disorders; heart disorders; birth disorders, such as extraction of the fetus, the birth of Siamese twins, blindness and idiocy; testicular atrophy; and various poisons.

One tablet pictures a man in an upright position with, what appears to be, worms falling from the anal region. The worms are called "earthworms," but are most likely roundworms, which are intestinal parasites of man and other animals, and which may be passed, in entirety, from the anus. The patient, having the worm infection, is also described as being jaundiced, exhausted, sleepless and weary. Roundworms may enter the pancreatic and bile ducts, causing jaundice and abscesses of the liver. Apparently, in some cases in infection, an attempt was made by the physicians to treat the liver abscess because one inscription directs the cutting of an incision between the eighth and ninth ribs. The possibility of such an operation is supported by the "Code of Hammurabi" which states "If a physician performed a major operation on a seignor with a bronze lancet, and has saved the seignor's life. . . ." How frequently such major operations were performed in antiquity is unknown but in Mesopotamia, Hammurabi's "Code" states that if the patient died, the physician was to have his hand cut off. Unless the technique had been perfected, and some methods had been developed to prevent infection, it would seem highly unlikely that a physician would undertake such a major operation which could easily result in the death of the patient.

The intestinal roundworm, *Ascaris lumbricoides,* has been known since antiquity, probably because of its large size, of perhaps 35 centimeters, which allows it to be easily seen in the feces of an infected person, if voided. The distribution of the infection is worldwide, but is dependent upon the lack of sanitary disposal of fecal material. Infection is common in areas where human feces are utilized as a fertilizer.

After copulation, the female roundworm produces ova which are passed with the feces. Infective larvae develop within the eggs. The ova may be conveyed to the mouth by dirty fingers, contaminated water and contaminated vegetables or other foods. The larvae are released in the small intestine and penetrate the intestinal wall, reaching the blood or lymphatic systems. They are carried to the lungs where they eventually penetrate from the capillaries into the air sacs, and pass through the bronchioles, bronchi and trachea to the epiglottis, where they are swallowed; in the small intestine they mature into adult male and female worms, and live for about one year.

The effects of an *Ascaris* infection vary with the age of the patient and the numbers of worms present. The presence of large numbers of worms may cause intestinal obstruction, the blockage of liver and bile ducts, hemorrhaging, pneumonia and abscesses in any organ into which they happen to wander. In extreme cases, surgery may be required to save the life of the patient but generally, the worms can be expelled with administration of an antihelminthic, such as hexylresorcinol, followed by a purgative. This treatment has no effect on migrating larvae. The disease is prevented by sanitary disposal of fecal material.

It is believed that epilepsy is described in some cuneiform tablets. Epilepsy was thought to be caused by a demon of the roof or roof beams, Bel Uri. An attack is described as an inturning or rolling upwards of the eyes, accompanied by a clenching of the hands and feet and labored breathing; the patient cries like an animal, saliva flows from his mouth, and his neck is pressed down to the left. A major attack will overtake him in the open country, not built up with houses, or in the corner of the house.

Epilepsy is a chronic functional disease which is characterized by fits or attacks in which there is a loss of consciousness, with a succession of interrupted or continuous convulsions. The length of the time of the attack varies with the patient, as does the frequency. A fit in which there are severe convulsions and loss of consciousness is termed "grand mal." The mild form which does not exhibit convulsions is termed "petit mal." Today, epilepsy is treated very effectively with drugs such as Dilantin and Mesantoin. The use of these, and similar drugs, controls the seizures in about 50 percent of the cases; for the remainder, the number and severity of the seizures are greatly reduced. Approximately four million Americans have some form of epilepsy. Although epilepsy is not considered an hereditary disease, proper prenatal care can help prevent some cases. In 1977, it was reported, by Dr. Tanaka of St. Mary's Hospital in Montreal, that pregnant women with a deficiency of the mineral manganese may give birth to epileptic children. Other commonly attributed causes of epilepsy are birth injuries, accidents that cause brain damage, diseases that starve the brain of oxygen and cerebral surgery. Recently, the FDA gave approval for the marketing of a new anti-convulsive drug, valproic acid, which is chemically similar to sodium valproate, a drug which had been available in Europe for years. The drug will be marketed under the brand name of Depakene.

An infectious disease which was, and still is, prevalent in the region of Mesopotamia is typhoid fever. It was thought to be caused by a demon, small of hand but with long fingers, who slipped into the house and stabbed the patient in the stomach with her fingers. The treatment was the administration of a spell which caused the demon to withdraw her fingers. A manifestation of the infection is the appearance of red spots on the abdomen of the patient from which is derived the common name, rose spot fever.

The causative agent is a bacterium, *Salmonella typhi*, which generally is consumed in water or foods which have been contaminated with fecal material containing the microorganism. The onset of the infection is gradual, with malaise, headache and a fever, which increases to about 104°F. Prostration, with diarrhea or constipation, occurs during the first week of the disease. This is frequently followed by abdominal tenderness and distension, and a cough and bronchitis. Rose spots on the abdomen frequently appear during the first two weeks of the infection. The bacteria multiply in the lymphoid tissue of the intestinal wall and regional lymph nodes and may gain access to the body and appear in various tissues, and be excreted in the urine or feces. Unsanitary disposal of body wastes leads to the spread of the infection to other hosts. Death may occur and is due to intestinal hemorrhages or perforations. In some cases, about three percent, a carrier state develops in the host who continues to excrete the microorganisms in the urine and feces for long periods of time and becomes a continual source of infection in the community. The most notorious of all typhoid carriers was Mary Mallon, known as Typhoid Mary, of New York City. She was the source of the 1903 outbreak with 1,300 cases. Because of her refusal to leave employment, often under assumed names, involving the handling of food, she was placed under permanent detention from 1915 until her death in 1938. One attack of typhoid fever generally confers immunity on the recovered patient. Although the disease was described by Budd, in 1856, the organism was not observed until 1880, by Eberth, or isolated until 1884, by Gaffky. Soon after its isolation by Gaffky, killed microorganisms were injected into humans for the purpose of immunization. Today, extracts of the organisms are utilized which result in a higher level of immunity and less toxic reaction. Infected persons are treated with sulfonamides, chloramphenicol, streptomycin and other antibiotics but administration of the drugs may not clear the body of the microorganisms. The disease can be controlled by the elimination of the sources of infection and sanitary sewage disposal.

Another bacterial disease which is believed to be described in cuneiform tablets is diphtheria, or commonly, Egyptian or Syrian ulcers. Described, is a child showing signs of suffocation which will not feed at the breast and which has a high temperature and has a fetid breath. The causative agent is the bacterium, *Corynebacterium diphtheriae.* Infection of man usually results in an acute disease or toxicosis which is due to the presence of the microorganisms in patches of pseudomembranes in the throat or other mucous surfaces and the absorption of the diphtheria toxin by the body. The disease is attended with swelling of the larynx, the pharynx, labored breathing, difficulty in swallowing and loss of the voice. General symptoms are fever, heart problems, anemia and prostration. Unless treated, the disease frequently results in death. The microorganism was first described by Klebs, in 1883, and was isolated in 1884 by Loeffler. The toxin was discovered by Roux and Yersin in 1888, and in 1890, and antitoxin was developed in animals by Kitasato and von Behring which, shortly after, was used in the treatment of human cases of diphtheria. In 1923, Ramon developed a formalin-treated toxin, called toxoid, that was, and is now, used in the immunization of man. People contracting the disease are now treated with antitoxin and antibiotics, such as penicillin. As in typhoid fever infections, carriers may develop who harbor the microorganisms in mucous membranes for several months which necessitates the quarantine of the patient until the organism has been eliminated from the host. Today, in progressive nations, the disease is controlled by vaccination of the population with the previously mentioned toxoid and elimination of carriers.

Other parasitic or bacterial diseases which are believed to be described in the cuneiform tablets are: Leishmaniasis; tuberculosis; pneumonic plague; and leprosy. The Mesopotamians regarded leprosy in the same manner as did the Hebrews, later, in the Old Testament. Boundary stones were placed around the villages and cities, and anyone having an unyielding skin infection could not pass the stones and enter the environs of the city. One tablet indicates that anyone having white patches or spots on his skin has been rejected by his God, and should be rejected by mankind.

ancient india

Approximately 1800 miles to the east of the junction of the Tigrus and Euphrates Rivers, in the country now called Pakistan, is the valley of the Indus River. Here, archeologists have unearthed the buried remains of another river culture of the ancient world. It is believed that the early immigrants into the Indus valley originated, as did the early settlers of Mesopotamia, from the mountain valleys of the regions now occupied by Iran and Iraq. Within one thousand years, the people established communal farming of the fertile lands with irrigation and flood control; planned cities with storehouses, wells, baths and sewerage systems; writing; and an extensive trade with other cultures. The earliest level of culture has been dated to about 2500 B.C. These people, the Dravidians, established many centers or cities, the two best known being Harappa and Mohenjo-daro. In about 1500 B.C., Indo-European invaders, the Aryans, entered from the north, conquered the Dravidians, and settled throughout the land. One of their gods was Indra, from whom the country took its name. A saga of the Aryans, the Rig-Veda, frequently refers to Indra as the "fort-destroyer" and he is described as having destroyed ninety forts. During the excavation of Mohenjo-daro, archeologists came upon piles of skeletons of its inhabitants who had apparently been massacred and left where they had fallen. The Aryans were nomadic and did not utilize the cities of the Dravidians; nor did they construct any of their own, as far as is known. Until the excavation of Harappa, in 1921, there was no known building in India that could be dated earlier than 500 B.C.

The Dravidians, an agricultural people, worshipped fertility gods and goddesses which were associated with successful crops and the breeding of domesticated animals. The worship of the "mother-goddess" was accompanied by human sacrifices. The male deity was represented by the worship of the phallus and the bull. Later Hindu deities, Shiva and Kali, resemble this primitive worship in that Shiva is associated with the bull, and Kali with human and animal sacrifices.

Animal sacrifices are still carried out in the Hindu religion today and, although illegal, human sacrifices still occur. In 1973 the Times of India reported that at the town of Manwat, near Bombay, 14 persons were arrested in the investigation of the sacrifice of eleven women and girls as a fertility offering so that the mistress of one of the suspects could become pregnant. The village sorceress was said to have advised him to offer the blood of virgins to the goddess of fertility in order to have his wishes granted.

The Aryans, being nomadic, worshipped gods of celestial natures, which are described in the "Vedas," a collection of hymns which attained their present form in about 800 B.C. The Rig-Veda is the oldest of the collection, is written in archaic Sanscrit and may be dated to about 1500 B.C. In this collection, primitive man, in the form of a cosmic giant, was consumed by fire at the time of the First Sacrifice and from the limbs of this creature came man and animals. Sacrifice was the center of the Vedic religion which, through fire, brought the celebrant into contact with the divine world. "Soma," plants and animals were the main articles utilized in the rituals. There were no temples or idols, although there were priests. Private rites were performed by the head of the family. Commentaries on the Vedas, the Brāhamanas, and later, the Upanisads, led to the development of the popular Hinduism. The eruption of the religion was brought about by the Indian Epics, the Māha-Bhārata and the Bhagavad-gītā. Other works are the Purānas, the Samhitās, the Āgamas and the Tantras.

The earliest sacred books of the Hindus are called "the Vedas" meaning "books of holy knowledge." Not one word of these books may be changed nor may one word of them be doubted. The Vedas are still so treasured that the Hindu priests memorize them and pass them, orally, from generation to generation. The Rig-Veda is the oldest in the collection; modern Hindu scholars claim it has an antiquity of from eight to twelve thousand years, while European scholars, tracing it to about 1200 B.C., set its beginning at about 2000 B.C. The following excerpts from the Rig-Veda were obtained from "The Sacred Books and Early Literature of the East," edited by Charles F. Horne.[1]

"I worship by hymns Agni, the high-priest of the sacrifice, the deity, the sacrificial priest who presents oblations to the deities and is the possessor of great riches. Aswins, destroyers of diseases, shorn of falsehood, leaders in the van of heroes, come to the mixed libations of Soma, extracted and placed on lopped Kus'a-grass. (The Aswins are healing gods of physicians.) Let us not incense thee, O Rudra, by our worship, not by bad praise, O hero, and not by divided praise! Raise up our men by thy medicines, for I hear that thou art the best of all physicians. O Rudra, where is thy soft stroking hand which cures and relieves? Thou, the remover of all heaven-sent mischief, wilt thou, O strong

---

1. "The Sacred Books and Early Literature of the East," edited by Charles F. Horne, 1917, Parke, Austin and Lipscomb, New York and London, pgs. 16, 17, 40-44.

hero, bear with me. O Rudra, a boy indeed makes obeisance to his father who comes to greet him: I praise the lord of brave men, the giver of many gifts, and thou, when thou hast been praised, wilt give us thy medicines. O Maruts (storm gods), those pure medicines of yours, the most beneficent and delightful, O heroes, those which Manu, our father, chose—those I crave from Rudra, as health and wealth. Soma and Rudra, draw far away in every direction the disease which has entered our house. Drive far away Nirriti, and may auspicious glories belong to us. Soma and Rudra, bestow all these remedies on our bodies. Protecting us, come to our protecting doors, be without illness among our people, O Rudra. A thousand medicines are thine, O thou who art freely accessible; do not hurt us in our kith and kin."

The Atharva-Veda is a collection of prayers or hymns, some magical in nature, dealing with a variety of subjects. Some describe diseases and were utilized as a charm to cure the disease. The following excerpts were obtained from "Hinduism," edited by Louis Renou.[2]

"May Agni drive the fever away from here, may Soma, the Press-stone, and Varuna, of tried skill; may the alter, the straw upon the alter, and the brightly flaming fagots drive him away! Away to naught shall go the hateful powers. Thou that maketh all men sallow, inflaming them like a searing fire, even now, O Fever, thou shalt become void of strength: do thou now go away down, aye, into the depths."

"The fever that is spotted, covered with spots, like reddish sediment, him thou, O plant of unremitting potency, drive away down below." (This red-spotted fever could be typhus fever)

"When thou, being cold, and then again deliriously hot, accompanied by cough, didst cause the suffer to shake, then O Fever, thy missiles were terrible: from these surely exempt us. Destroy the fever that returns on each third day, the one that intermits each third day, the one that continues without intermission, and the autumnal one; destroy the cold fever, the hot, him that comes in summer, and him that arrives in the rainy season." (Malaria)

"Born of the wind, the atmosphere, the lightning, and the light, may this pearl shell, born of gold, protect us from straits. With the shell we conquer disease and poverty; with the shell, too, the demons. The shell is our universal remedy; the pearl shall protect us from straits."

Typhus fever is an acute infectious disease caused by the rickettsia, *Rickettsia prowazeki,* and transmitted to man by the body louse, *Pediculus humanus corporis* and the head louse, *Pediculus humanus capitis.* The disease is characterized by a high fever, headache and generalized rash with a fatality rate of about 20 percent. The disease was first clearly described by Fracastoro in 1546. Epidemics of the disease have generally occurred during wars and famines: In Ireland, between 1816-19, over 700,000 people died; in Russia, between 1918-22, 3 million died; there are many other examples of the danger of this infection.

---

2. "Hinduism," edited by Louis Renou, 1961, Washington Square Press Inc., N.Y., pgs. 52-54.

After an incubation period of about two weeks, the host develops and sustains a high temperature of about 104°F., and develops a "mulberry" rash which spreads over the entire body. During the second or third week, increasing prostration develops and the patient is unable to eat or drink. Involvement of the lungs, heart and kidneys may lead to coma and death. Gangrene of the toes, fingers, ears, nose, penis and scrotum may occur. Infection is now treated, dramatically, with the tetracyclines and chloramphenicol, improvement occurring within two to three days. The disease is prevented by vaccination and delousing procedures. It is interesting that in the Sashruta Samhita, a patient is described as dying, when lice are seen crawling freely about on the head of the patient.

In the Vedas, Prithivi, the earth, and Dyaus, the sky, produced all the Gods and man. There was no particular supreme god but each had a specific place in the order of the functioning of the religion. Some of the better known deities are: Indra; Tvashtri; Agni; Soma; and Vishnu.

Indra was the storm god and wielder of the thunderbolt who protected the other gods and man against demons representing the harsh aspects of nature, especially drought. He is of an extremely violent nature and has an insatiable thirst for "Soma," an intoxicating drink. Tvashtri, brother of Indra, is endowed with magical powers, rather than strength. He was responsible for the generative powers of mankind and the production of children, and guarded religious sacrifices. He fashioned a magical bowl which remains constantly filled with "Soma." Another brother, Agni, fire god, originated the use of clarified butter in sacrificial fires. He represents the spark of life in all living things and can consume anything and yet remains pure. This is the old ritual of purification by fire. Vishnu was a minor deity of the Aryans who, in Hinduism, is one of the major deities and is noted for his incarnations, the last one being Buddha. Soma was the name of the fermented milky juice of the "soma" plant which nourished all the gods and was of an intoxicating nature. Later, the drink was worshipped as the god Soma, who was all powerful, healed all diseases and was a bestower of riches.

Scholars have speculated about the "soma" plant for many years. The Vedas describe it as a plant, without seeds, flowers or roots, that cannot be cultivated. Recently, Wasson has theorized that the "soma" plant is the fly agaric mushroom, *Amanita muscaria.* This mushroom contains, among other compounds, mycoatropine, an alkaloid which is soluble in alcohol and has mydriatic and narcotic effects when ingested by man. It stimulates the heart and breathing rates and causes dilation of the pupil of the eye. The eyes also lose their ability to focus on various objects. Consumption of the alkaloid may result in delirium, coma and death. If Wasson's postulation is correct, it may be that the mushroom was consumed for religious purposes and the production of an euphoric state in the priests. Mushrooms were, and still are, utilized by certain peoples of the Americas.

The daughter of Tvashtri, Saranyu, was fertilized by the rising sun, Visvasvat, and produced the first man and woman, twins, Yama and Yami. Yama was therefore the first man to die and became established as the "Ruler of the Dead." The route from life to death was presided over by his grandfather, the fire-god, Agni, which established the ritual of the cremation of the corpse. The ashes from the cremation represented all that was evil and impure, while the fire carried aloft all that was good and pure. In order to attain the "heaven" that awaited the pure spirits, certain sacrifices had to be performed by the offspring of the deceased which stimulated the production of large families and, today, overpopulation. Those who did not enter "heaven" were sent to an area of hundreds of thousands of hells ruled by Yama. These unfortunates were reborn as worms, moths or serpents. The good people attained fusion with the universal spirit, which was without beginning or end.

Later, Brahma, first of the gods, framer of the universe and guardian of the world came into prominence in the religious beliefs. During the Brahmanic period it was formulated that time was a never ending cycle of creation and destruction, each cycle being represented by one hundred years in the life of Brahma. One day in the life of Brahma is equivalent to 4,320 millions of earth years.

At the end of the period, the universe, Brahma, and everything else are dissolved in a great cataclysm, Mahapralaya. This is followed by 100 years of chaos, after which another Brahma is born and the cycle begins anew. At the present time, we are in the "Kaliyuga," or "Age of Degeneration" in which "men are wicked and beggarlike; they are unlucky because they deserve no luck; they value what is degraded, overeat, and live in cities filled with thieves; they are dominated by their women who are shallow, garrulous and lascivious, bearing too many children. They are oppressed by their kings and by the ravages of nature, famines and wars. Their miseries can only come to an end with the coming of Kali, the Destroyer."

The destruction is preceded by 100 years of drought; seven suns will appear in the sky and evaporate all the water. Fire, swept by winds will consume the earth. Rains, lasting for 12 years, will submerge the earth. Brahma, contained within a lotus blossom, sleeps until the time of awakening and renewed creation. During this time, the Gods and man are resorbed into Brahma, the universal spirit.

Ruling, with Brahma, are two other major gods, Shiva and Vishnu. Shiva is frequently referred to as the supreme god because of his power as the Creator or Destroyer. His power is obtained from yoga. He is worshipped as the god of cattle and medicine. His long hair represents the seven sacred rivers of India. He is accompanied by a bull, the crescent moon and serpents. He is perhaps most frequently portrayed as "Dancing Shiva," performing the "Tandava," the dance which will bring about the destruction of the world.

86   *Magic, Myths and Medicine*

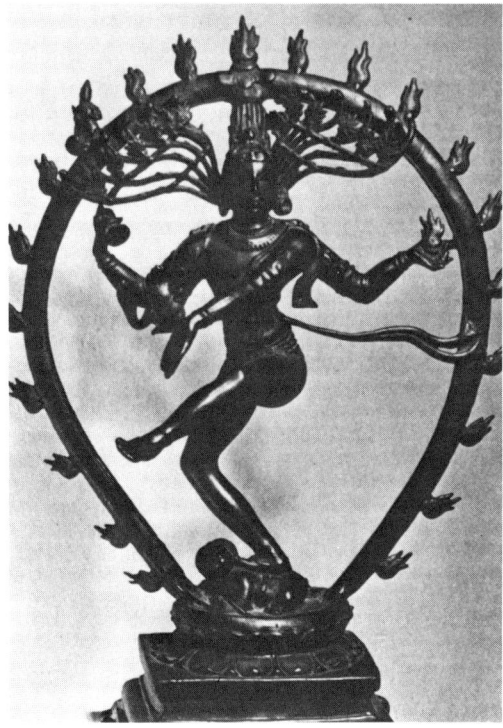

Shiva.

Vishnu is the cosmic ocean, Nara, which was everywhere before the creation of the universe. He is pictured as sleeping in a human form on the coiled serpent, Shesha (Ananta). Brahma is sometimes pictured as arising as a lotus from the navel of Vishnu. The incarnations of Vishnu, or Avatars, are numerous, the more recent ones being, Rama, Krishna and Buddha.

The social order that was established by the Aryans has had a great effect on the culture of that area and resulted in the caste system that, although it has been declared illegal, still exists today. The social order of the Aryans was: hereditary nobles at whose head was the chief or Raja; priests; citizens; conquered people, inferior to all others. After some time, the priests raised themselves into the highest position by giving a new importance to religious rituals. At first, the caste system was flexible, but later, it became extremely rigid and towards the end of the Vedic era, dramatic protests were made against Hinduism by such men as Gautama Buddha, with little result, except for the formation of a new religion, Buddhism.

Gautama Buddha was born in Nepal in about 563 B.C., and established a doctrine that spread all through India and Asia. In the doctrine, man is continually afflicted with illness and suffering; the suffering will end when desire ends; the cessation of desire is the state of Nirvana, the goal of all Buddhists. Jivaka, the physician who attended Buddha, has been credited with great skill in surgery, and was reported to have performed trepanations as a remedy for certain types of blindness.

For about two hundred years, India came under the influence of the Persians. Cyrus of Persia invaded India and his nephew, Darius conquered the Indus valley and Punjab, in 518 B.C. Indian troops served with Xerxes when his armies invaded Greece in 479 B.C. Alexander of Greece invaded India in 327 B.C., and the conquered regions of India were included in the Seleucid Empire at the death of Alexander. In 305 B.C., Chandragupta defeated the Seleucid army and established a central rule under which the apogee of Indian culture has been claimed to have reached its height.

The grandson of Chandragupta, Ashoka, ruled from 269-232 B.C., and consolidated the Gupta Empire. He caused hospitals to be established for man and animals and ordered medicinal herbs to be planted so as to be available for everyone. He accepted Buddhism and forbade the killing of animals that were not used for eating purposes. In western history, hospitals were first established by the Bishop Basil, in Caesarea, between 330-379 A.D.

Under Ashoka, and later rulers, the Empire established universities which attracted students from Asia and the Middle East. Nalanda, in the north, had eight colleges and three libraries. Mathematics were taught using Arabic numerals and the value "zero" was utilized. Astronomy, algebra, were utilized. The earth was thought to be a globe which rotated on an axis. Techniques were developed for working with iron, textiles and dyes. These techniques were later brought to Europe. Literature from this era includes the well-known, "Thousand and One Nights."

The Gupta Empire was conquered by the Huns in about 467 A.D., who ruled as the Rajputs for about 400 years. In the Thirteenth Century, Moslem rulers built a new empire in India and introduced a new religion into India, which would later cause the division of the land into India and Pakistan. In about 1524, Mongols, the descendants of Timur and Genghis Khan, invaded India and established the Moghal Empire which lasted until 1707.

There is an abundance of literature which has survived from ancient India, mainly religious in nature in its earliest forms, and becoming more scientific in later times. The Vedas are believed to have been compiled between 1500 and 1200 B.C. The later medicinal works of Charaka and Sashruta are believed by some scholars to have been written as early as the Sixth Century B.C., or as late as the Fifth Century A.D. The Sashruta Samhitá was mentioned in writings in the Fourth Century B.C., and in the Bower Manuscript of 400 A.D. Oral tradition makes the Sashruta Samhita very old, but the original text has not been uncovered. Most current texts are based upon the revision made by Nágárjuna, in the Second Century, B.C.

According to legend, the material contained within the Sashruta Samhitá was disclosed to him by the sage Dhanvantari, a mighty celestial, incarnated in the form of Divodása, the king of Kási. The information concerning medical science was incorporated into the Áyur-Veda, which originally formed one of the subsections of the Atharva-Veda.

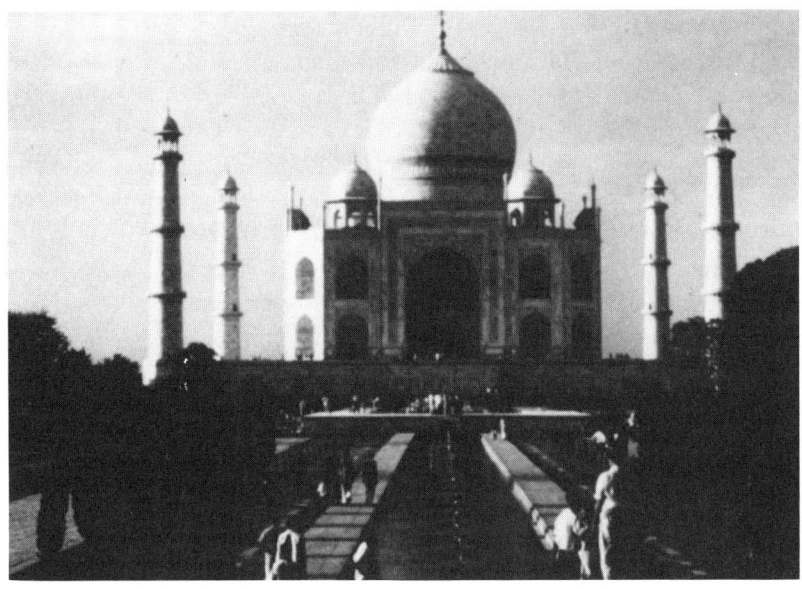

The Taj Mahal, Agra, India.

The Áyur-Veda is divided into eight different branches: (1) the removal of foreign substances from the body, description of surgical instruments, the use of cauterization; (2) the treatment of diseases of the eyes, ears, nose and throat; (3) the treatment of general diseases such as fevers, dysentery, insanity, hysteria, leprosy; (4) incantations and modes of exorcising evil spirits; (5) management of children; (6) toxicology of the bites of snakes, spiders and worms; (7) science of rejuvenation; (8) science of aphrodisiacs.

Sashruta, instructed by the king of Kási in the ways of medicine and surgery, compiled the Sashruta Samhitá, as a guide for other physicians and surgeons. The Sashruta Samhitá deals mainly with the problems of surgery and midwifery. The members of the healing art were divided into five groups; the physicians, the surgeons, the poison curers, the demon doctors and the magic doctors. Since Sashruta was a surgeon, the book deals mainly with surgery. Sashruta divided surgical operations into five areas; extraction of solid objects, incising, excising, puncturing, suturing and the evacuation of fluids. This work also describes 101 surgical instruments and instructs the surgeon to construct others, when necessary. Sashruta is credited with the first attempts at plastic surgery and the discovery of cataract-couching. In the Samhitá are also described the amputation of limbs, abdominal sections, the treatment of hernias and ruptures, the removal of hemorrhoids and fistula, the removal of bladder and urethral stones, the use of anaesthetics, problems of birth including the use of forceps and craniotomy, the dissection of dead bodies for the instruction of medical students and surgical practice for surgeons. It is interesting that the corpses used in anatomical studies were usually children because of the Hindu religious law which required the cremation of all dead bodies of persons over two years of age.

The following quotations of the Sashruta Samhitá were obtained from an edition edited by Kunja Lal Bhishagratna.[3] "Surgical instruments number one hundred and one in all, of which the hand is the most important, in as much as they all depend on the hand and as none of them can be handled without it. Appliances should be made neither too large nor too small, and their mouths or edges should be made sharp and keen. They should be made with a special eye as to strength and steadiness, and they should be provided with convenient handles."

"In cases that require incising, excising and scraping, alkalies are of greater importance than surgical instruments since their property is of corroding or destroying the skin and flesh where such an effect is desired."

"A fire is better than an alkali as far as its healing property is concerned. A disease burnt with fire is cured and does not return. Diseases which baffle the surgeon and physician, never yielding to medicinal or surgical remedies, are found to yield to fire."

"Leeches should be applied where the patient would be found to be old or imbecile, or a woman, or an infant, or a person of an extremely timid disposition, or a person of a delicate constitution, and as such, is not fit to be surgically operated upon, since this mode of bleeding is the gentlest that can be possibly devised. Blood can be sucked through a horn, through a gourd appliance, or by leeches or with whichsoever of them is available at the time."

"The food is fully digested with the help of the internal heat and ultimately assimilated into the system, giving rise to blood which is extremely thin in its consistency and which forms the essence of the assimilated food. The blood, running through the whole organism, has its primary seat in the heart. whence it flows through the twenty-four vessels which branch off from the latter to the remotest parts and extremities of the body. The blood is transformed into the catamenial flow in women which commences at the age of twelve and ceases at fifty."

"Now I shall deal with the process of affixing an artificial nose. First the leaf of a creeper, long and broad enough to fully cover the whole of the severed off part, should be gathered, and a patch of living flesh, equal in dimension to the preceding leaf, should be sliced of from the region of the cheek and, after

---

3. "Sashruta Samhitá," edited by Kunja Lal Bhishagratna, 1907, The Chowkhamba Sanskrit Series Office, Varanosi-1, India, Vol. I–pgs. 56, 78, 88, 98, 106, 152, 153. Vol. II–pgs. 333-336, 400-401, 40-42. Vol. III–pgs. 76-78.

scarifying it with a knife, swiftly adhered to the severed nose. Then the cool-headed physician should steadily tie it up with a bandage and should make sure that the adhesion of the severed parts has been fully effected. Then insert two small pipes into the nostrils to facilitate breathing and to prevent the adhesioned flesh from hanging down. After that, the adhesioned part should be sprinkled with powders and the nose should be enveloped in cotton and sprinkled over with the refined oil of pure sesamum. Adhesion should be deemed complete after the incidental ulcer has been perfectly healed up, while the nose should be again scarified and bandaged in the case of a semi or partial adhesion. The adhesioned nose should be tried to be elongated where it would fall short of its natural and previous length, or it should be surgically restored to its natural size in the case of the abnormal growth of its newly formed flesh."

Removal of a Bladder Stone

"A person of strong physique and unagitated mind should be first made to sit on a level board or table as high as the knee joint. The patient should then be made to lie on his back on the table, placing the upper part of his body in the attendant's lap, with his waist resting on an elevated cloth cushion. Then the elbows and knee joints of the patient should be contracted and bound up with fastenings or with linen. After that, the umbilical region of the patient should be well rubbed with oil or with clarified butter and the left side of the umbilical region should be pressed down with a closed fist so that the *stone* comes within the reach of the operator. The surgeon should then introduce into the rectum, the second and third fingers of his left hand, duly anointed and with the nails well pared. Then the fingers should be carried upward towards the rope of the perineum, in the middle line so as to bring the stone between the rectum and the sexual organs, when it should be so firmly and strongly pressed, as to look like an elevated tumor, taking care that the bladder remains contracted, but at the same time, even."

"An operation should not be proceeded with nor an attempt made to extract the stone in a case where, the stone on being handled, the patient would be found to drop down motionless with his head bent down, and his eyes fixed in a vacant stare like that of a dead man, as an extraction in such a case is sure to be followed by death. The operation should only be continued in the absence of such an occurrence."

"An incision should then be made on the left side of the raphe of the perineum (midway between the sexual organs and the anus) at the distance of a barley-corn and of sufficient width to allow the free egress of the stone. Several authorities recommend that the opening be on the right side of the raphe of the perineum for the convenience of the operation. Special care should be taken in extracting the stone from its cavity so that it may not break into pieces or leave any broken particles behind, however small, as they would, in case, be sure to grow larger again. Hence the entire stone should be extracted with the help of an Agravaktra Yantra (a forceps with blunted points)."

"After the extraction of a stone, the patient should be made to sit in a Droni (cauldron) full of warm water and be fomented thereby. In doing so, the possibility of an accumulation of blood in the bladder will be prevented; however, if blood be accumulated therein, a decoction of the Kshira-trees should be injected into the bladder with the help of a Pushpa-netra (urethral syringe)."

Removal of a Urethral Stone

"A seminal stone or gravel spontaneously brought down into the urethral passage should be removed through the same passage. The urethra should be cut open and the stone should be extracted with a hook or any other instrument in the case of its not being expelled out by the passage. The patient should refrain from sexual intercourse, riding on horse back or on the back of an elephant, swimming, climbing on trees and up mountains and partaking of indigestible substances for a year even after the healing of the ulcer."

Intestinal Surgery

"The patient should be first treated with emulsive measures and fomentations and then anointed with a "sneha." Then an incision should be made on the left side of the abdomen below the umbilicus and four fingers to the left of the line of hair which stretches downward from the navel. The *intestine* to the length of four fingers should be gently drawn out; any stone, any dry hardened substance or any hair found stiffing to the intestine should be carefully examined and removed. Then the intestine should be moistened with honey and clarified butter. It should then be gently replaced in its original position and the mouth of the incision in the abdomen should be sewn up." "In cases of the Parisrávi (blockage) type, the obstructing matter should be similarly removed from the intestines as in the preceding case, and the secreting intestine should be purified. The two ends of the severed intestines should be firmly pressed and adhered together and large black ants should be applied to these spots to grip them fastly with their claws. Then the bodies of the ants having their heads firmly adhering to the spots, as directed, should be severed and the intestines should be gently reintroduced into their original position, with the severed heads of the ants adhering to the ends of the incision, and sutured up, as in the preceding case. A union or adhesion of the incidental wound should then be duly effected. The seam should now be plastered with black earth mixed with Yashtimadhu and duly bandaged."

Removal of a Cataract

"Now we shall describe the surgical measures to be employed for curing a case of Linganáśa (obstruction or choking up at the pupil with a cataract) due to the action of the deranged Kapha. In cases where the deranged Dosha in the organ, that is the affected part of the organ does not appear semicircular, or thin in the middle, nor fixed, nor irregular, nor marked by a large number of lines or a variety of tints, or where it does not resemble a pearl or a drop of water in shape, or if it does not become painful and red coloured, the patient should be first treated with Sneha and Sveda at a season of the year which is neither too cold nor too hot for the purpose. Then the hands of the patient should be secured with proper fastenings and he should be made to sit, looking simultaneously, with his two eyes, at the tip of his nose. Then the intelligent surgeon, leaving off two portions of the white part of the eyeball from the end of the eye, and having fully and carefully drawn apart the eyelids with his thumb and the index and the middle fingers, should insert the Yava-vaktra (needle of copper) instrument through the sides of the natural apperaturelike point near the external angles of the eye, neither above nor below, care being taken not to pierce the veins. The left eye should be pierced with the right hand and the right with the left. The satisfactory nature of the operation should be presumed from the characteristic report or sound, and the emission of a drop of water from the affected region, following upon the perforation. The region of the Drishti-mandala should be subsequently scraped with the pointed end of the Sáláká. The part should be regarded as properly scraped when it would assume the glossiness of a resplendent cloudless sun and would be free from pain. Then the Sáláká (rod) should be gently withdrawn as soon as it would be able to perceive vision, and then the affected eye should be sprinkled over with clarified butter and bandaged with a piece of linen. The bandage should be removed on every fourth day and the organ should be washed with the decoction of the drugs of Vayu-subduing (infection-subduing) properties and bandaged again with a fresh one. This rule should be followed for ten days, as it would impart a fresh vigor to the sight."

These examples of medicine and surgery from the Sashrurá Samhita indicate the high quality of Indian medicine in antiquity. A controversy does exist over the possibility of the influence of medicinal beliefs of the Mediterranean region having been introduced into India between 300-500 B.C. Conversely, it may be that Indian medicinal treatments were introduced into the Mediterranean region during this same period. It is interesting that surgery was held in high esteem in India but apparently was not by the Greeks. Hippocrates, the Greek physician, to whom is accredited the famous "Oath," is thought to have lived in the Fifth Century B.C. In the Hippocratic Oath is stated "I will not cut persons laboring under the stone, but will leave this to be done by men who are practitioners of this work." Sashruta also described a method for replacing or repairing the nose. Historically, this procedure is next utilized by Professore Tagliacozzi, of Bologna University, in the Sixteenth Century, A.D., and later, in 1814, by Carpue, the pioneer of modern plastic surgery. These two examples seem to indicate the independent development of surgery in the Indian subcontinent.

Many diseases are also described in the Sashrutá Samhita which are too numerous to discuss since the document consists of approximately 1700 pages. In the past, and today, there are several diseases which have infected large numbers of the population and some have been the cause of millions of deaths.[4] These diseases are: malaria, more than 1,000,000 deaths per year; typhoid fever, epidemic but the death rate is low; cholera, 200,000 per year but may be in the millions during epidemics; dysentery, amebic and bacillary, epidemic; respiratory diseases, 400,000 per year; influenza, in 1918, claimed 20,000,000 lives; tuberculosis, 500,000 deaths per year; maternal mortality, 200,000 per year; leprosy, endemic.

Descriptions of leprosy (Hansen's Disease) are found in the literature of many ancient civilizations, including India. The following description of the disease is found in the Sashruta Samhitá:

"A preponderance of the deranged Vayu in a case of Kushtham (leprosy) is indicated by a contraction of the skin, local anaesthesia, a copious flow of perspiration, swelling, and a piercing or cutting pain in the affected part, together with a deformity of the limbs and hoarseness. Similarly, an excess of the deranged Pittam in a case of Kushtham, should be presumed from the suppuration of the affected part, from the breaking of the local skin, from the falling off of the fingers, from the sinking of the nose and ears, from the redness of the eyes and from the germination of parasites in the incidental ulcer. As a tree, full grown in the course of time, has driven its roots deeper and deeper into the successive strata of the soil, so this disease, first affecting and confining itself to the upper layers of the skin, will invade the deeper tissues and organs of the patient, if unchecked. A child, which is the offspring of the contaminated semen and ovum of its parents afflicted with Kushtham (leprosy), should be likewise regarded as a Kushthi (leper). Kushtham is a highly contagious disease; the contagion being usually communicated through sexual intercourse with a Kushthi, or by his touch or breath, or through partaking of the same bed, and eating or drinking out of the same vessel with him, or through using the wearing apparel, unguents and garlands of flowers previously used by a person afflicted with this terrible disease."

The earliest effective treatment for leprosy was derived from an Indian legend concerning King Rama of Benares, which many scholars date to 1000 B.C. In the legend, Rama contracted leprosy and left the city to live in the jungles, where his diet consisted mainly of herbs, fruits and berries. He was befriended by wild animals who instructed him to eat the seeds of the kalaw tree. The symptoms of leprosy subsided and he was eventually cured of the disease. One day, he rescued a girl, from a tiger, who was greatly disfigured by leprosy and he gave her the seeds of the kalaw tree, restoring her to good health. Rama then discovered that she was the Princess Piya. They returned to Benares, were married, raised 16 sets of twins, and lived happily ever after.

---

4. "Village Life in Northern India," Oscar Lewis, 1958.

The kalaw or chaulmoogra tree is found in southern Asia and India and the seeds of the tree contain an oil, chaulmoogra oil, which has been used in the treatments of leprosy, arthritis, skin diseases and syphilis. The Ayur-veda states that chaulmoogra oil is effective in the treatment of leprosy and recommends a dosage of 10-20 drops of the oil after meals for at least three months. The oil may also be used externally on the affected parts.

In 1950, the U.S. Leprosarium, at Carville, La., utilized the following treatment for leprosy: "Treatment is usually begun with gelatin capsules containing five drops of Chaulmoogra oil, taken daily after meals. The dosage is increased until the patient's tolerance is reached. Chaulmoogra is frequently used locally, in ointments or liniments."

Leprosy (Hansen's disease) is a bacterial infection caused by *Mycobacterium leprae*, a microorganism so fastidious in its growth requirements that it has not been successfully cultivated outside of living tissues. The microorganisms grow very slowly in the host so that following infection, it may take years before the first signs of leprosy appear. One of the first indications of infection is the thickening of the flesh at the bridge of the nose which is followed by an enlargement of the lobes of the ears. Leprous tubercles appear on the body and face as pale, colored spots or, the skin may take on a silvery sheen or, may be covered with large red bumps. The eyebrows are gradually destroyed and the face becomes puffed, resulting in the classic leonine face of the leper. When the nerves are invaded, white patches may develop all over the body. Gradually, the loss of sensation occurs in the extremities. Appendages may be deformed or lost entirely and, in rare cases, the case terminates with sudden paralysis and death. Children are more susceptible than adults and males are more susceptible than females. It is estimated that there are approximately 3-5 million lepers in the world today, the majority being found in Asia and Africa.

The use of chaulmoogra oil was introduced to the western world by Dr. F.J. Mouat of the Indian Medical Service. In 1901, Dr. Hopkins of the Tulane Medical School introduced the use of the oil in the treatment of lepers at Carville, La. In 1904, a refined oil which produced less toxic side effects was prepared by Dr. Power, of London, England. The refined chaulmoogra oil was administered to patients at the Hawaiian leper colony which resulted in the release of approximately 200 persons as cured. Unfortunately, there was no assured supply of chaulmoogra oil, since the tree grew in India and southern Asia. In 1920, Dr. Rock, of the University of Hawaii, set out to obtain seeds of the chaulmoogra tree which he found in north Burma. The seeds were shipped to Hawaii and within one year, thousands of seedlings were growing. By 1930, enough oil was being derived from the plantations to supply Molokai, Hawaii and Carville, La. Today, an effective oil can be obtained from two trees, *Taraktogenos kurzii* and *Hydnocarpus wightiana*.

Chaulmoogra oil was the basis for all therapy of leprosy until the sulfone drugs were utilized and later, streptomycin. More recently, the drug dapsone and related compounds have been found to be very effective in the treatment of Hansen's disease, although the drugs are known to cause cancer in test animals. Specialists believe that the benefits of the drugs outweigh any known cancer risk. The drug was tested on thousands of American soldiers in Vietnam for its effects on a resistant strain of malaria. Remissions of the disease frequently occur which indicate that the disease may be arrested, rather than cured. However, today, in many of the underdeveloped parts of the world, chaulmoogra oil is the only treatment available. In other areas, no treatment is available.

The causative agent of leprosy was first found in diseased tissue by Dr. Hansen of Norway, in 1874. In 1962, Dr. Shepard, CDC, Atlanta, Georgia, cultivated the microorganisms outside the human body, in the footpad of mice. At the present time, attempts are being made to cultivate the organism in tissue cultures.

Cholera has been endemic in India since antiquity and there have been frequent epidemics. Since 1817, epidemic waves have started in India, some of which have spread, reaching Europe in 1830 and America in 1832. In 1830, over 300,000 deaths occurred in India and in 1950, over 200,000 cases were reported. In 1977, in the Middle East, an outbreak of cholera occurred. It was thought to have originated in Syria and rapidly spread to Jordan, Lebanon, Kuwait, Iraq and Saudi Arabia. More than 3000 cases with about 80 deaths were reported in a two month period. Officials of Saudi Arabia, fearing a major epidemic during the pilgrimage to Mecca, stated that Moslems without valid vaccination certificates would not be admitted. The importation of fruits and vegetables from countries where cholera existed was banned. Cholera is

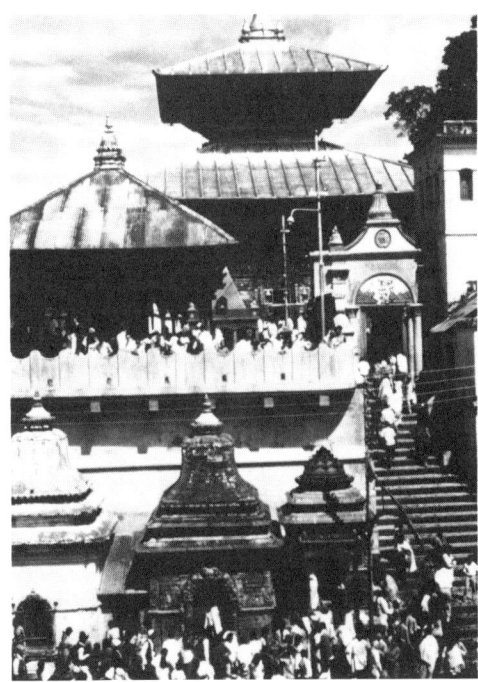

Lunar holiday celebration at the Pashupatinath Temple on the bank of the sacred River Bagmati. The temple has a two-tier golden roof and silver doors. The cremation areas are in the foreground.

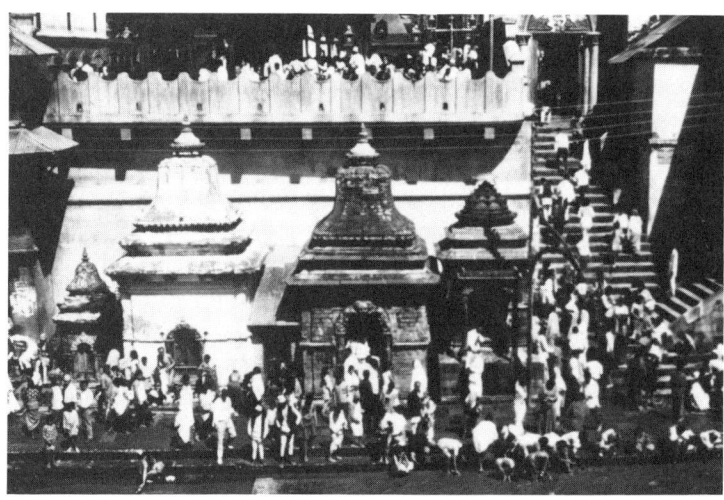

Cremation area at the Pashupatinath Temple.

spread by contaminated water and food, by flies, and by direct contact. The religous purification rites of the Middle East, India and southern Asia aid in the dissemination of the disease, and it is apt to flouish in the late summer, particularly when crowds gather at pilgrimage centers. Formerly, the disease followed pilgrimage routes, caravan routes and shipping lanes. Today, with rapid air travel, outbreaks of the infection may occur any place in the world where proper precautions are not taken.

The disease is described in the Sashruta Samhita as follows: "Now we shall discourse on the chapter which deals with the symptoms and medical treatment of Vishu-chika type of cholera. The disease, in which the deranged and incarcerated bodily Vayu produces, owing to the presence of indigestion, a pricking pain in the limbs is called Visuchika by the physicians. Men well-versed in the dietetic principles and temperate in their diet, enjoy an almost absolute immunity from its attack, whereas fools, who are greedy and intemperate and eat like gluttons, fall an easy victim to it. Fainting, diarrhea, loose motions, vomiting, thirst, pain, cramps, vertigo, yawning, a burning sensation in the body, discoloring or paleness of the complexion, cramps at the heart, and a breaking pain in the head are the symptoms of cholera. A patient exhibiting such symptoms as a blackish-blue color of teeth, nails and lips, diminished consciousness, vomiting, eyes sunk in their sockets, feeble voice and looseness of all joints should be regarded as not returning from his journey to the eternal home. In the curable types, cauterization of the regions of the heels, dry heat applications, exhibition of strong emetics and such like measures are recommended. Fasting should be observed at the time of the digestion of the food. Digestive remedies as well as purgatives should also be prescribed. The patient gets instantaneous relief in cases of fainting, diarrhea, and others, on the cleansing of his body with the medicinal emetic or purgative remedies. Intestinal injections may be likewise applied in all cases of the present disease."

The bacterium, *Vibrio cholerae,* is the causative agent of cholera in man. The microorganism was discovered by Koch in 1883, but its association with contaminated water was established by Snow, in 1854, in the Broad Street Well epidemic, in London, England. The vibrios are ingested and multiply rapidly in the intestine, which irritates the gut walls and results in an out-pouring of fluids. This is accompanied by diarrhea and causes a massive dehydration of the body which results in shock and death, unless proper treatment is undertaken. The stools of the host lose their normal character and are called "rice-water stools." Death may occur after a few hours once the symptoms have set in. The patients are treated with antibiotics, sulfonamides and are administered subcutaneous or intravenous injections of fluids to combat the dehydration. Recovery from cholera usually confers immunity which lasts for years. A carrier state may exist in the recovered patient, for a month, but this is unusual. Today, immunization is accomplished with killed vibrios and immunity is reported to last for six months to one year. The disease can be controlled by isolation and cure of the infected hosts; sanitary disposal of sewerage; and the purification of water supplies.

In about 100 B.C., the Indian physician, Charaka (Caraka), compiled a medical text which had probably been transmitted orally for approximately one thousand years, and which today is called the Charaka Samhita. The drug collection noted in Charaka's text outnumbered that of ancient Egypt and Mesopotamia. The Greek physician, Dioscorides, of about 50 A.D., wrote a five volume book on medicinal plants and drugs, which drew heavily from the work of Charaka, and was regarded as a most valuable medicinal text until the Seventeenth Century. In Charaka's text is mentioned an Indian plant which was used to lower the blood pressure and was administered as a tranquilizer. The plant, *Rauwolfia serpentina,* was rediscovered in the west in 1558 A.D., and is now known to contain alkaloid compounds. Reserpine, the drug from the "snake root" was found to have too many unpleasant side effects which has led to the formulation of the many tranquilizing drugs that are now available on the medicinal market. In the United States, in 1956, 30 millions of prescriptions for tranquilizing drugs were filled! By 1979, it was estimated that about 15% of the adult population of the United States would take a tranquilizer, and and among the drugs used, approximately 50 million prescriptions would be for Valium, at a cost of about $250 millions of dollars. According to the National Institute on Drug Abuse, tranquilizers which contain benzodaizepines, when mixed with alcohol and/or other drugs, contributed to 54,000 emergency room visits and 900 deaths between May, 1976 and April, 1977.

The Charaka Samhita is an extremely lengthy work compiled in six volumes with approximately 600-700 pages per volume in its modern printed form. The following quotations are from a printing of the Charaka Samhita edited and published by the Shree Gulabkunverba.[5]

---

5. "Charaka Samhita," edited and published by Shree Gulabkunverba, Ayurvedic Society, 1949, Jamnagar, India, Vol. I, pgs. 84, 162-164, 245, 250-253, 255, 257-259, 307, 308, 327, 328, 331, 601, 606.

98 *Magic, Myths and Medicine*

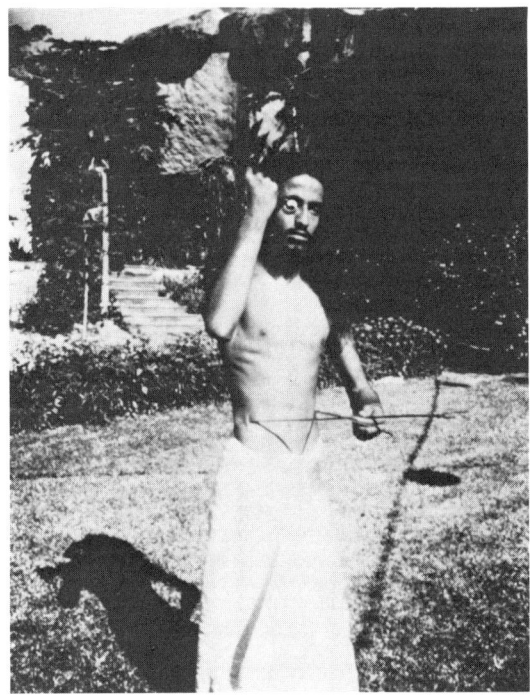

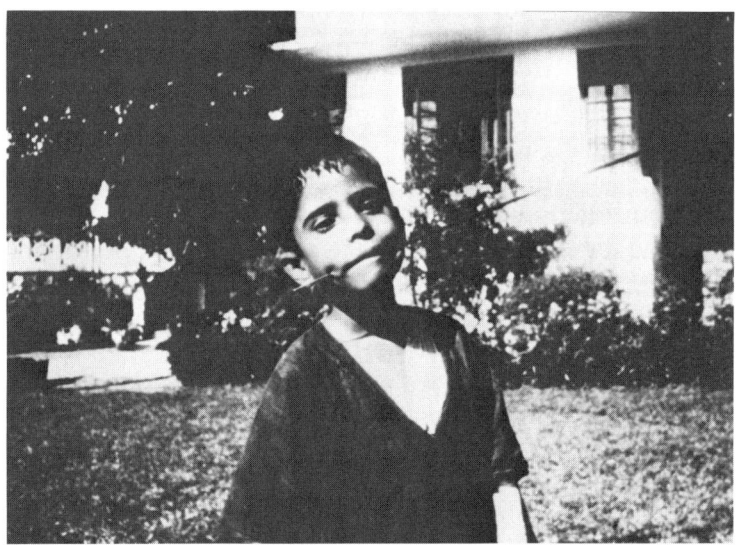

The complete control over various portions of the body can apparently allow these Indians to puncture themselves with long metal swords. (Photograph courtesy of Steven Krolik, San Francisco, Calif.)

"Sesa, the king of serpents, who is versed in the Vedas and the Ayur Veda, which is a sub-Veda of the Atharva Veda, took his birth in the world as the son of a sage versed in the Vedas and the sciences, and went about as a peripatetic (traveling) teacher. Thus from the word "cara," a perigrinator, he came to be known as Caraka, the last syllable being added without altering the sense. He took up the text of the teaching of Atreya, as codified by Agnivesa, and redacted it, and made it popular in the world."

The Oath of Initiation (compare with Oath of Hippocrates).

"The teacher then should instruct the disciple in the presence of the sacred fire, Brahmanas and physicians saying, Thou shalt lead the life of a bachelor, grow thy hair and beard, speak only the truth, eat not meat, eat only pure articles of food, be free from envy and carry no arms. There shall be nothing that thou oughtest not do at my behest except hating the king, or causing another's death or committing an act of great unrighteousness, or acts leading to calamity."

"Thou shalt dedicate thyself to me and regard me as thy chief. Thou shalt be subject to me and conduct thyself forever for my welfare and pleasure. Thou shalt serve and dwell with me like a son or slave or a supplicant (humble person). Thou shalt behave and act without arrogance and with care and attention, and with undistracted mind, humility, constant reflection, and with ungrudging obedience. Acting either at my behest or otherwise, thou shalt conduct thyself for achievement of thy teacher's purposes alone, to the best of thy abilities."

"If thou desirest success, wealth and fame as a physician, and heaven after death, thou shalt pray for the welfare of all creatures, beginning with the cows and Brahmanas."

"Day and night, however, thou mayest be engaged, thou shalt endeavour for the relief of patients with all thy heart and soul. Thou shalt not desert or injure thy patient even for the sake of thy life or thy living. Thou shalt not commit adultery even in thought. Even so, thou shalt not covet other's possessions. Thou shalt be modest in thy attire and appearance. Thou shouldst not be a drunkard or a sinful man, nor shouldst thou associate with the abettors of crimes. Thou shouldst speak words that are gentle, pure and righteous, pleasing, worthy, true wholesome and moderate. Thy behavior must be in consideration of time and place and heedful of past experience. Thou shalt act always with a view to the acquisition of knowledge and the fullness of equipment."

"No persons who are hated of the king or who are haters of the king or who are haters of the public shall receive treatment. Similarly, those that are very unnatural, wicked and miserable character and conduct, those who have not vindicated their honor and those that are on the point of death, and similarly, women who are unattended by their husbands or guardians, shall not receive treatment."

"No offering of gifts by a woman without the behest of her husband or guardian shall be accepted by thee. While entering the patient's house thou shalt be accompanied by a man who is known to the patient and who has his permission to enter and thou shalt be well clad and bent of head, self-possessed and conduct thyself after repeated consideration. Thou shalt thus properly make thy entry. Having entered, thy speech, mind, intellect and senses shall be entirely devoted to no other thought than that of being helpful to the patient and of things concerning him only."

"The peculiar customs of the patient's household shall not be made public. Even knowing that the patient's span of life has come to its close, it shall not be mentioned by thee there, where if so done, it would cause shock to the patient and to others."

"Though possessed of knowledge, one should not boast very much of one's knowledge. Most people are offended by the boastfulness of even those who are otherwise good and authoritative."

The Individual and Medicine

"The object of the science of medicine is two-fold. Firstly, it is for the preservation of good health and prolongation of life, for this task demands all the diligent effort man is capable of, and secondly, the combatting of disease."

"The knowers of the principles of homologation consider it desirable to acquire homologation regarding food and behavior to things which are antagonistic to the characteristics of the country and the causative factors of the diseases prevalent there. These and other diseases occur in those who do not observe the rules of healthful living. Hence the healthy man should be diligent in the observance of the rules of healthful living. One should eliminate the accumulated morbid matter in the months of Caitra, Sravana and Margasirsa. The wise physician should, after preliminary preparation of the body with the oleation and sudation procedures, carry out the purification procedures of vomitation, purgation, enemata and errhines (nasal) according to the season. Thereafter, the physician skilled in the science of climatology should administer alterative and virilific remedies of tested efficacy systematically and as indicated. Thus, the body elements being restored to the normal state, susceptibility to disease disappears, the body elements get aggrandised and the pace of age is slackened. . . . He who rightly observes the rules of health laid down here will not be deprived of the full measure of the hundred years of diseaseless life."

"The woman should know what such and such a thing is delectable to the man or detestable or is wholesome or unwholesome to him in diet. She must know and give to her husband articles which are liked by him and are wholesome to him. She must know articles to be such or otherwise. Thus rare drugs and salt, oil, fragrant drugs and pungent drugs, and pot-herbs, should be preserved in the house. Drugs difficult to obtain must be collected and stored.

Radish, peach, spinach, Damanaka, Indian hog-plum, phut, cucumber, common cucumber, brinjal, ash-gourd, bottle-gourd, telinga, potato, lin, cowage, sambo, wind-killer, garlic and onion etc., the seeds of these and such other medicinal plants should be collected and sown in their proper season. . . . On special occasions people shall be allowed to manufacture white liquor or medicated wine for use in diseases and other kinds of liquor."

"A village should not be constructed where the country abounds in disease, where there is no physician, where there is no leader to guide and protect, where the number of irreligious people is great, and where the country is situated near a mountain. People should reside in a place which bears plenty of water, medicinal herbs, sacrificial sticks, flowers, grass, and firewood, and which yields abundant food, where there is complete safety of property and person, where the outskirts are beautiful and pleasing and lastly which is adorned by the presence of learned people."

"The king shall provide the orphans, the aged, the infirm, the afflicted and the helpless with maintenance. He shall also provide subsistence to helpless women when they are carrying and also to the children they give birth to. The king shall avoid taking possession of any country which is liable to the inroads of enemies and wild tribes, and which is harrassed by frequent visitations of famine and pestilence."

"Such medicinal herbs as grown in marshy grounds are to be grown not only in grounds suitable for them, but also in pots. One who uselessly cuts medicinal herbs planted in cultivated soil or grown wildly, should, in order to absolve himself of the sin, follow a cow and subsist on milk alone for one day."

"One suffering from wounds should be first taken to the surgical ward, and that ward should be built according to the rules of the architectural science. In a ward built thuswise, which is auspicious, clean and protected from the sun and wind, one is free from diseases—psychic or somatic, or diseases caused by external factors. The physician desiring to perform any of the surgical measures should keep in readiness beforehand the following appurtenances; appliances, instruments, caustic alkalies, fire, probes, horns, leeches, sucking gourd, Jambavaustha, swabs, suturing thread, leaves, bandages, honey, ghee, fat, milk, oil, soothing lotions, ointment, paste, fan, cold and hot water, basin, etc., and attendants who are affectionate, steadfast and strong."

Pharmacy. "Now medicine is of two kinds: one kind is promotive of vigor in the healthy, the other destructive of disease in the ailing. Abundance, applicability, usability in multifarious modes and richness of quality—these four are said to be the tetrad of desiderata in drugs. The physician, the drugs, the attendant and the patient constitute the four basic factors of treatment."

"The art of prescription depends upon the knowledge of dosage and time, and on this art, in return, depends success; hence the skillful physician stands ever superior to those possessing merely a theoretical knowledge of drugs. Though treating with the right prescriptions, yet if the physician be ignorant of the knowledge of place etc., he cannot achieve success in treatment. There exist many differences in the nature of men as regards age, vitality, constitution, etc."

"Just as the seed lies dormant in the soil and germinates in season, in the same manner the toxic matter lies quiescent in the body-element and flares up when the time is right. Thus the morbific factor gathering strength and biding the propitious time, manifests itself as the tertain or quartan fever as soon as the disease-resisting power in the body is lowered. In this manner, the disease-generating factors, having worked themselves out, lapse into quiescence and retire to their respective stations in the body; then, mustering up their strength, once again, these toxic elements afflict the patient with fever at their own ripe times."

"The physician who knows the differential diagnosis between the curable and the incurable diseases and begins treatment with full knowledge of the case and in time, obtains success for his effort without fail. The curable diseases are of two kinds: those that are easily cured and those that are cured with difficulty. The incurable diseases also fall into two categories: those that are palliable and those that are absolutely irremediable."

Although a variety of diseases were known in ancient India, and various surgical and medicinal treatments were prescribed, these were not available to the majority of the population. In 1952,[6] according to official government figures, there was one doctor for every 6300 people; one nurse for every 43,000 people and one dentist for every 300,000 people. Seventy-five percent of the doctors lived in the cities which left the country with few to go around. Only six percent of the towns had protected water supplies; while three percent of the population was provided with a sewerage disposal system. The above figures have been improved by the Five Year Plans.

---

6. "Village Life in Northern India," Oscar Lewis, 1958.

Ancient India   103

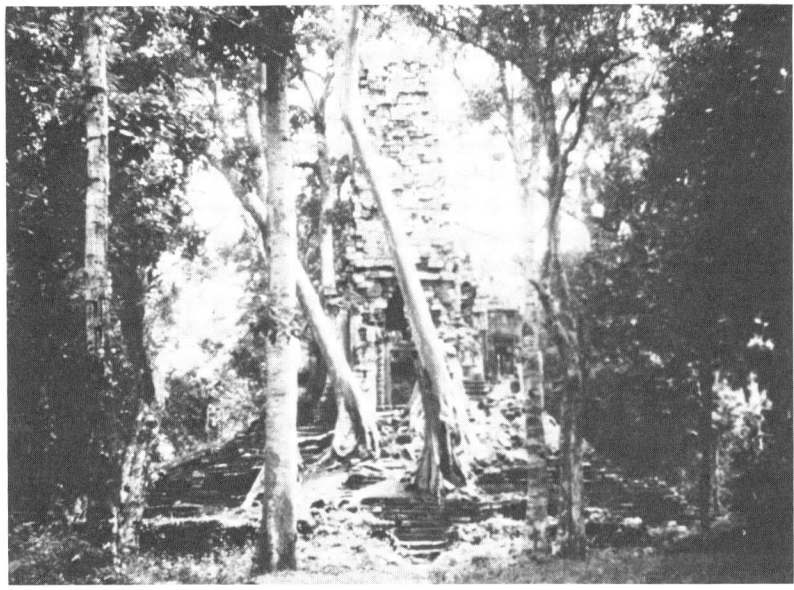

Unrestored Khmer ruins in the dense forests of Cambodia. The culture reached its height during the Middle Ages.

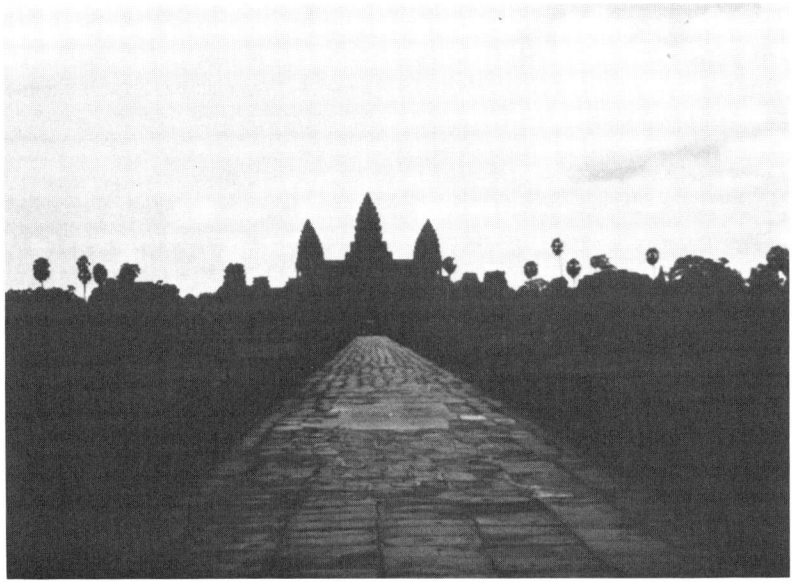

The Grand Causeway of Angkor Wat, a temple complex covering approximately 500 acres near Siem Reap, Cambodia.

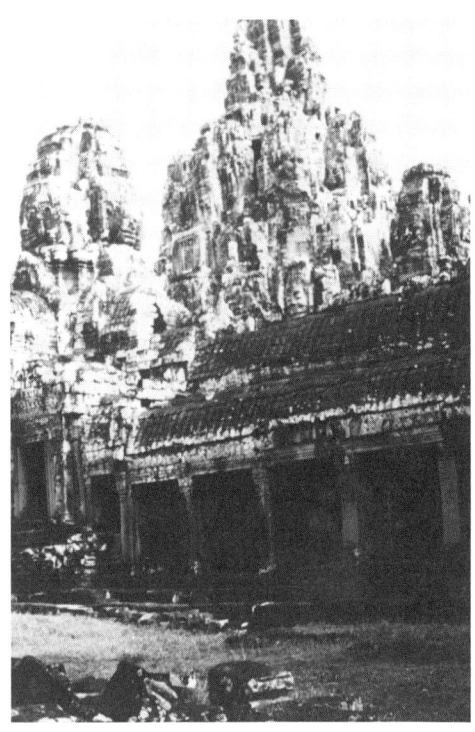

The Angkor Tom temple complex near Angkor Wat.

These statues were collected from the temples of the Angkor Wat complex and were stored in this hall to prevent people from stealing them. However, the author observed that many of them had fallen down and were exposed to the elements in the "Hall of a Thousand Buddhas."

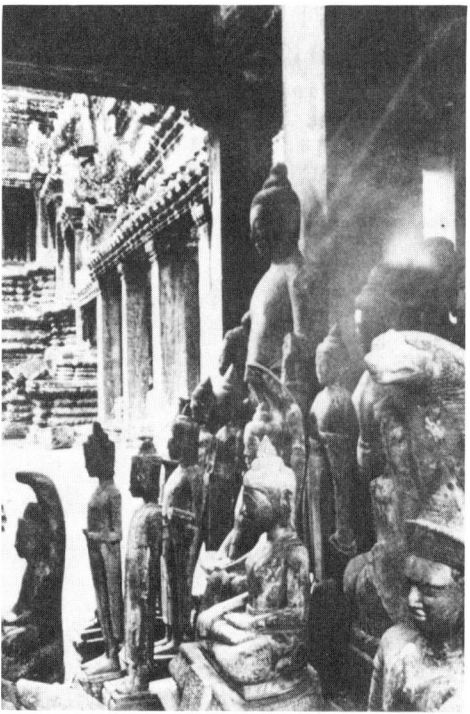

Ancient India   105

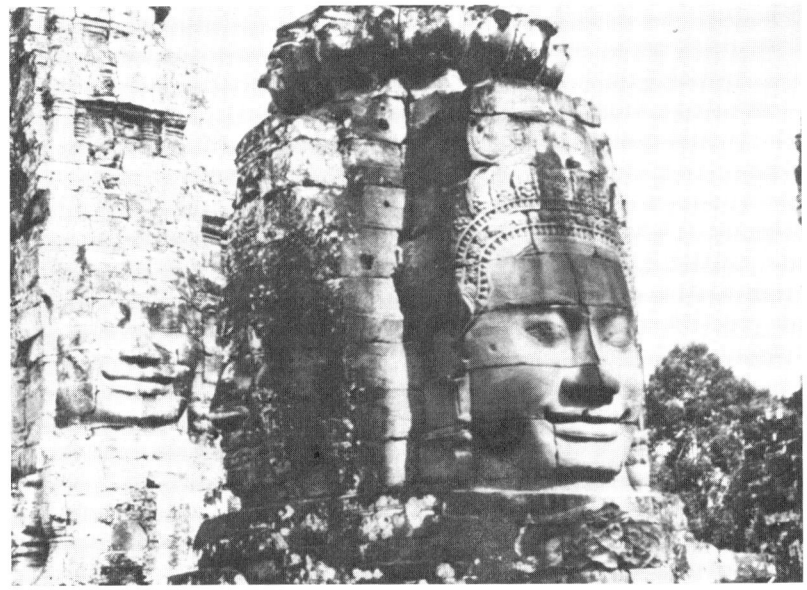

The towers of Angkor Tom are actually beautifully sculptured faces.

ancient china

The central plain of China, watered by the Yellow River and its tributaries, provides the setting for another great civilization which, as was observed in Egypt, Mesopotamia and India, arose in close association with the development of agriculture, or specifically, in the cultivation of millet, and later, rice. The beginnings of this civilization are lost in antiquity but at some early date, between 2000-3000 B.C., the agricultural society was ruled by a class of nobles and a monarch, or monarchs, whose chief purpose was to protect the people from nomadic raiders and to ensure the concordance of the seasonal cycles with the agricultural cycles.

Primitive Chinese religion was based upon a celestial order, which was governed by the "Sovereign on High" (Shang-ti), and a human order, which was based upon an earthly king, the "Son of Heaven" (T'ien-tzu). Many sacrifices, of animals and humans, were necessary throughout the year to insure its proper continuance and a successful harvest. In the second month of summer, during the dry season, sacrifices and prayers for rain were made which, if unsuccessful, were succeeded by the sacrificing of all the sorcerers whose incantations had been unsuccessful. Recently, in Honan Province, near Anyang, the capital of the Shang Dynasty, Chinese scientists discovered 250 pits containing the remains of slaves killed as human sacrifices. Most of the 1000 skeletons had their heads chopped off, but some had been tied up and buried alive. The slaves had been buried as sacrifices together with pigs, horses, dogs and birds.

Associated with the celestial and human orders, was the worship of ancestors, at first adopted by the nobles, and later by the entire population of China. It was believed that a person possessed two spirits; one which ascended to heaven at death, and another, which stayed with the corpse on earth. The spirit which remained on the earth was nourished by the offerings of the family and was thus able to continue to take part in the life of the family.

The agricultural society of ancient China, due to climatic conditions, was divided into two seasons; the agricultural portion of the year which was dominated by the male population who were engaged in the planting, care and harvesting of crops; and the winter season, which was dominated by the work of the female population.

Everything was divided into two analogous groups which were based on the male principle, Yang (light, heat, expansion, dryness), and the female principle, Yin (dark, cold, contraction, wetness). The two principles, although opposites, could be modified, altered, transformed or mutated, because of their interdependence on each other for the maintenance of the order of the universe and society. This classification was to dominate all systems of Chinese philosophy up to the present times.

Much literature exists concerning ancient China which must be viewed with caution for the following reason. Between the years 246-210 B.C., the first emperor of the Ch'in Dynasty, Ch'in Shih-huang-ti (Tsin Chi-huang-ti), unified the territory of China and established a rule which was to last, under various dynasties, until 1912 A.D. He centralized the government; divided China into 36 areas, each with its own governors; standardized the writing; completed the great "Wall of China"; and most important to us, in 213 B.C., ordered the destruction of the classics of literature, especially the books of the school of Confucius. Therefore, the authenticity of many books which have been dated, by legend or history, prior to 213 B.C., is in doubt. It is also possible that the ancient writings were hidden by scholars which were later "found" when the atmosphere was favorable.

The list of rulers who were supposed to have reigned over China begins in about 2900 B.C., in the Age of the Three Sovereigns, with the rule of Fu Hsi. His mother had conceived him by stepping in the footprint of a giant. He was born with the head of a human and the body of a dragon and showed mankind how to use nets in the capture of animals and fish. (This legend probably originated in preagricultural China.) His wife and sister, Nu Wa, used ashes to soak up the waters of the flood; stones of five colors to mend a hole in the sky and raised it firmly in the atmosphere on four pillars made from the legs of a giant turtle. She was the goddess who controlled the rains and floods.

The Age of the Three Sovereigns and of the Five Rulers was succeeded by various dynasties which ruled China from about 2000 B.C., until 1912 A.D., and, with the exception of the first dynasty, are well-documented:

Hsia Dynasty—from about 2200 to 1500 B.C.; of which little is known; Time of Legendary flood.

Shang Dynasty—from about 1500 to 1050 B.C.; also called the Yin Dynasty, and verified by excavations at An-yang, in northern Honan.

Chou Dynasty—from about 1050 to 246 B.C.; confirmed by written history and includes a partial building of the great "Wall."

Ch'in Dynasty—from about 246 to 210 B.C.; Emperor Ch'in Shih-huang-ti established the Empire, completed the "Wall" and ordered the writings destroyed.

Ancient China 109

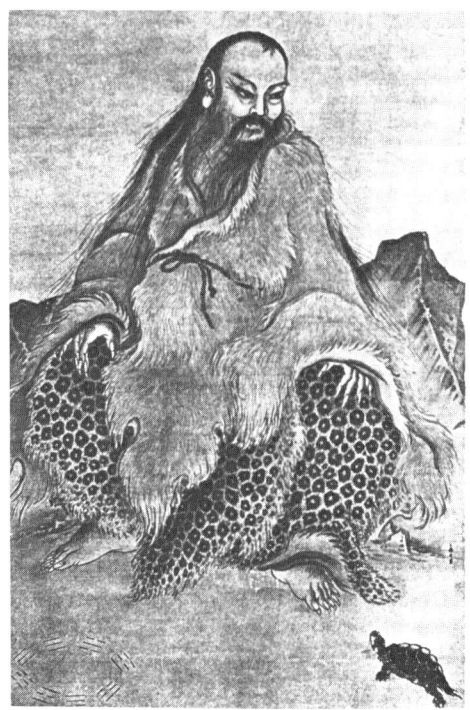

Fu Hsi, the legendary first ruler of China. (Photograph courtesy the National Palace Museum, Taipei, Taiwan)

Han Dynasty—about 210 B.C., to 220 A.D.; completed the unification of China to about its extent today, but was followed by a period of division and invasion.
Wei Dynasty—424 to 581 A.D.: division and invasion.
Sui Dynasty—581 to 618 A.D.; unification.
T'ang Dynasty—618 to 907 A.D.; period followed by anarchy.
Sung Dynasty—960 to 1279 A.D.; period of invasion.
Genghis Khan—1215 to 1251 A.D.; invaded China.
Yuan Dynasty—1251 to 1368 A.D.; Kublai Khan and Timur.
Ming Dynasty—1368 to 1644 A.D.; Portuguese arrive in China in 1514.
Manchu Dynasty—1644 to 1912 A.D.; also called Ch'ing Dynasty, period of weakening and great European influence.
Republic of China—established in 1912 after the fall of the Manchu Dynasty.

The "Legend of Hou Chi" (Fu Hsi) which follows, was obtained from "Sacred Books and Early Literature of the East," edited by Charles F. Horne.[1]
"Chiang Yuan was the first of our race; she lived in the days of yore;

Now list to the wondrous tale of her and the son she bore.
She brought an offering pure to the gods, and prayed them to bless
The mother, who fain would be freed from the curse of her barrenness.

1. "Sacred Books and Early Literature of the East," edited by Charles F. Horne, 1917, Parke, Austin and Lipscomb, Inc., N.Y. and London, Vol. II, pgs. 179-182.

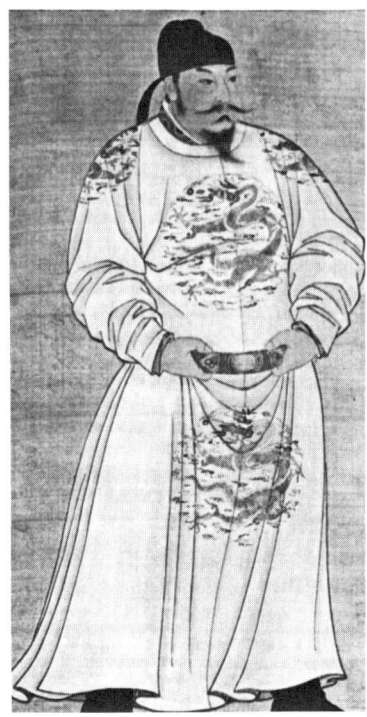

A portrait of the Emperor T'ai Tsung of the T'ang Dynasty. (Photograph courtesy the National Palace Museum, Taipei, Taiwan.)

And it came to pass that she stepped on the footprint a god had made,
And thus in a marvelous way was answered the prayer she prayed.
She conceived; so she dwelt retired, till she brought forth her son; and he,
Whom she bore and nourished there, was the wonderful child, Hou Chi.
So kind were the gods that when the months ere his birth were run,
The mother was spared all pangs in bearing her first-born son.
As a lamb without hurt or pain is dropped on the flowering lea,
So without distress of throe did his mother bring forth Hou Chi.
Yet the new-born babe was laid in a narrow lane to die, (by her husband)
'Neath the feet of oxen and sheep, who would crush him in passing by.
But oxen and sheep forebore, and with tender and loving care
They fostered and saved the life of the child that was lying there.
Men left him then, to starve in a wilderness vast and wild,
But woodcutters passed that way who found and preserved the child.
So they placed him naked on ice, to be killed by the winter's cold;
But the wings of a wild swan clasped the child in their soft, warm fold.
When the wild swan flew at last, the boy so bewept the bird,
Through the country far and near was the sound of his wailing heard,
While yet he crawled on the ground, unable to stand up-right,

Men marveled to see a child, so majestic, so wise and bright.
And when he became a lad, who himself could supply his needs,
It was his delight to plant large beans on the level meads.
Right well did his tillage thrive, his beans formed a glorious show,
And his light green tufts of rice were shining row upon row.
And strong and close did his crops of hemp and of wheat upshoot,
    (hemp-*Cannabis sativa*-provides a tough fiber and narcotic)
And the trailing gourds, which yielded abundance of yellow fruit.
And what was the rule he learnt as his guide in his husbandry?
He transgressed not Nature's laws, but assisted reverently.
Though heaven has boons in store, and rich is the bountiful soil,
Yet the gifts of both shall be lost, if man shall forbear to toil.
Thus the folk of T'ai rejoiced in the plenty the fields afford;
And they praise Hou Chi and choose him to be their king and their lord.
He gave them beautiful grain that his people might well be fed;
The double-kerneled millet, the black, the white and the red.
They planted them far and wide through the country side around.
And in autumn they reaped the harvest, and stacked the sheaves on the ground;
Or heaped upon backs and shoulders they carried the crops away,
To be used for the solemn offering Hou Chi was the first to pay.
And now of the Sacrifice. 'Tis thus that the rites begin:
In a mortar the grain is hulled and cleared of the husk and skin.
It is sifted and winnowed clean, and shaken in water until
It is fit to make purest spirit, whose vapor may float and fill
The hall where the worship is paid. The omens are duly learnt
From herbs which are mixed with the fat of a victim devoutly burnt.
For a lamb must be slain to furnish the broiled and the roasted meat,
That a new year's blessing be won by an offering made complete.
The earthen and wooden stands with gifts must be loaded high,
That a sweet and fragrant steam may ascend from earth to the sky.
The gods in their home above delight in a grateful smell,
And gifts at their proper season are needed to please them well.
This sacrifice Hou Chi founded. From him to the present day
Is there ever a man to grudge it, regret it, or wish it away."

    The Legend of Hou Chi is from the "Shih King," a collection of ancient poetry, some dating to the seventeenth century, B.C., which, by tradition, was compiled by Confucius. In this poem, Hou Chi (Fu Hsi) is credited with teaching man the arts of farming. However, a later legendary emperor, Shen Nung, is usually referred to as the Patron of Agriculture and Herbal Medicine. To Fu Hsi is credited the "I-Ching, the Canon of Changes, said to have been written in about 2900 B.C. To Shen Nung is credited an herbal, which bears his name, and contains 365 herbs and drugs, and is dated to about 2700 B.C.

112   *Magic, Myths and Medicine*

The "I-Ching" is a book used to foretell the future by describing the meaning of various groups of lines as they may appear on burned tortoise shells or in the grouping of millet or milfoil stalks. This method of divination was used by Chinese sages to resolve the doubts of the mind of mysteries of the universe. The method is ascribed to the legendary Fu Hsi but modern scholars attribute it to the Chou Dynasty, or about 1000 B.C.

The original body of the "I-Ching" is composed of the "Eight Trigrams," which are formed from various combinations of straight lines and are arranged in a circle as follows:[2]

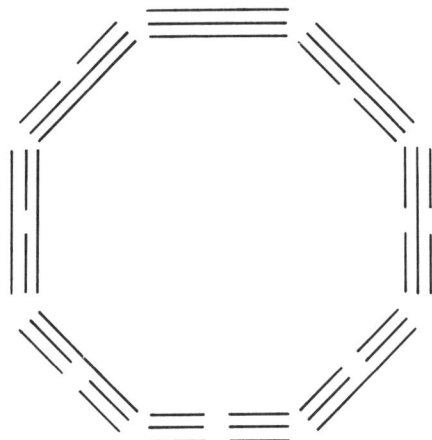

The continuous lines represent the male, or positive principle and the divided lines represent the female, or negative principle; Yang and Yin. Various combinations were made by combination of the trigrams forming 64 hexagrams. It is from these combinations of lines that divinations were, and are, made. An explanation of one of the combinations possible follows:[3]

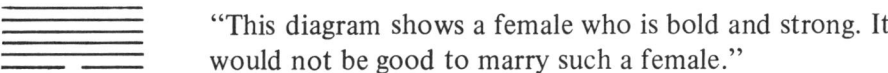

"This diagram shows a female who is bold and strong. It would not be good to marry such a female."

"The first six, divided, shows how its subject should be fixed to a heavy object which, with a firm hand, will result in good fortune. If the subject moves in any direction, there will be bad luck. The second nine, undivided, shows the subject with a bag of fish. There will be no error but the first subject should not be allowed to greet guests. The third nine, undivided, shows one whose buttocks have been stripped of skin, giving a perilous position but no great error. The fourth nine, undivided, shows the subject with an empty bag which

2. "I-Ching" or "Book of Changes," trans. by James Legge, 1964, University Books, New Hyde Park, N.Y., pg. 27.
3. *op. cit.*, pg. 154.

foretells evil. The fifth nine, undivided, shows a tree growing over a gourd meaning the subject should keep his qualities concealed if he wishes to go to heaven. The sixth nine, undivided, shows the subject meeting other with his horns. At times there will be bad luck but no errors."

The following poem, "Chang Fa," is found in the "Shih King" or Classic of Poetry, translated in "Sacred Books and Early Literature of the East,"[4] and dated to the seventeenth or eighteenth century, B.C., the time of the Hsia-Shang Dynasty. In it, there is reference to a great flood:

"Profoundly wise were the lords of Shang, and long had there appeared the omens of their dignity. When the waters of the deluge spread vast abroad, Yu arranged and divided the regions of the land, And assigned to the exterior great States their boundaries, with their borders extending all over the kingdom. Even then, the chief of Sung was beginning to be great, and God raised up the son of his daughter, and founded the line of Shang."

Actually, Yu is the legendary founder of the Hsia Dynasty of 2200 B.C., so there is some confusion as to time and dynasty involved.

The reign of the "Three Sovereigns," Fu Hsi and others, from 2900-2700 B.C., was followed by the "Age of the Five Rulers," from 2700 B.C., to about 2200 B.C. The first ruler of this group, Huang-ti, has a name which means "Yellow Emperor" and which is also the name of the Supreme God who ruled among the Gods of China. Huang-ti is credited as the creator of ritual and of medicine and is the legendary author of the "Nei-ching," the Canon of Medicine. Another ruler of this group, Shen Nung, is the patron of agriculture and herbal medicine and is the Chinese "Father of Medicine." To Shen Nung is accredited the "Pen-Ts'ao," the "Treatise on Medicine," an herbal containing 340 plant remedies and 25 other drugs.

From the "Age of the Five Rulers" comes a creation myth which concerns "P'an Ku," who is described as being a dog-of-many-colors and who was born from primeval chaos. The dog, P'an Ku, gave birth to China and the surrounding universe. He aided one of the Five Rulers, Kao Hsin, in the defeat of the southern barbarians and married the Emperor's daughter.

The "Nei-ching," or Canon of Medicine, ascribed to the legendary Huang-ti, 2700 B.C., is known from recensions of the work completed by various authors after the first century A.D., to which were added the ideas and knowledge of the "new authors." Although there are portions which, due to archaic language use, might be ascribed to the fifth century B.C., the present form of the "Nei-ching" should be viewed as a composite work of Chinese scholars from the fifth century, B.C., to the ninth century, A.D.

It is believed that the "Nei-ching" was of one structural composition until about 200 B.C., when it was divided into two sections: the first section, "Su-wen," reveals the questions of Huang-ti and the answers of his advisers in nine

---

4. "Sacred Books and Literature of the East," edited by Charles F. Horne, 1917, Parke, Austin and Lipscomb, N.Y. and London, Vol. II, pgs. 196, 197.

chapters, and is mainly theoretical in its medicinal concepts; the second section, "Ling-shu" is also composed of nine chapters, but discusses practical medicine, mainly acupuncture.

The Chinese system of diagnosis, as presented in the "Nei-ching" and other works, classifed disease symptoms into six areas based upon their relations to the six tracts (ching) which were followed by the pneuma (chhi) as it flowed in the body. Utilizing the Yang-Yin principles, three of the tracts were allotted to each principle, and each tract ruled one of the six days. The six tracts are similar to those utilized in acupuncture, but in acupuncture, the tracts are composed of two six-tract systems which are interrelated. The internal viscera also came under the principles of Yang-Yin: the Yang viscera are the small and large intestines, the gall-bladder, stomach and urinary bladder; the Yin viscera are the uro-genital tract, the liver, heart, lungs and spleen.

The following excerpts are from a translation of the "Huang Ti Nei Ching Su Wen," The Yellow Emperor's Classic on Internal Medicine, by Ilza Veith.[5] This work is considered, by legend, to be the oldest document on Chinese medicine, and consists of a series of questions posed by the Yellow Emperor which are answered by the physician Ch'i Po.

Book I

Treatise on the Natural Truth in Ancient Times

In ancient times when the Yellow Emperor was born he was endowed with divine talents; while yet in early infancy he could speak; while still very young he was quick of apprehension and penetrating; when he was grown up he was sincere and comprehending; when he became perfect he ascended to Heaven.

The Yellow Emperor once addressed T'ien Shih, the divinely inspired teacher: "I have heard that in ancient times the people lived to be over a hundred years, and yet they remained active and did not become decrepit in their activities. But nowadays people reach only half of that age and yet become decrepit and failing. Is it because the world changes from generation to generation? Or is it that mankind is becoming negligent of the laws of nature?"

Ch'i Po answered: "In ancient times those people who understood Tao patterned themselves upon the Yin and the Yang and they lived in harmony with the arts of divination.

"There was temperance in eating and drinking. Their hours of rising and retiring were regular and not disorderly and wild. By these means the ancients kept their bodies united with their souls, so as to fulfill their allotted span completely, measuring unto a hundred years before they passed away.

---

5. "Huang Ti Nei Ching Su Wen," translated by Ilza Veith, 1966, University of California Press, Berkeley and Los Angeles.

"Nowadays people are not like this; they use wine as beverage and they adopt recklessness as usual behaviour. They enter the chamber (of love) in an intoxicated condition; their passions exhaust their vital forces; their cravings dissipate their true essence; they do not know how to find contentment within themselves; they are not skilled in the control of their spirits. They devote all their attention to the amusement of their minds, thus cutting themselves off from the joys of long life. Their rising and retiring is without regularity. For these reasons they reach only one half of the hundred years and then they degenerate."

"If Yin is healthy then Yang is apt to be defective, if Yang is healthy then Yin is apt to be sick. If the male element is victorious then there will be heat, if the female element is victorious there will be cold.

"Cold injures the body while heat injures the spirit."

"When the spirit is hurt severe pains ensue, when the body is hurt there will be swellings. Thus in those cases where severe pains are felt first and the swellings appear later, one can say that the spirit has injured the body. And in those cases where swellings appear first and severe pains are felt later, one can say that the body has injured the spirit.

"Nature has four seasons and five elements (metal, wood, water, fire, and earth). In order to grant a long life the four seasons and the five elements store up the power of creation within cold, heat, excessive dryness, moisture and wind.

"Man has five viscera (liver, heart, stomach, lungs, and kidneys) in which these five climates are transformed to create joy, anger, sympathy, grief and fear."

"The emotions of joy and anger are injurious to the spirit. Cold and heat are injurious to the body. Violent anger is hurtful to Yin, violent joy is hurtful to Yang. When rebellious emotions rise to Heaven, the pulse expires and leaves the body.

"When joy and anger are without moderation, then cold and heat exceed all measure and life is no longer secure. Yin and Yang should be respected to an equal extent.

"It is said: When people are injured through the severe cold of Winter, the sickness will recur in Spring. When people are hurt through the wind in Spring, they will not be able to retain their food in Summer. When people are hurt through the extreme heat of Summer, they will get intermittent fever in the Fall. When people are hurt through the humidity of Fall, they will get a cough in Winter."

The Yellow Emperor said: "It is said that in former times the ancient sages discoursed on the human body and that they enumerated separately each of the viscera and each of the bowels. They talked about the origin of the blood vessels and about the vascular system, and said that where the blood vessels and the arteries (veins) meet there are six junctions. Following the course of each of the arteries there are the (365) vital points for acupuncture.

"Each of these points has a place and a name, just as 'hollow' refers to the bones, and they all have sections which set them apart from each other."

Book II

The Great Treatise on the Interaction of Yin and Yang.[6]

The Yellow Emperor said: "The Principle of Yin and Yang is the basic principle of the entire universe. It is the principle of everything in creation. It brings about the transformation to parenthood; it is the root and source of life and death; and it is also found within the temples of the gods.

"In order to treat and cure diseases one must search into their origin.

"Heaven was created by an accumulation of Yang, the element of light; Earth was created by an accumulation of Yin, the element of darkness.

"Yang stands for peace and serenity, Yin stands for recklessness and turmoil. Yang stands for destruction and Yin stands for conservation. Yang causes evaporation and Yin gives shape to things.

"Extreme cold brings forth intense heat (fever) and intense heat brings forth extreme cold (chills). Cold air generates mud and corruption; hot air generates clarity and honesty.

"If the air upon earth is clear, then food is produced and eaten at leisure. If the air above is foul, it causes dropsical swellings.

"Through these interactions of their functions, Yin and Yang, the negative and positive principles in nature, are responsible for diseases which befall those who are rebellious to the laws of nature as well as those who conform to them.

"The pure and lucid element of light represents Heaven and the turbid element of darkness represents Earth. When the vapors of the earth ascend they create clouds, and when the vapors of Heaven descend they create rain. Thus rain appears to be the climate of the earth and clouds appear to be the climate of Heaven.

"The pure and lucid element of light is manifest in the upper orifices and the element of darkness is manifest in the lower orifices.

"Yang, the element of light, originates in the pores. Yin, the element of darkness, moves within the five viscera.

"Yang, the lucid element of life, is truly represented by the four extremities; and Yang, the turbid element of darkness, restores the powers of the six treasuries of nature.

"Water represents Yin, and fire represents Yang. Yang creates the air and Yin creates the flavors. The flavors belong to the physical body. When the body dies the ethereal spirit is restored to the air, having thus undergone a complete metamorphosis.

"The ethereal spirit receives its nourishment from the air and the body receives its nourishment from the flavors."

6. *op. cit.*, pgs. 115, 116, 117, 118, 65, 68.

Acupuncture and moxibustion: "The complicated relationship of the dual power with the various parts of the body can function smoothly only if the flux of Yin and Yang is uninterrupted. When there is stagnation in certain parts of the body and hence a deficiency in others, the result is disease. The twelve ducts are the supposed carriers of the two cosmic forces, and if stagnation occurs it takes place within these channels. It is thought that by puncturing the channels at those points which are connected with the diseased organ, the evil air that caused the stagnation is forced to escape and circulation can set in again. The needles, whether of gold, silver, iron, chrome or other metal, are from the Yin-Yang point of view of the elements, charged with the activity of Yin . . . that is to say, dilatory, centrifugal, relaxing, calming, by the system of the ducts. They restore all cells and organs by giving the stimulus of Yin. Consequently, acupuncture is primarily recommended for all excess of Yang. But through the equilibrium of Yang, which it gives to the organism, it restores the energy of Yin and indirectly gives favorable results in maladies of Yin, in addition to its direct stimulating action on Yin."

"Moxa, or moxibustion has a purpose similar to acupuncture, that is, to bring into proper balance the flow of Yin and Yang. Moxibustion which is based on heat is therefore of the nature of Yang. It is very highly recommended in all diseases which are caused by the excess of Yin. Activity of the blood, production of albuminoids, congestion, etc., are all Yang by nature.

"The practice of moxabustion consists of the application to the skin of combustible cones of powdered leaves of *Artemisia vulgaris.* (*Artemisia* plants are used as tonics, stimulants, vermifuges, and in the healings of wounds.) These cones are placed on particular spots and are ignited; they are extinguished only after they burn down to the skin and a blister is formed. There are separate charts for moxibustion which usually show a symmetric pattern, for the most part applied to the back; but moxa can sometimes also be applied to the acupuncture points after the needle has been withdrawn."

"In order to find an auspicious moment for the application of acupuncture and moxa, the physician must establish the position of the heavenly bodies, their relation to the prevailing season, and the weather conditions resulting therefrom."

In 1939, Kirlian photography, or radiation field photography, was invented which today is causing disturbances in the scientific world. The electrophotographs show that certain points on the human body radiate light flares more forcibly than the areas around them and claims have been made that these points correspond to the points of acupuncture utilized by the acupuncturists. Even more puzzling is the reduction in size of the emanations from "healers" fingers after they have touched a "patient" and the increase in the size and intensity of the emanations from the "patient" after they have been touched, which seems to indicate a transfer of energy from the "healer" to the "patient."

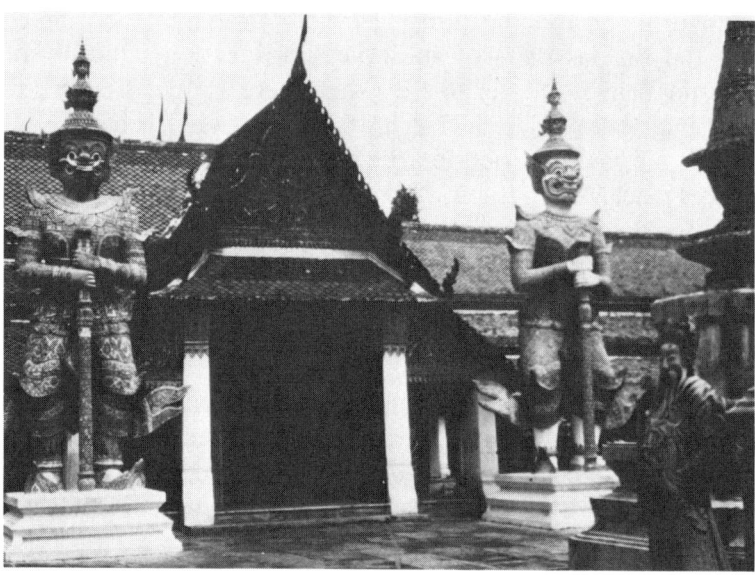

Demon Guards at the Grand Palace, Bangkok, Thailand.

The Chinese physicians, utilizing the theories of the Yang-Yin tracts and organs, internal and external factors, the five elements, diagnostic principles, meteorology, divination, spirits, and accumulated knowledge, were able to formulate an unusual theory of the diagnosis and treatment of diseases.

The oldest indications of medicine in ancient China are found on bone and turtle shells utilized by the sorcerer-physicians in their divinations associated with diseases which can be dated to the Hsia-Chang Dynasties of about 1500 B.C., and where a disease is depicted by the drawing of a bed. Different diseases were depicted by additions to the basic bed-picture. Similar inscriptions were later depicted on bronze ceremonial vessels of the Chou Dynasty. Scholars believe that the following diseases are described by these pictographs: general epidemic disease; itching epidemic (scabies); infectious fever with a rash; eczema, alopecia or psoriasis; arthritis; diseases of the eyes and ears; dental troubles; abdominal diseases; deficiency diseases; pregnancy abnormalities; diseases of women and children; schistosomiasis; speech defects; ulcers; edema; leprosy; typhus fever; tetanus; tonsillitis; pneumonia; malaria; tuberculosis; rickets; dysentery and others.

One of the most annoying diseases of man is "the Itch" or scabies, which is caused by infestation of the skin with the itch or mange mite, *Sarcoptes scabiei*. Scabies is transmitted from person to person by close contact with the infected individual or articles utilized by infected persons such as towels, clothing or bed linen. The mites burrow beneath the skin, excavating small tunnels, in which the female deposits 40-50 eggs. Larvae hatch from the eggs in about one week and excavate new areas in which they mature in about two weeks.

Copulation usually occurs on the surface of the skin from which the mites may be transferred to another person or fomite. The excretions of the mites in the tunnels in the skin, warmth and perspiration bring about an intense itching. This causes scratching and dissemination of the infection and a possible secondary bacterial infection. After several weeks of infection, the skin becomes sensitized which results in a red, itching eruption. Scabies is treated by applications of insecticides such as lindane, benzyl-benzoate or DDT. The infection is controlled by the treatment of infected individuals and the sterilization of fomites. Today, care must be taken when traveling, due to the use of sanitary facilities, hotel rooms, and amusement areas by large numbers of people. Toilets, bedspreads and furniture are not sterilized each time they are used.

The earliest medical texts are commentaries on the "Chhun-chhiu," Annals of the State of Lu, 722-481 B.C., the greatest being the commentary, "Tso-chuan," dated to about 540 B.C. More than forty-five diseases and consultations are mentioned in these records which also include the lectures of the physician Ho to the Prince of Chin. The lectures include the fundamental principles of medicine at that time and the division of all diseases into classifications. The illness of the Prince was diagnosed by Ho as exhaustion and melancolia due to excessive sexual intercourse. Other things of interest mentioned in the "Tso-chuan" are: the denunciation of the burning of a witch as a remedy for drought; cases of human deformities; beri-beri; leprosy; death due to heart disorders; chronic disorders; rabies; and a reference to the belief that the only good leech was one who had broken his arm three times.

The separation of physicians (Yi) from the priests and sorcerers (Wu) appears to have occurred between 300-400 B.C., the period of organization of administration and ritual. The "Nan-ching," concerned with difficult medical problems, was composed at this time by Pien Ts'io, who utilized the pulse rate in the diagnosis and prognosis of diseases.

Another text from this period, the "Shan Hai-ching," describes herbs, stones and animals which can be used to ward off diseases and spirits, and describes such diseases as; trachoma, lymphangitis, intestinal worms, influenza, schistosomiasis, nephritis, tuberculosis, liver flukes, peritoneal abscess, hepatitis and others.

In about 250 B.C., Tsou Yen introduced into medicine, the idea of the five elements (earth, fire, water, metal and wood) and their mutual birth and destruction. This idea originated in the medicinal beliefs of India, Persia and the Greeks and brought alchemy into Chinese medicine. This led to experimentation with poisons, herbs and minerals and the discovery of some beneficial treatments.

The period from 246 B.C. to 220 A.D. covers the Ch'in and Han Dynasties and marks a period of consolidation of power and an expansion in foreign trade which led to an exchange of ideas. The cultivation of silk worms was attributed to the legendary Huang-ti, who showed the people how to make cloth so that they would not have to wear the skins of animals or plant materials. Silk was in much demand in India and the Mediterranean region, so maritime routes were developed and the famous silk caravans traveled overland to the edges of the Persian and Roman Empires. The Alexandrian geographers, in 90 A.D., described a sea route down the Persian Gulf, around Malacca, to the capital of the Han Empire in China, where silk could be obtained. Chinese historians recorded, in 166 A.D., the arrival of an envoy of the emperor, Marcus Aurelius (Antoninus). By these two routes, foreign religions also entered China, including Buddhism, which was to greatly influence the future of China.

While silks, spices and other commodities were the main items that traveled these routes, microorganisms also traveled with their hosts and frequently caused local epidemics wherever the ship or caravan stopped. Three diseases, easily transported from one area to another, and from one host to another, are bacillary and amebic dysenteries and smallpox.

References to dysenterylike diseases can be found in the records of most early civilizations. Herodotus, the Greek historian, reported that the defeat of the Persian Army, in 380 B.C., was due, in part, to many of the Persians contracting dysentery. Later, the Greek Physician Hippocrates furnished epidemiologic descriptions if the infection. However, it was not until the late nineteenth century that the causative agents of dysentery were separated, one being an ameba, *Entamoeba histolytica;* and the other, a bacterium, *Shigella dysenteriae.*

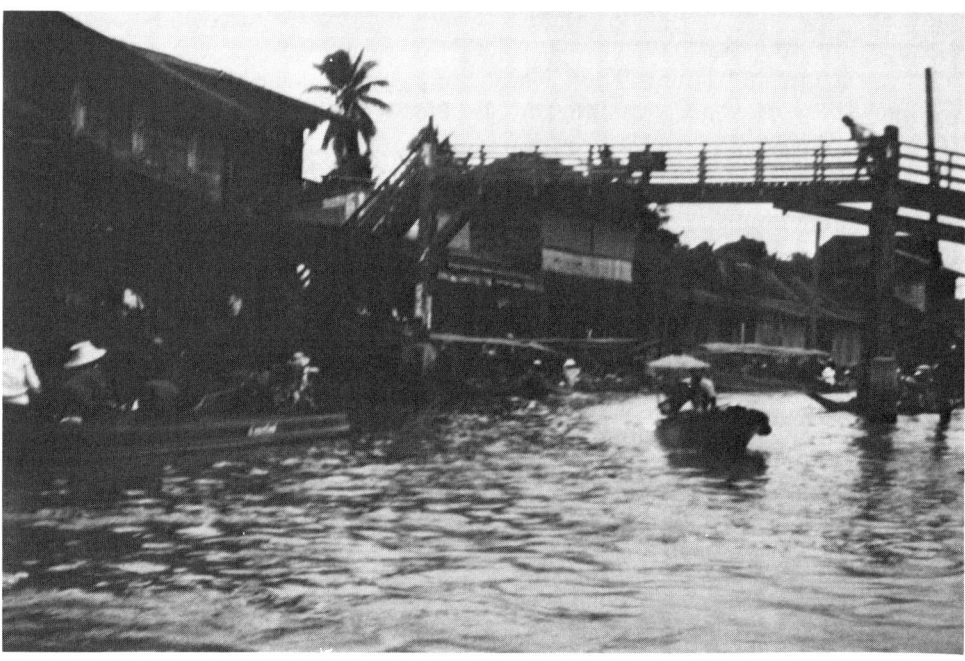

In some parts of Asia, rivers are the highways, water supply, sewerage systems and bathing and washing sites for the people.

Dysentery is the general term for a number of disorders of the intestines, especially of the colon, and attended by pain in the abdomen, tenesmus, and frequent stools containing blood and mucus. The ameba or bacteria causing the infection enter the body through contaminated water, food or fingers. Inflammation of the bowel wall is followed by necrosis and, in severe cases, ulceration. Hemorrhaging may easily occur with resulting bloody stools. The causative agents, in the stools of the host, can be passed to other hosts, by the contamination of water, food and fomites. Control measures therefore are directed at the source of infection and prevention of the spread of the diseases. A proper sewerage disposal system would virtually eliminate the diseases in any area. Water purification systems and personal hygiene also play an important role in the prevention of infection. Development of the carrier state is rare in bacillary dysentery but the chronic patient or asymptomatic carrier is prevalent in amebic dysentery.

Immunization against bacillary dysentery has not shown evidence of significant protection and there is no immunization against amebic dysentery. An active infection of bacillary dysentery may be treated with antibiotics, such as the tetracyclines and chloramphenicol, with a prompt disappearance of clinical symptoms. Amebic dysentery is treated with several drugs such as the iodohydroxyquinolines or arsenic acid derivatives, which are alternated in the treatment. Extra-intestinal amebiasis is treated with antimalarial drugs, such as chloroquine, which are effective against the ameba-form, and Emetine, a drug obtained from a Central American plant, *Cephaelis ipecacuanha,* commonly called ipecac.

Smallpox, or Variola, is an acute, infectious viral disease which is characterized by vomiting, lumbar pains, fever, and the development of a rash, first papular, then vesicular and later, pustular. The pustules increase in size, dry and break, forming soft, yellow crusts which have an offensive odor. After about a week, the scabs fall off, leaving pitted scars or pock-marks. In severe cases, death occurs in the first or second week of illness, and is usually due to encephalitis, heart failure or pneumonia, accompanied by hemorrhaging.

Historically, the disease is very old. The mummy of Ramses V, who ruled Egypt in about 1100 B.C., is said to reveal the scars of a smallpox infection. Later, in 165 A.D., Marcus Aurelius and the Roman Army, fighting in Mesopotamia, developed an epidemic of smallpox which caused them to withdraw. The viral disease was then spread throughout the Roman Empire. The disease was described by Galen at this time, according to the Arabic Physician, Rhazes, in his commentary on the infection in the tenth century, A.D. Variolation, the deliberate introduction of the smallpox pustular-material, from mild cases of the disease to uninfected persons, in the hope of developing a mild infection rather than a severe infection, is believed to have been developed in the Middle East, and gradually spread throughout Asia and Europe. This same method was also developed for use in Leishmaniasis infections.

The first description of smallpox in China was by Ko Hung, in about 300 A.D., who stated that the disease was introduced into China by the Huns. In 1798, Jenner announced the use of cowpox material in the prevention of smallpox, rather than the smallpox material which actually caused the disease and had a death rate of about 1:200. Today, the disease has been brought under control in the Western countries by vaccination procedures but is still endemic in India and parts of Asia. The U.S. Public Health Department has recently dropped its requirement of smallpox vaccination. However, a recent outbreak in Great Britain, caused by the transfer of an infected person from the Middle East to Great Britain by airplane, indicates that great care should be taken when traveling outside of the United States. Immune gamma globulin can be used to treat active infections and antibiotics may prevent secondary bacterial infections.

During the Han Dynasty, from about 200-400 A.D., a number of medical works were produced in China which have survived which are classics in Chinese Medicine.

The "Shang-han lun," a work concerned with ailments caused by cold, or fevers, was compiled by the encyclopedist, Chang Chung-ching, sometimes called the "Chinese Hippocrates" because of his codification of symptomatology and therapeutics. He was the first Chinese Physician to clearly differentiate the symptoms of Yang and Yin.

Living, at approximately the same time as Chang Chung-ching was the famous surgeon, Hua T'o (Yuan Hua). Several books exist which are ascribed to him, but apparently, some were restorations which were completed at a much later date. Hua T'o is credited with remarkable surgical operations in which he used Indian hemp as the general anaesthetic. These include trepannings, rhinoplasty, removal of stones, grafting of organs, intestinal resections and others. These surgical procedures are reminiscent of those performed in the Sashruta Samhita of India. He is also credited with charts of the human anatomy and acupunctural procedures, hydrotherapy and medicinal baths, sutures, antiseptics, ointments, antihelminthics, and others.

In about 250 A.D., Huang-Fu Mi produced his classic work on acupuncture. Acupuncture is a procedure used to treat the stoppage of body fluids and to restore the normal flow of fluids and pneuma by phlebotomies or by a manual clearing of the ducts with needles, or in some instances, massage or moxas (burnings). The number of acupuncture points on the body differs in various writings, but 365 is frequently used. Various researchers in France, Japan and China have reported that the points of acupuncture on the skin have a greater permeability to electrical current than do the surrounding areas of skin. It has been claimed that many infectious bacterial and parasitic diseases have been cured through acupuncture, but these cases have been frequently treated also with medical therapy. Functional disorders such as pains, vomiting, hiccups and related malfunctions are, apparently, easily treated with this method. Acupuncture is currently being viewed with great interest in countries of the West and many experiments testing the procedures are currently being conducted in major universities and medical schools. Recently, at a meeting of the American Society of Anesthesiologists[1] a detailed experiment with 199 patients who received a total of 1100 acupuncture treatments was reported. The patients had been randomly divided into groups. In some, the needles were inserted into the classical Chinese body points and either rotated by hand or stimulated electrically with a device made in the People's Republic of China. In others, the needles were inserted in other parts of the body where the Chinese texts say they would do no good at all, and there, the needles were stimulated by hand or by electricity. The results were that there was no significant difference at all in the results among the various groups of patients.

Dr. Ronald Melzack, who has conducted research on the physiology of pain, has recently suggested that the "Gate-Control Theory of Pain" of Melzack-Wall, 1965, offers an explanation as to how acupuncture works. This theory suggests that the transmission of pain to the brain and spinal cord from various parts of the body is not a stationary, unchangeable process, but rather, is an energetic one that is capable of variation and change. The theory suggests a gatelike mechanism in the pain transmission system which may be open, partially open, or completely closed, in which case signals from bodily injuries would never be detected by the brain. The sensory nerves, extending from the body's surface to the central nervous system, are composed of large and small fibers. The large fibers, when stimulated, as in the use of acupuncture, tend to "close the gate" and therefore the level of pain diminishes or is eliminated. Stimulation of the small fibers, in the same nerve, results in the transmission of signals that "open the gate" and produce the sensation of pain. Stimulation of the brainstem can also eliminate pain from large portions of the body and the duration of the reaction frequently extends beyond the time of stimulation. Psychologically, the suggestion that the procedure will reduce or eliminate pain aids in the actual decrease in the level of perceived pain, by relieving anxiety, which produces higher pain levels. It is hoped that the current interest in acupuncture will bring about the recognition that health, as viewed by the Chinese, is a balance of various elements of the body, rather than, as viewed in the West, an absence of disease.

Egypt has long been associated with excavations of ancient tombs and burial grounds, the discovery of treasures, such as that of the Pharaoh Tutankhamon, and the mummification of animal and human bodies. Some early excavations in China revealed burial procedures in antiquity that resemble the "pit-tombs of Ur," in Mesopotamia. However, recently, in 1968 and 1972, excavations in China have revealed two rather startling discoveries: those of the tombs of a Prince of the Han Dynasty and his consort; and the tomb of the Lady Li of Tai, all dated to approximately 100 B.C.

---

1. San Francisco Chronicle, Thursday, October 14, 1976.

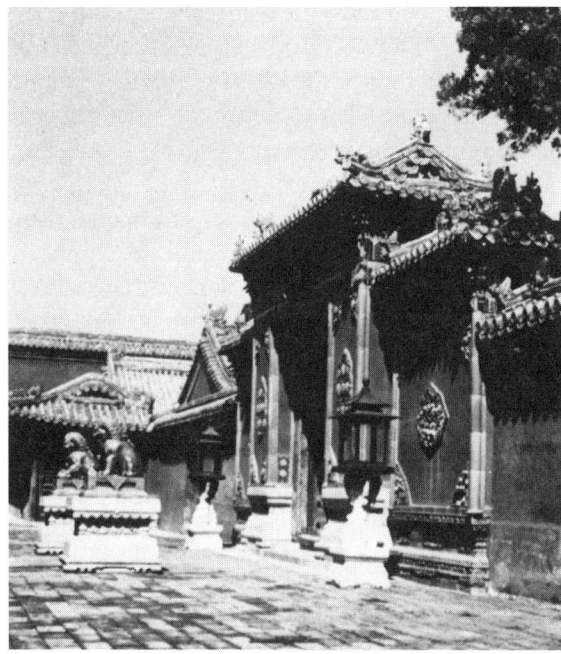

Ming Dynasty lions guard a temple entrance outside the Forbidden City, Beijing (Peking). (Photograph courtesy the National Palace Museum, Taipei, Taiwan.)

The tombs of the Prince and his consort were undisturbed for approximately 2000 years and when excavated, were found to contain about 2800 funerary objects along with the jade-encased bodies of the deceased royalty. The tomb was hewn out of a rock cliff and was sealed with iron and rock walls which, according to reports, took two months to break through, even with the use of dynamite. The tomb of the Prince contained 12 chariots and the remains of sacrificed horses still in their harnesses. Pottery for foods and drinks, furniture, silk materials, glass, lacquer, silver and gold objects and others. The body of the Prince and consort were completely clothed in wafers of jade sewn together with gold thread.

The tomb of the Lady Li was found buried under approximately sixty feet of earth. The burial site was surrounded by white clay, inside of which were tons of charcoal, inside of which were a series of six boxes. The innermost box was an airtight coffin which contained the silk-wrapped body of Lady Li and which was preserved in an acidic fluid containing mercurial compounds. The fluid had preserved the body and moisture content so that the flesh was still moist, rather than dry, as in the case of most mummified remains.

Specialists were able to determine that Lady Li had type A blood; and produced children; had broken her right arm; had had tuberculosis; had a severe case of gall stones; had died of atherosclerosis. The hair was still well-attached; the body joints were still flexible; the internal organs were in excellent condition and, although the brain had collapsed, this body is the best preserved subject autopsied from antiquity.

Ancient China 125

Ko Hung, a Taoist physician and alchemist, who lived about 280 to 340 A.D., wrote under the name of "Pao-p'u Tzu" and composed several medicinal works; "The Medications of the Golden Box" (Chin-kuei-yo-fang), first aid measures, "Chou-hou pei-tsi fang," and the remarkable work concerned with magic, dietetics and alchemy, "Pao-p'u Tzu nei-wai-p'ien." Ko Hung spent much of his time seeking an elixer which would prolong life and in doing so, formulated a life style which, if followed, would prevent diseases and result in longevity. It was basically a diet-drug-exercise regimen formulated from the beliefs of Taoism. Taoism was, by legend, founded by the sage Lao Tzu in the fifth century, B.C., and has retained some ancient magical practices where, by use of respiratory exercises, the practitioner reaches a state of ecstasy similar to that of the practitioners of yoga. Ko Hung is credited with he first known description of smallpox and also made observations concerning tuberculosis, beri-beri (vitamin B_1 deficiency), hepatitis, bubonic plague, acute lymphangitis, rabies, glanders, and Tsutsugamushi fever.

Tsutsugamushi fever, or scrub typhus, is an infectious disease transmitted by the larvae of mites, *Trombicula akamushi,* to rodent and human hosts. The causative agent is *Rickettsia tsutsugamushi.* Following infection, illness begins

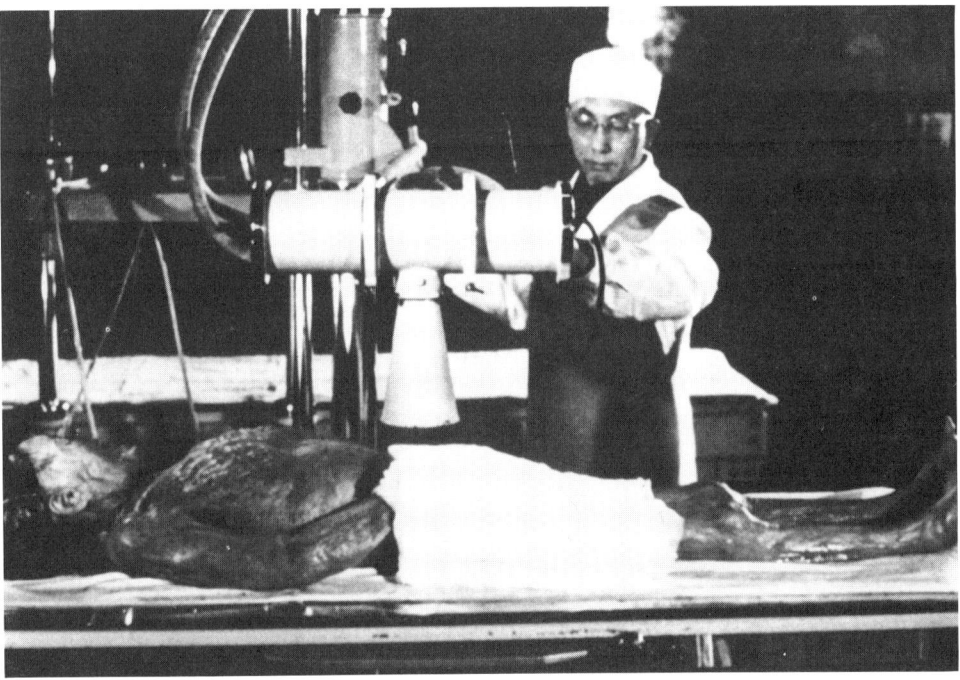

The body of a Chinese noblewoman of the Han Dynasty, approximately 2100 years old, under examination at the Hunan Medical College, China. It was determined that she had group A blood; tuberculosis scars; a fracture of the right forearm; gallstones; whipworms; pinworms; schistosomiasis; and had died of a heart attack. (Photograph courtesy of National Geographic Magazine, Vol. 145, No. 5, May, 1974; page 662) and China Pictorial, Beijing (Peking).

126   *Magic, Myths and Medicine*

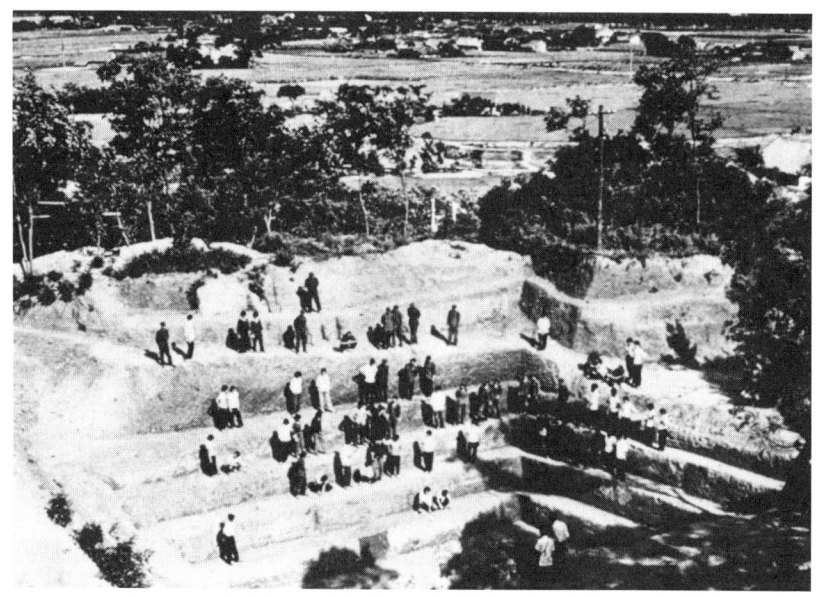

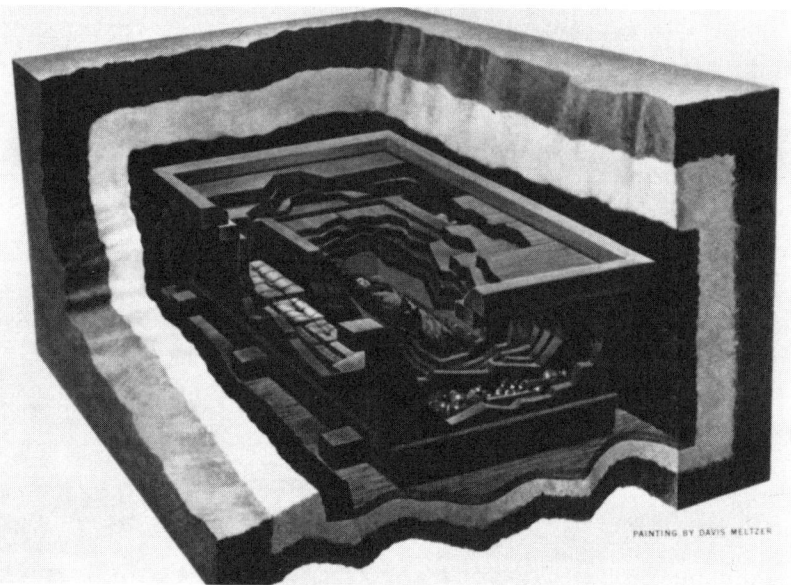

The tomb of the Chinese noblewoman was found at the bottom of an excavation approximately 52 feet deep, in the Ch'angsha area of China. Tomb painting by Davis Meltzer. (Photographs courtesy of National Geographic Magazine, Vol. 145, No. 5, May, 1974; pgs. 664-665 and China Pictorial, Peking.)

with a fever and the patient develops chills and a severe headache and a rash. The mortality rate varies from 1-60 percent in untreated cases where death is generally due to pneumonia, encephalitis or circulatory failure. Dramatic recovery generally occurs with the administration of antibiotics such as chloramphenicol, aureomycin or terramycin. The disease is controlled by the elimination of mites in an area with insecticides or by spraying of clothing. Persons in endemic areas can be vaccinated against the disease.

Ko Hung also formulated an "Immortality Pill" utilizing gold, yellow arsenic, mercuric sulphide, sulphur, jade and mercury and advised the use of henbane in the treatment of dementia. Henbane is a plant of the Genus *Hyoscyamus*. Some members of this group, and others such as *Atropa belladonna* and *Datura stramonium*, contain hyoscyamine, known in the alkaloid form as atropine, and used as a hypnotic, pain reliever and antispasmodic in the treatment of mental disorders, epilepsy and colic.

In 624 A.D., the study of medicine came under the control of the Grand Medical Service (T'ai-i-shu) which tested physicians by examination. This is an extremely early example of the state supervision of medicine which is today, virtually worldwide. This led to a great organization of medicine, a consolidation of medical observations, and the production of numerous documents and books. In 659 A.D., the work of Su Kung mentions the use of a mixture of mercury, silver and tin, a paste, which was used to fill dental cavities. This technique did not become well-known in Europe until the early 1800s (Regnart and Taveau). Recently, several investigators are predicting the use of barnacle cement in the filling of dental cavities because of its strength, resistance to temperature variations and nonsolubility. The replacement of lost teeth has also been a problem to man and the dentists. The implantation of new "teeth" often results in infection and deterioration of the jawbone. A new technique developed at the University of Southern California replaces the empty socket with vitreous carbon to which the false tooth is fastened. The carbon is compatible to the human body and there is no rejection and does not readily break down under chewing pressures. Dentistry in the People's Republic of China includes a method not used in the West. On finding a decaying tooth in a patient's mouth, the Chinese dentist will extract the tooth, repair it, and replace it in the patient's mouth. According to the China News Agency, a hospital in the Shanxi Province replanted 250 teeth in the past three years, with a 90 per cent rate of success. Replaced teeth are ready for normal, hard chewing within three weeks.

In 1305 A.D., the Imperial College of Medicine was established which led to further reforms and stricter examinations for its member physicians. There were, of course, still soothsayers, geomancers, fortune tellers, herbalists, cuppers and quacks who also treated people. Organized medicine rarely reached into the country until the present time.

The last work that shall be considered in the area of Chinese medicine is the "Materia Medica" of Li Shih-chen (1518-93), the only scientific work of the sixteenth century of importance that is outside of the influence of Western scientists. Included in this work are portions dealing with pathology, therapeutics, a classification of vegetable, animal and mineral products, chemistry and many others. It also refers to syphilis, which appeared in China in the early 1500s, as it had in the west, and prescribed a treatment with mercurial compounds and ginseng. This great work has been translated into the principal languages of the world, and should be consulted, along with later works, by those interested in a further study of Chinese medicine.

In 1965, in a directive on health work, Chairman Mao criticized the Ministry of Health because most of its work had been concerned with urban areas and he wanted a change in medical and health work directed toward the rural areas of the country. Thousand of medical workers left the cities and went to the rural and mountainous areas to bring medicine to the masses. A socialistic medical service system, suited to rural needs, was set up throughout the country staffed by "barefoot doctors" who are combining traditional Chinese medicine with Western medicine. This combination and herbal medicine is being used for the prevention and treatment of the common and recurrent diseases, and the medical and health picture in these areas is rapidly changing. These medical assistants in the rural areas are also learning from the people, old remedies which have been utilized for ages in their families; they are gathering the herbs or materials and are testing their efficiency in the treatment of diseases. This exchange of medical ideas may prove of great benefit to the people and the medical profession.

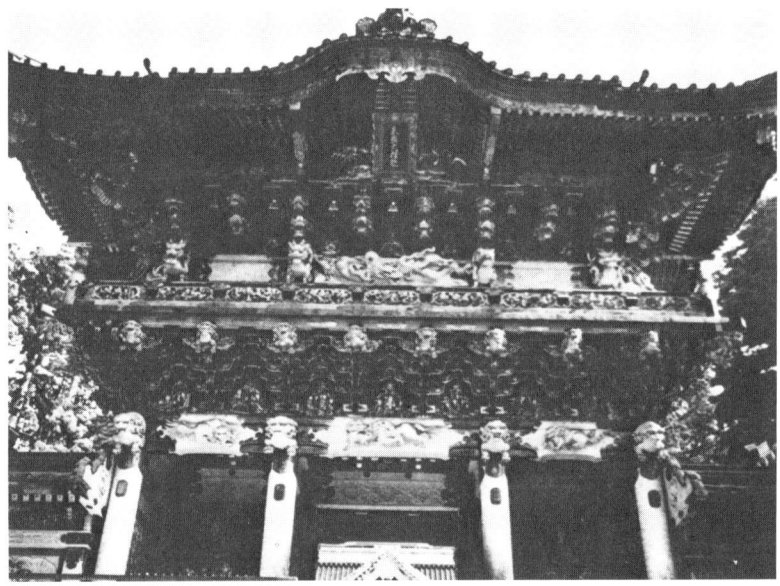

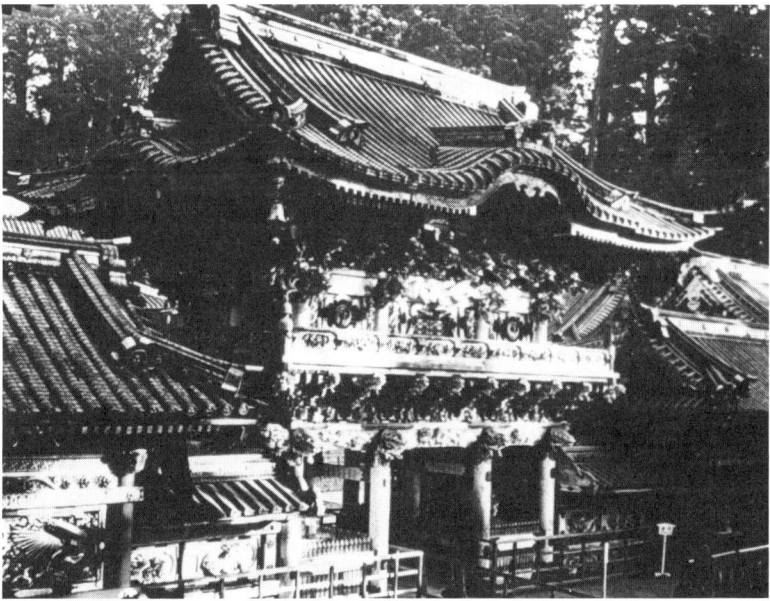

A fusion of Buddhism and Shintoism led to the construction of these beautiful buildings in the temple complex of Nikko, Japan.

CRETE~MYCENAE~ GREECE~ROME

The island of Crete in the Mediterranean Sea is located approximately midway between Greece, Turkey and Africa, in a north-south line, and between Italy and the Fertile Crescent in an east-west line. Here, an early civilization developed, aided by trading contacts with the surrounding mainland cultures of the Fertile Crescent, Egypt, Mycenae and others. The culture of Crete spread to Athens and Sparta and later to Rome, which conquered much of the known world, spreading the culture across Europe to the British Isles. For these reasons, Crete is frequently called the "Cradle of Western Civilization."

During the period between 3000 and 1100 B.C., there were two chief cities representative of the culture, Knossus on the island of Crete and Mycenae, on the mainland, near the entrance to the Aegean Sea. Eventually Mycenae conquered Crete and in about 1200 B.C., led the Greeks in a war against Troy.

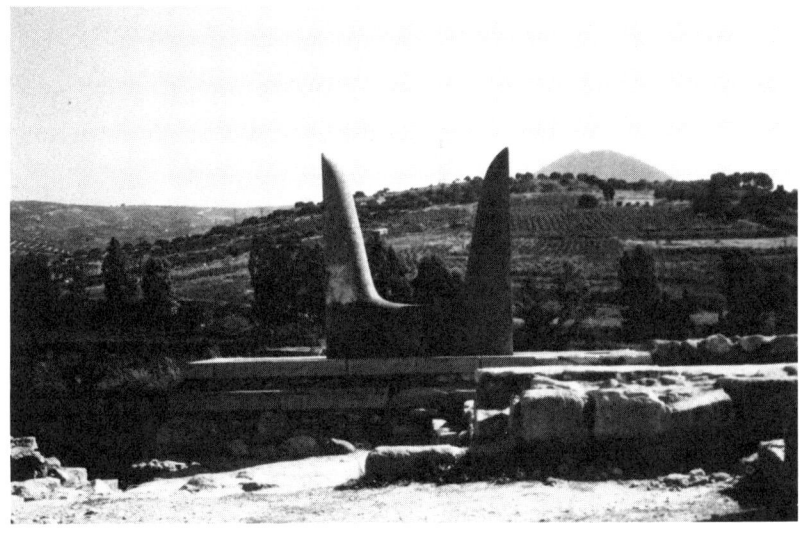

Ruins of the Palace of Knossus, Crete.

The height of the Cretan civilization was reached between the seventeenth and fifteenth centuries, B.C., and was ruled from the Palace of Knossus by the legendary King Minos. From this period come the legends concerning Minos, Queen Pasiphae, the Minotaur, Theseus, Ariadne, Phaedra, Daedalus, Icarus and others. Sometime between 1550 and 1450 B.C., the island of Thera (Santorini) suffered a volcanic eruption and explosion that destroyed much of the island and resulted in the fall of the Cretan Empire, only 70 miles away. The palace of Knossus was apparently rebuilt but soon after was destroyed by fire. Many believe that the Greeks conquered Crete after the eruption of Thera, Thereafter, the center of rule moved to Mycenae. Towards the end of the thirteenth century, B.C., Mycenae and other centers were destroyed by peoples moving into the area from the north and in the eleventh century, B.C., the Dorian Greeks entered in the same manner. Homer's "Iliad and Odyssey" tells of the downfall of this early culture which ended with the conquest by the Dorians. Dorian Greece gradually assumed the political configuration which lasted until the time of Alexander the Great. The basis of the Greek civilization was the city-state and colonization, which led to great trade throughout the Mediterranean. The Greek culture was brought to the Etruscans in Italy, the forerunners of the Roman civilization.

Around 1876 A.D., Schliemann excavated Troy and Mycenae and later, Evans excavated the palace of Knossus on Crete. In addition to the various art works and treasures found in the ruins, the palace of Knossus revealed public health constructions found in no other culture at this time in the West. The palace was very large and on several levels so that air shafts were included in the construction to bring light and air to the lower levels. Water was brought in by aqueducts and a drainage system allowed the flow of waste waters out of the palace. In the so-called "Queen's Chamber" was found a chairlike object placed over a drain which is believed to be the forerunner of the present day flush-toilet.

The mythology of Crete, Mycenae and Greece is so intertwined and lengthy that it cannot be reviewed here in detail. The earth (Gaea) was created from Chaos by its separation from the sky (Uranus). From the union of earth and sky, Gaea and Uranus, were produced the twelve Titans, the Cyclops and three giants whom Uranus imprisoned in the depths of the Earth. A Titan, Cronus, aided by Gaea, castrated Uranus, freed the Titans and assumed the rule. Cronus wedded with Rhea, but devoured their children as they were born, so as to escape the curse of Uranus. Rhea, pregnant, fled to Crete where she hid in a cave until the birth of her son, Zeus. Rhea assigned the care of the child to the King of Crete and returned to Cronus, presenting a stone wrapped in swaddling clothes as her child, which Cronus immediately swallowed, believing it to be the child. Zeus meanwhile, grew to manhood on Crete and finally, aided by Gaea and Rhea, overthrew Cronus and forced him to vomit up the children and the stone and he ruled thereafter from Mount Olympus. Zeus

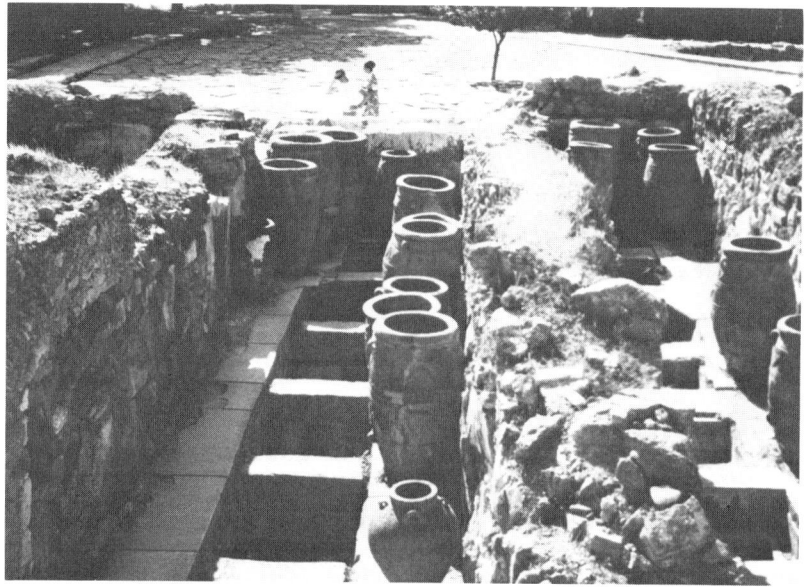

Foods, beverages and oils could have been stored in these large jars in the storerooms of the palace of Knossus.

carried the stone to Mount Parnassus and placed it in the shrine of the Delphi Oracle, in the care of the Pythoness. She was a priestess who sat over a cleft in the earth, through which vapors drifted from below of an intoxicating nature. From her trancelike state, the Pythoness pronounced oracular prophecies and was sought out by many people in the legends of Greece. Later, Zeus became enamored of Europa and disguised as a bull, carried her off to Crete where she produced three sons, the most famous being Minos I. The son of Minos I, Minos II married Pasiphae who produced several children, including Ariadne and Phaedra. Pasiphae, under a spell by Poseidon, mated with a bull and produced the Minotaur, a monster with a human body and the head of a bull, whom Minos imprisoned in the Labyrinth beneath the palace of Knossus. Later, Theseus of Athens killed the Minotaur with the help of Ariadne. Another child of Minos and Pasiphae, Aerope, married Crateus and produced Atreus, whose sons, Menelaus and Agamemnon, later journeyed to Troy in search of the beautiful Helen.

Returning now to the creation of the Earth and the release of the Titans by Cronus, plants and animals were placed on the Earth, but a nobler animal was wanted so Prometheus, one of the Titans, took some earth, mixed it with water, and fashioned man in the image of the Gods. With the aid of Minerva, Prometheus lighted a torch from the sun chariot and gave fire to man, which gave them domination over the animals. For this desecration, Prometheus was chained to a mountain rock where each day an eagle devoured his liver, in

134   *Magic, Myths and Medicine*

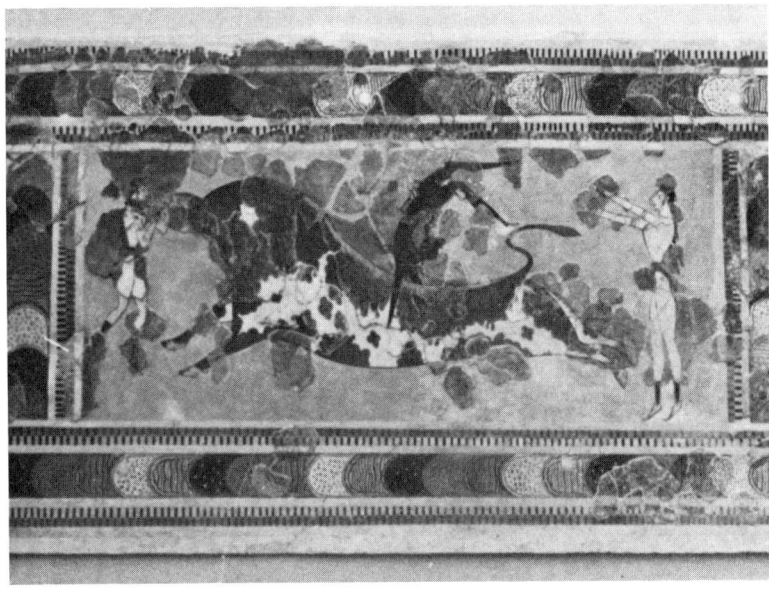

Minoan Bull Leapers, from the palace of Knossus, Crete. (Photograph courtesy of the Heraklion Museum, Heraklion, Crete)

which organ was believed to be located the seat of life. To punish man for having the use of fire, woman was created and placed on the Earth. This woman was Pandora who later opened a box which loosed the plagues that thereafter afflicted mankind.

Eventually the Earth became populated with people who became corrupt and neglected the Gods so Jupiter caused Neptune to flood the Earth, saving two righteous people, Deucalion and Pyrrha, on Mount Parnassus. After the deluge, Deucalion and Pyrrha visited the oracular priestess, the Pythoness, who told them to create man again by throwing the bones of their ancestors behind them. The riddle of the priestess was finally solved by Deucalion who remembered that Prometheus had created man from earth, so they threw rocks behind them. Those thrown by Deucalion became men, and those thrown by Pyrrha became women.

The God of Sun, Apollo, was also recognized as the God of Medicine by the Greeks. The son of Apollo, Aesculapius, was raised by the centaur, Chiron, who taught him the secrets of medicine. Aesculapius became so adept in medicinal arts that he could restore the dead to life. Pluto, king of the Underworld, resented the interference of Aesculapius and asked Jupiter to intercede. Jupiter struck Aesculapius with a bolt of lightning and elevated him to the company of the gods where he became the popular God of Medicine. A son of Aesculapius, Machaon, appeared in the "Odyssey" of Homer where he is described as a surgeon and warrior and is wounded by an arrow shot by Paris. Homer also mentions the medicine of the Egyptians whose God of Medicine, Imhotep, was recognized by the Greeks as being Aesculapius.

Many temples were dedicated to Aesculapius and his daughters, Hygeia and Panacea, the most celebrated being at Epidaurus. There, the sick sought oracular responses, refuge and the recovery of their health by visiting and sleeping in the temples. The temples were built on scenic grounds with natural springs, bathing pools, theatres and stadiums. Serpents were sacred and were kept in the temples. Accounts indicate that the treatments resembled animal magnetism or mesmerism. The patients, after purification, slept in the temples at which time they were visited by Aesculapius and his daughters who prescribed drugs and performed surgery. Temple tablets have been found which list the miraculous cures that had been effected there. The worship of Aesculapius was brought into Rome, at the request of the Romans, during a plague.

From the time of Homer, and later, the literature mentions physicians who were not connected with temple medicine. Qualified physicians were those who had undergone a period of training under a master physician. It was the custom of communities to appoint official physicians whose duty it was to treat the poor, relieve epidemics and give testimony in the courts. The candi-

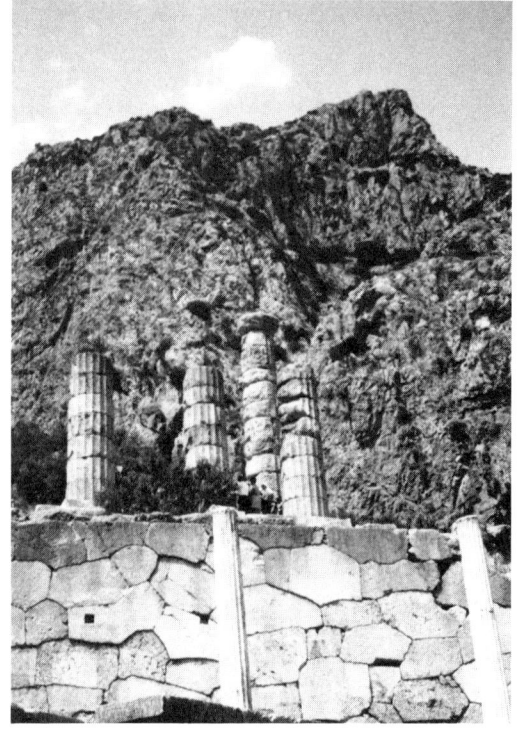

The temple of Apollo, Delphi, Greece, on the slopes of Mount Parnassus. Nearby, the Pythia uttered her oracles in an ancient sanctuary from which vapors arose from deep within the earth.

dates were chosen by popular assembly after presentation of proof of their training and abilities. The physicians practiced in their homes or traveled in a circuit. The patients were treated at home or in medical homes. Such places for treatment were established by physicians or scholars or were provided for by the communities. The medical homes were utilized chiefly for surgical operations during which students and scholars were allowed to observe or assist the master physicians, and thus obtain the necessary experience and training. When traveling, the physicians carried their instruments, bandages, and drugs with them in cases, some of which have survived until today. Eventually schools were developed in association with the temples of Aesculapius which were derived from the physicians rather than the temple priests, the most famous being at Rhodes, Cnidos and Cos. The school of Cnidos was interested in diagnosis and treatment with diet, herbs and drugs. The school of Cos specialized in the treatment of the patient rather than the treatment of the disease. A guild was formed which upheld the veneration of Aesculapius, promoted scientific views, supported a high standard of medicine and ethics. The members were bounded together by an oath. They believed in passing the profession from father to son but would allow strangers to become members. Instruction included the structure and function of the body, causes of diseases, and different diseases and their treatments. From this school came the famous "Oath of Hippocrates."

In the fifth century B.C., medicine began to sever its connection with religion and its control by the priesthood. Guilds were established for the physicians who passed their knowledge on to their sons or disciples and were bound together by an oath. According to legend, into such a guild, on the island of Cos, in 460 B.C., was born Hippocrates, who later, was to become one of the best remembered physicians in the world. Little is actually known about Hippocrates but many stories have survived, true or false, concerning this great teacher and physician.

The father of Hippocrates, Heraclides, was a physician and the first teacher of his son. Later teachers were Herodicus, Gorgias the sophist, and Democritus the philosopher. Hippocrates traveled widely and effected remarkable cures in Athens, Argos, Abdera and Thessaly and was sought after as the court physician for Artaxerxes of Persia. He died in Thessaly at the age of 104 years. About 200 years later, the Greeks who founded the library at Alexandria, Egypt, attempted to gather all the ancient knowledge together for their students, including medicine. The scholars found a group of writings, several of which were attributed to Hippocrates, which described sick people, careful descriptions of their appearances, and a history of the onset, course, and outcome of the specific diseases. This differed greatly from the usual fatalistic attitude of diseases which were caused by gods or demons or evil spirits and which were cured by spells or charms or incantations. The majority of the

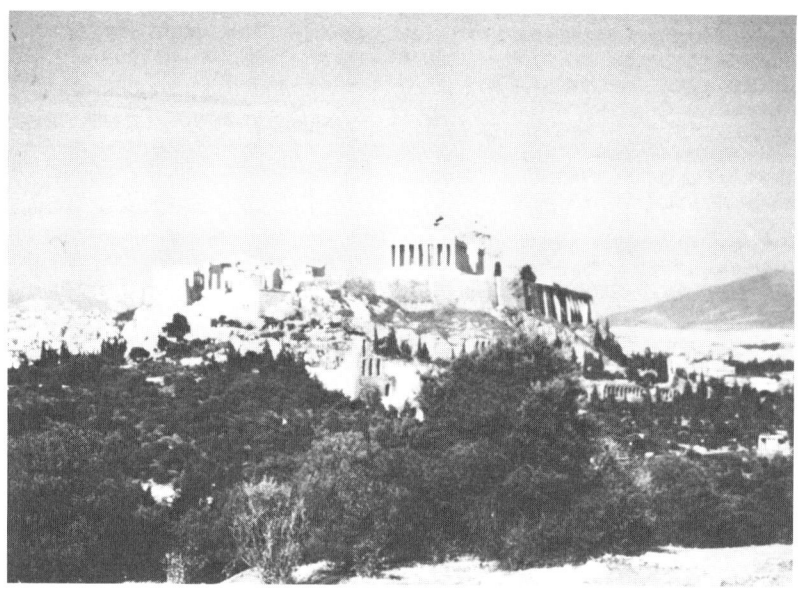

The Acropolis, Athens, Greece.

medical writings which were similar to those attributed to Hippocrates, were classified under his name. It is not important who wrote the observations but it is important that at this time man made a beginning toward the scientific study of diseases. The following quotations are from "The Genuine Works of Hippocrates," translated by Francis Adams.[1]

THE OATH

I swear by Apollo the physician, and Aesculapius, and Health, and All-heal, and all the gods and goddesses, that, according to my ability and judgment, I will keep this Oath and this stipulation—to reckon him who taught me this Art equally dear to me as my parents, to share my substance with him, and relieve his necessities if required; to look upon his offspring in the same footing as my own brothers, and to teach them this art, if they shall wish to learn it, without fee or stipulation; and that by precept, lecture, and every other mode of instruction, I will impart a knowledge of the Art to my own sons, and those of my teachers, and to disciples bound by a stipulation and oath according to the law of medicine, but to none others. I will follow that system of regimen which, according to my ability and judgment, I consider for the benefit of my patients, and abstain from whatever is deleterious and mischievous. I will give no deadly medicine to anyone if asked, nor suggest any such counsel; and in like manner I

---

1. "The Genuine Works of Hippocrates," translated by Francis Adams, ©1939, The Williams and Wilkins Co., Baltimore, Md.

will not give to a woman a pessary to produce abortion. With purity and with holiness I will pass my life and practice my Art. I will not cut persons laboring under the stone, but will leave this to be done by men who are practitioners of this work. Into whatever houses I enter, I will go into them for the benefit of the sick, and will abstain from every voluntary act of mischief and corruption; and, further, from the seduction of females or males, of freemen and slaves. Whatever, in connection with my professional practice or not, in connection with it, I see or hear, in the life of men, which ought not to be spoken of abroad, I will not divulge, as reckoning that all such should be kept secret. While I continue to keep this Oath unviolated, may it be granted to me to enjoy life and the practice of the art, respected by all men, in all times! But should I trespass and violate this Oath, may the reverse be my lot!

On Ancient Medicine

"I hold that the diet and food which people in health now use would not have been discovered, provided it had suited with man to eat and drink in the manner as the ox, the horse, and all other animals, except man, do of the productions of the earth, such as fruits, weeds and grass; for from such things these animals grow, live free of disease, and require no other kind of food. And, at first, I am of opinion that man used the same sort of food, and that the present articles of diet had been discovered and invented only after a long lapse of time, for when they suffered much and severely from this strong and brutish diet, swallowing things which were raw, unmixed, and possessing great strength, they became exposed to strong pains and diseases, and to early deaths. It is likely, indeed, that from habit they would suffer less from these things then, than we would now, but still they would suffer severely even then; and it is likely that the greater number, and those who had weaker constitutions, would all perish; whereas the stronger would hold out for a longer time, as even nowadays some, in consequence of using strong articles of food, get off with little trouble, but others with much pain and suffering. From this necessity it appears to me that they would search out the food befitting their nature, and thus discover that which we now use: and that from wheat . . . they formed bread; and from barley they formed cake; they boiled, they roasted, they mixed, they diluted those things which are strong and of intense qualities with weaker things, fashioning them to the nature and powers of man, and considering that the stronger things Nature would not be able to manage if administered, and that from such things pains, diseases and death would arise, but such as Nature could manage, that from them food, growth, and health would arise. To such a discovery and investigation what more suitable name could one give than that of Medicine? since it was discovered for the health of man, for his nourishment and safety, as a substitute for that kind of diet by which pains, diseases, and deaths were occasioned."

"Let us inquire then regarding what is admitted to be Medicine; namely, that which was invented for the sake of the sick, which possesses a name and practitioners, whether it also seeks to accomplish the same objects, and whence it derived its origin. To me, then, it appears, as I said at the commencement, that nobody would have sought for medicine at all, provided the same kinds of diet had suited with men in sickness as in good health."

"What other object, then, had he in view who is called a physician, and is admitted to be a practitioner of the art, who found out the regimen and diet befitting the sick, than he who originally found out and prepared for all mankind that kind of food which we all now use, in place of the former savage and brutish mode of living."

"But I wish the discourse to revert to the new method of those who prosecute their inquiries in the Art by hypothesis. For if hot, or cold, or moist, or dry, be that which proves injurious to man, and if the person who would treat him properly must apply cold to the hot, hot to the cold, moist to the dry, and dry to the moist—let me be presented with a man, not indeed one of a strong constitution, but one of the weaker, and let him eat wheat, such as it is supplied from the thrashing-floor, raw and unprepared, with raw meat, and let him drink water. By using such a diet I know that he will suffer much and severely, for he will experience pains, his body will become weak, and his bowels deranged, and he will not subsist long. What remedy, then, is to be provided for one so situated? Hot? or cold? or moist? or dry? For it is clear that it must be one or other of these. . . . But the surest and most obvious remedy is to change the diet which the person used, and instead of wheat to give bread, and instead of raw flesh, boiled, and to drink wine in addition to these; for by making these changes it is impossible but that he must get better, unless completely disorganized by time and diet. . . . Whoever pays no attention to these things, or, paying attention, does not comprehend them, how can he understand the diseases which befall a man?"

"Wherefore it appears to me necessary to every physician to be skilled in nature, and strive to know, if he would wish to perform his duties, what man is in relation to the articles of food and drink, and to his other occupations, and what are the effects of each of them to everyone."

"And it appears to me that one ought also to know what diseases arise in man from the powers, and what from the structures. What do I mean by this? By powers, I mean intense and strong juices; and by structures, whatever conformations there are in man. For some are hollow, and from broad contracted into narrow; some expanded, some hard and round, some broad and suspended (diaphragm?), some stretched, some long, some dense, some rare and succulent (mammary glands?), some spong and of loose texture (spleen, lungs?)" . . .

"And thus, too, the instruments which are used for cupping are broad below and gradually become narrow, and are so constructed in order to suck and draw in from the fleshy parts."

On Airs, Waters and Places

"Whoever wishes to investigate medicine properly, should proceed thus: in the first place to consider the seasons of the year, and what effects each of them produces, for they are not at all alike, but differ much from themselves in regard to their changes. Then the winds, the hot and the cold, especially such as are common to all countries, and then such as are peculiar to each locality. We must also consider the qualities of the waters, for as they differ from one another in taste and weight, so also do they differ much in their qualities."

"Having made these investigations, and knowing beforehand the seasons, such a one must be acquainted with each particular, and must succeed in the preservation of health, and be by no means unsuccessful in the practice of his art. And if it shall be thought that these things belong rather to meteorology, it will be admitted, on second thoughts, that astronomy contributes not a little, but a very great deal, indeed, to medicine. For with the seasons, the digestive organs of men undergo a change."

"Men become affected with the stone, and are seized with diseases of the kidneys, strangury, sciatica, and become ruptured, when they drink all sorts of waters, and those from great rivers into which other rivulets run, or from a lake into which many streams flow, and such as are brought from a considerable distance. For it is impossible that such waters can resemble one another, but one kind is sweet, another saltish and aluminous, and some flow from thermal springs; and these being all mixed up together disagree, and the strongest part always prevails.... There must be deposits of mud and sand in the vessels from such waters, and the aforesaid diseases must be engendered by them when drunk, but why not to all I will now explain. When the bowels are loose and in a healthy state, and when the bladder is not hot, nor the neck of the bladder very contracted, all such persons pass water freely, and no concretion forms in the bladder; but those in whom the belly is hot, the bladder must be in the same condition; and when preternaturally heated, its neck becomes inflamed; and when these things happen, the bladder does not expel the urine, but raises its heat excessively. And the thinnest part of its is secreted, and the purest part is passed off in the form of urine, but the thickest and most turbid part is condensed and concreted, at first in small quantity, but afterwards in greater; for being rolled about in the urine, whatever is of a thick consistence it assimilates to itself, and thus it increases and becomes indurated. And when such persons make water, the stone forced down by the urine falls into the neck of the bladder and stops the urine, and occasions intense pain; so that calculous children rub their privy parts and tear at them, as supposing that the obstruction to the urine is situated there."

"I will pass over the smaller differences among the nations, but will now treat of such as are great either from nature, or custom; and, first, concerning the Macrocephali. There is no other race of men which have heads in the least resembling theirs. At first, usage was the principal cause of the length of their head, but now nature cooperates with usage. They think those the most noble who have the longest heads. It is thus with regard to the usage: immediately after the child is born, and while its head is still tender, they fashion it with their hands, and constrain it to assume a lengthened shape by applying bandages and other suitable contrivances whereby the spherical form of the head is destroyed, and it is made to increase in length. Thus, at first, usage operated, so that this constitution was the result of force: but, in the course of time, it was formed naturally; so that usage had nothing to do with it.... But now these things do not happen as they did formerly, for the custom no longer prevails owing to their intercourse with other men. Thus it appears to me to be with regard to them."

The Book of Prognostics

"It appears to me a most excellent thing for the Physician to cultivate Prognosis; for by foreseeing and foretelling, in the presence of the sick, the present, the past, and the future, and explaining the omissions which patients have been guilty of, he will be the more readily believed to be acquainted with the circumstances of the sick; so that men will have confidence to intrust themselves to such a physician."

On Regimen in Acute Diseases

"Acute diseases are those which the ancients named pleurisy, pneumonia, phrenitis, lethargy, causus and other diseases allied to these, including the continual fevers. For, unless when some general form of pestilential disease is epidemic, and diseases are sporadic and not of a similar character, there are more deaths from these diseases than from all the others taken together. The vulgar, indeed, do not recognize the difference between such physicians and their common attendants, and are rather disposed to commend and censure extraordinary remedies. This, then, is a great proof that the common people are most incompetent, of themselves, to form a judgement how such diseases should be treated: since persons who are not physicians pass for physicians owing most especially to these diseases, for it is an easy matter to learn the names of these things which are applicable to persons laboring under such complaints. For, if one names the juice of ptisan, and such and such a wine, and hydromel, the vulgar fancy that he prescribes exactly the same things as the physicians do, both the good and the bad, but in these matters there is a great difference between them."

(Ptisan is a drink made from boiled barley; hydromel is liquid honey, which, if acidified, is called oxymel.)[3]

"A Draught for a Dropsical Person: Take three cantharides, and removing their head, feet and wings, triturate their bodies in three cupfuls of water, and when the person who has drunk the draught complains of pain, let him have hot fomentations applied. The patient should be first anointed with oil, should take the draught fasting, and eat hot bread with oil."

(Dropsy is the condition in which fluids accumulate in the body. Cantharides are insects (*Cantharis vesicatoria*) whose bodies contain cantharidin, an anhydride of cantharidic acid. When taken internally, it causes pain and vomiting and externally, it is a rubefacient and vesicant.)[4]

"A Styptic: Apply the juice of the fig inwardly to the vein; or having moulded biestings into a tent, introduce up the nostril, or push up some chalcitis (brass dust) with the finger, and press the cartilages of the nostrils together; and open the bowels with the boiled milk of asses; or having shaved the head, apply cold things to it if in the summer season."

(A styptic is a substance that checks hemorrhage by causing the contraction of the blood vessels. Among other compounds, the fig contains ficin, a proteolytic enzyme, which is also used as an active vermicide for various intestinal worms. A variety of copper compounds are used as astringents or caustics.)[5]

"The sesamoides purges upwards when pounded in oxymel to the amount of a drachm and a half, and drunk; it is combined with the hellebores, to the amount of the third part, and thus it is less apt to produce suffocation."

(Sesamoides refers to either sesame seeds or something resembling the seeds, such as the sesamoid cartilages in the nose which are pounded in acidified honey and combined with hellebores. Hellebores are plants of the Genera *Helleborus* or *Veratrum* and may contain a number of alkaloids which, when taken internally, reduce the respiration and pulse and reduce the blood pressure. Therefore, the use of this plant would reduce the blood pressure and stop the bleeding. It is diluted here in order to prevent the death of the patient.)[6]

3, 4, 5, 6. Author's notes.

"For Persons Affected with Empyema: Having cut some bulbs or squill, boil in water, and when well boiled, throw this away, and having poured in more water, boil until it appears to the touch soft and well-boiled; then triturate finely and mix roasted cumin, and white sesames, and young almonds pounded in honey, form into an electuary and give; and afterwards sweet wine. In draughts, having pounded about a small acetabulum of the white poppy, moisten it with water in which summer wheat has been washed, add honey, and boil. Let him take this frequently during the day. And then taking into account what are to happen, give him supper."

(Empyema is a disease in which various body cavities accumulate pus. The treatment prescribed utilizes the plant bulb of *Urginea maritima* or *U. indica*, which have been found to contain the glycosides, scillaren A and B. These glycosides, when ingested, cause vomiting, retard the pulse, and cause a ventricular fibrillation and cardiac arrhythmia. The acetabulum of the white poppy, *Papaver album*, would yield alkaloids, the main one being morphine, which would relive pain.)[7]

"For watery eyes: Take one drachm of ebeny and nine oboli of burnt copper, rub them on a whetstone, add three oboli of saffron; triturate all these things reduced to a fine powder, pour in an Attic hemina of sweet wine, and then place in the sun and cover up; when sufficiently digested, use it."

"For violent pains in the eyes: Take of chalcitis, and of raisin, of each one dr., when digested for two days, strain; and pounding myrrh and saffron, and having mixed must, with these things, digest in the sun; and with this anoint the eyes when in a state of severe pain. Let it be kept in a copper vessel."

(It is interesting that both of the treatments for the eys utilize copper in some form. The ancient Egyptians utilized copper compounds in their eye make-up and its use is mentioned in various medical papyri.)[8]

Of the Epidemics: "The physician must be able to tell the antecedents, know the present, and foretell the future—must meditate these things, and have two special objects in view with regard to diseases, namely, to do good or to do no harm. The art consists in three things—the disease, the patient and the physician. The physician is the servant of the art, and the patient must combat the disease along with the physician."

Of the Epidemics

"Early in spring, along with the prevailing cold, there were many cases of erysipelas, some from a manifest cause, and some not. They were of a malignant nature, and proved fatal to many; many had sore-throat and loss of speech. There were many cases of ardent fever, phrensy, aphthous affections of the mouth, tumors on the genital organs; of ophthalmia, anthrax, disorder of the bowels, anorexia, with thirst and without it; of disordered urine, large in

---

7, 8. Author's notes.

quantity, and bad in quality; of persons affected with coma for a long time, and then falling into a state of insomnolency. There were many cases of failure of crisis, and many of unfavorable crisis; many of dropsy and of phthisis. Such were the diseases then epidemic. There were patients affected with every one of the species which have been mentioned, and many died. The symptoms in each of these cases were as follows: In many cases erysipelas, from some obvious cause, such as an accident, and sometimes from even a very small wound, broke out all over the body, especially in persons about sixty years of age, about the head, if such an accident was neglected in the slightest degree; and this happened in some who were under treatment; great inflammation took place, and the erysipelas quickly spread all over. In the most of them the abscesses ended in suppurations, and there were great fallings off of the flesh, tendons and bones; and the defluxion which seated in the part was not like pus, but a sort of putrefaction, and the running was large and of various characters. Those cases in which any of these things happened about the head were accompanied with falling off of the hairs of the head and chin, the bones were laid bare and separated, and there were excessive runnings; and these symptoms happened in fevers and without fevers. But these things were more formidable in appearance than dangerous; for when the concoction in these cases turned into a suppuration, most of them recovered; but when the inflammation and the erysipelas disappeared and when no abscess was formed, a great number of these died. In like manner, the same things happened to whatever part of the body the disease wandered, for in many cases both forearm and arm dropped off; and in those cases in which it fell upon the sides, the parts there, either before or behind, got into a bad state; and in some cases the whole femur and bones of the leg and whole foot were laid bare. But of all such cases, the most formidable were those which took place about the pubes and genital organs. Such was the nature of these cases when attended with sores, and proceeding from an external cause; but the same things occurred in fevers, before fevers, and after fevers. But those cases in which an abscess was formed, and turned to a suppuration, or a seasonable diarrhea or discharge of good urine took place, were relieved thereby: but those cases in which none of these symptoms occurred, but they disappeared without a crisis, proved fatal. The greater number of these erysipelatous cases took place in the spring, but were prolonged through the summer and during the autumn."

Erysipelas is a disease caused by hemolytic streptococci, bacteria which cause the hemolysis of mammalian erythrocytes. They were first described in 1874, by Billroth, as globular chains of microorganisms in erysipelas and wound infections, and later by Pasteur, Ogston and Koch. When the skin becomes infected with these streptococci, the infection spreads in all directions in the subepidermal tissues from the original site of infection. Complications of the infection may result in acute rheumatic fever, acute hemorrhagic glomerulonephritis and erythema nodosum. The microorganisms are generally transmitted from the respiratory tract of an infected individual to another host, but transfer can be through contaminated food and other fomites. Recovery from infection may result in the formation of the carrier state, but many people carry the organisms as the normal flora of the respiratory tract. In antiquity, there was little that could be done to cure the patient but with the advent of the sulfa drugs, treatment was available. The sulfa drugs retard the multiplication of the streptococci which allows the body defence mechanisms of the host to control the infection. Penicillin, and other antibiotics, destroy the streptococci and are the drugs of choice today.

Trepanning

"With regard to trepanning, when there is a necessity for it, the following particulars should be known. If you have had the management of the case from the first, you must not at once saw the bone down to the meninx; for it is not proper that the membrane should be laid bare and exposed to injuries for a length of time, as in the end it may become fungous. And there is another danger if you saw the bone down to the meninx and remove it at once, lest in the act of sawing you should wound the meninx. But in trepanning, when only a very little of the bone remains to be sawed through, and the bone can be moved, you must desist from sawing, and leave the bone to fall out of itself. For to a bone not sawed through, and where a portion is left of the sawing, no mischief can happen; for the portion now left is sufficiently thin. In other respects you must conduct the treatment as may appear suitable to the wound. And in trepanning you must frequently remove the trepan, on account of the heat in the bone, and plunge it in cold water. For the trepan being heated by running around, and heating and drying the bone, burns it and makes a larger piece of bone around the sawing to drop off, than would otherwise do. And if you wish to saw at once down to the membrane, and then remove the bone, you must also, in like manner, frequently take out the trepan and dip it in cold water. But you must take care where you apply the trepan, and see that you do so only where it appears to be particularly thick, and having fixed the instrument there, that you frequently make examinations and endeavor by moving the bone to bring it up. Having removed it, you must apply other suitable remedies to the wound."

On the Surgery

"The things relating to surgery, are—the patient; the operator; the assistants; the instruments; the light, where and how; how many things, and how; where the body, and the instruments; the time; the manner; the place. The operator is either sitting or standing, conveniently for himself, for the person operated upon, for the light. Those about the patient must present the part to be operated upon as may seem proper, and they must hold the rest of the body steady, in silence, and listening to the commands of the operator."

On the Sacred Disease

"It is thus with regard to the disease called Sacred; It appears to me to be nowise more divine or more sacred than other diseases, but has a natural cause from which it originates like other affections. Men regard its nature and cause as divine from ignorance and wonder, because it is not at all like to other diseases. And this notion of its divinity is kept up by their inability to comprehend it, and the simplicity of the mode by which it is cured, for men are freed from it by purifications and incantations. Yet, if it were more divine than the others, this disease ought to befall all alike, and make no distinction between the bilious and phelgmatic. But in them, the brain is the cause of this affection, as it is of other very great diseases, and in what manner and from what cause it is formed, I will now plainly declare. The brain of man, as in all other animals, is double, and a thin membrane divides it through the middle, and therefore the pain is not always in the same part of the head; for sometimes it is situated on either side, and sometimes the whole is affected; and veins run to it from all parts of the body, many of which are small, but two are thick,—the one from the liver, and the other from the spleen. And it is thus with regard to the one from the liver: a portion of it runs downward through the parts on the right side, near the kidneys and the psoas muscles (loin), to the inner part of the thigh, and extends to the foot. It is called vena cava. The other runs upward by the right veins and the lungs, and divides into branches for the heart and the right arm. The remaining part of it rises upward across the clavicle to the right side of the neck, and is superficial so as to be seen; near the ear it is concealed, and there it divides; its thickest, largest, and most hollow part ends in the brain; another small vein goes to the right ear, another to the right eye, and another to the nostril. Such are the distributions of the hepatic vein. And a vein from the spleen is distributed on the left side, upward and downward, like that from the liver, but more slender and feeble. By these veins we draw in much spirit for they are the spiracles of our bodies inhaling air to themselves and distributing it to the rest of the body, and to the smaller veins, and they cool and afterwards exhale it. For the breath (pneuma) cannot be stationary, but it passes upward and downward, for if stopped and intercepted, the part where it is stopped becomes powerless."

The Hippocratic School also produced a disease theory based upon the four humors of the body which were regarded as physiological analogues of four principles of physics. The four humors are blood, phlegm, yellow bile and black bile (or bile and atrabile, urine and feces) which were described as being hot and wet, cold and wet, hot and dry, and cold and dry, and corresponded to fire, water, air and earth. The four humors, in different blends, composed the various parts of the body. A disarrangement of the humors could result in sickness which would be cured when the four humors were restored to normality.

Other Schools or groups which were involved in medicine included the Pythagoreans, the Sophists, the Empirics, the Gymnasts, the Rhizotomists, the midwives and quacks. Famous philosophers also contributed to medicine by stimulation of students and interest in the various sciences. The greatest among these were Socrates, Plato and Aristotle. Socrates was poisoned with hemlock, not the plant that we call hemlock today, but a plant belonging to the carrot family. Socrates was the teacher of Plato. These schools or groups were responsible for scientific works that would form the basis of later European science and medicine. Plato established the "Academy," an institution that was to last from about 387 B.C., to about 529 A.D., and in his writings, claimed that the "brain is man's most noble tool" and that "medicine is the art of understanding the love affairs of the organs of the body." Aristotle was one of the pupils of this school and he later instructed Alexander, who eventually conquered much of the Mediterranean area and the Middle East. Aristotle established the "Lyceum" in Athens in about 335 B.C., and may have influenced the ruler of Egypt, Ptolemy Soter (305-283 B.C.) in the establishment of the school and library at Alexandria. During the reign of Ptolemy Philadelphus the library contained approximately 500,000 books. The library was partially destroyed by the Romans and the remaining volumes were burned centuries later in order to heat the public baths under the Caliph Omar.

The most important Greek physician after Hippocrates was Galen. Galen was born at Pergamos in about 130 A.D., and was well-educated by his father, Nikon, an architect. He studied in a variety of Schools but never identified himself with any particular system. Eventually, he devoted his studies to medicine and traveled widely and visited many centers of learning in Asia Minor, Palestine and Egypt. The Alexandrian School was noted at that time for the study of the bones and the art of dissection and undoubtedly, Galen learned much there concerning anatomy and dissection. He returned to Pergamos and was appointed the physician to the gladiators where he became involved in surgery and made use of bandages soaked in wine to prevent infections in wounds. He went to Rome and quickly became established as an excellent physician and gave lectures on the structure and functions of the human body. He wrote many books including studies of diseases of the eyes, the anatomy of the uterus, the movement of the lungs, anatomy and physiology. His works, and those attributed to Hippocrates are extremely important in that they were later translated and studied by the Moslems and Europeans, forming the basis of their medicinal theories. Galen's work in human anatomy was for centuries the standard but unfortunately, contained many errors. Apparently, he did not carry out human dissections but based his observations on animals such as apes, bears, pigs and others, and applied his findings to man. The following example of his writing is a translation of Galen's "On the Best Constitution of our Body," by Penella and Hall.[9]

---

9. Galen's "On the Best Constitution of Our Body," translated by Robert J. Penella and Thomas S. Hall, Bulletin of the History of Medicine, Vol. XLVII, No. 3, May-June, 1973.

"What is the best constitution of our body? Is a perfectly tempered constitution the best, as was the opinion of many ancient physicians and philosophers? Or is it rather the case that, even though the best constitution is necessarily perfectly tempered, a (merely) perfectly tempered constitution is not necessarily the best? For a balanced mixture of hot, cold, dry, and wet is what constitutes the health of our body's homogeneous parts (homoiomerē). But the formation of a living creature out of all these homogeneous parts depends on the arrangement, size, shape, and number of the body's composites; and it would seem possible that, even though a body is composed of parts all or almost all of which are well-tempered, there could still be something wrong with the size of these or with their number, configuration, or arrangement in relation to one another.

"We must attempt, then, to treat all these matters in order, beginning with the terms that we need to use in this discussion; for there is disagreement even about them. Some think it proper to refer to the best 'constitution' (kataskeuē) of the body, whereas others prefer the term 'disposition' (diathesis) or 'state' (schesis) or 'nature' (physis) or whatever term a person may think is best. I find no fault with anyone's explaining a term as he pleases, but I would disapprove of his reproaching those who use it differently than he does; for I think that the fullest and greatest measure of attention should be given to the issues that constitute the subject-matter of a discussion rather than to its terms. Whether a person wishes to use the term best 'constitution' of the body or 'disposition' or 'state' or 'habit' or 'nature' or some other term—if, after deciding on the term, he begins with the commonly accepted notion of it and, as he proceeds to investigate its essence, carries out his research in an orderly and methodical manner, then I shall commend him far more than I would a person who gives the impression of being a master of terminology. So let us proceed in a similar fashion beginning with the generally accepted notion, and after defining it, we may advance methodically to the next step of our inquiry.

"What, then, is the generally accepted notion of the best constitution of the body? One can hear men differ with one another verbally about this matter, even though all in fact are thinking one and the same thing. (For example, all men praise the 'healthiest' (hygieinotaton) body, just as they praise the 'soundest' (euektikōtaton) body. In both cases they are focusing on the same thing and are directing their thoughts to it, though they have no clear conception of it nor can they explain it distinctly. For they think that the functions of all the body's parts must be strong and not easily overcome by the causes of disease. 'Health' (hygieia) is to be found when the functions of the parts are in accordance with nature; 'soundness' (euexia), when these functions have a certain robustness. But the condition common to both states is that the body is not easily overcome by diseases; so naturally the healthiest (hygieinotatē) condition—which all men long for—is a sound one (euektikē). It is also characterized by the proper working of the body's functions and a resistance to dissolution. This condition is quite rightly called 'soundness' (euexia); the term 'hexis' itself already denotes stability and resistance to dissolution, but the term 'euexia' denotes these qualities even better, since an ideal 'hexis' is predicted by it. Thus, whether we refer to the best constitution of the body as 'healthiest' or 'soundest,' we shall not be incorrect; and our criterion of this condition will be whether the body's functions are working properly and (so) resist dissolution.

"Now that this definition has been laid down, we must consider next what is the essence of such a state (hexis) of the body. Here, again, we may begin our inquiry by asking what the disposition of our body is when we are functioning best. To do this we must call to mind some principles already set forth in other treatises. The first point is that our bodies are composed of a mixture of hot, cold, dry and wet; these matters have been elucidated in the book entitled 'On the Elements according to Hippocrates.' Secondly, we must recall how the temperaments of the parts are defined; these matters have been discused in the treatise entitled 'On Temperaments.' Next, recall that each of the organic members of the body has one part in it that is the cause of its function, and that all the other parts making up the complete organ were produced for the sake of this one; these matters have been elucidated well enough in the work entitled 'On the Use of the Parts.' The best constitution of the body, then, will be that in which all the homogeneous parts—that, of course, is the name given to the parts that are uniform to our perception—have their own proper temperament, and in which the composition of each of the organic parts out of the homogeneous parts has been achieved with perfect proportion in respect to their size, number, configuration, and arrangement in relation to one another.

"It should not be hard to recognize that the body whose functions are all in perfect condition is also the least susceptible of all to disease. And any part that functions at its best is a product of the good temperament of the homogeneous parts and the well-balanced constitution of the organic parts—precisely the description of the body mentioned above. Thus, it is clear that such a body will function best of all. That it is also least susceptible to disease you can clearly understand in the following way.

"Of the things that harm our bodies, some come from external causes, while others arise from the residues (perittōmata) of food. Those that come from external causes affect bodies that have been heated and cooled or moistened and dried excessively; in this category should be placed fatigue, insomnia, distress, anxiety, and other such conditions. Those that come from residues of food are of two kinds (for the residues themselves are of two kinds, some troubling the body by their quantity, others by their quality), but they take many forms."

While in Rome, the Emperor, Marcus Aurelius learned of the excellent reputation Galen had achieved as a physician and asked him to join him on a campaign against the barbarians, who were threatening the boundaries of the Empire. In about 165, the Roman Army in Mesopotamia quelling a revolt, suffered an epidemic of smallpox, which, apparently, was brought back to Italy, because at this time, about 170, the pestilence broke out at court. Marcus Aurelius went off to fight the barbarians and Galen remained in Rome until his death in about 199. Galen's successors, in general, failed to carry out further research and relied on the writings of their predecessors, so his writings and theories concerning medicine, especially human anatomy, were accepted by most academicians until the sixteenth century, when Vesalius (1514-64), proved that Galen's writings were frequently in error.

The death of Galen is considered by many to indicate the end of the Greek-Roman era of science and the beginning of a general period of decline marked by religious wars, the invasions by the barbarians and later, the Moslem period of conquests.

The Roman Empire declined and finally fell, according to authoritative speculation, not because of the barbarian hordes, overextended colonization or moral decadence, but mainly as a result of lead poisoning. Eating and drinking from vessels containing lead and dabbing themselves with lead-laden cosmetics, the upper-class Romans unwittingly poisoned themselves, sapping their vitality and the vitality of the society which they headed. A study of ancient tombstones indicates a life expectancy of 22 to 25 years among upper-class Romans. Their birth rate was one-fourth of that needed to replace themselves. The poorer Romans used cheap earthenware vessels and could not afford the cosmetics.

In 324, Emperor Constantine declared Christianity the official religion of the Empire and made Constantinople the capital. By 527, Rome was under the control of Germanic tribes while Justinian ruled in the East. He closed Plato's Academy, which had been in existence since 387 B.C., and the teachers fled to Persia, with whom the Eastern Empire was at war. In 570, Mohammed was born in Mecca, who later formulated the Moslem religion, and while the Eastern Empire and Persia were battling, the Moslem forces were increasing in the south. By 717, the Moslems ruled from Afganistan to Spain, and their advances into Europe were not halted until 732, at Tours, France, by forces under Charles Martel.

When the Moslem Empire became settled, the Arabs noted the advances of the conquered civilizations and utilized them. Libraries, schools and hospitals were built and scientific books were translated into Arabic. Greek-Roman medicine replaced Arabic charms and amulets, and was ministered by school-trained physicians, two of the most famous being Rhazes and Avicenna.

Abu Bekr Mohammed ibn Zakkariya, Ar-Razi, (850-932), is the actual name of the Arabic physician known in the West as Rhazes. Little is known concerning his life except that he was a prolific writer of books on medicine, philosophy, chemistry, mathematics and astronomy. His fame among the Arabs is based upon an encyclopedia of medical knowledge of the time, compiled by his pupils after his death, and contains observations by Rhazes on diseases with their case histories and treatments. His treatise concerning smallpox and measles is regarded as one of the first monographs on specific diseases. During the Middle Ages, many physicians in the West utilized one of his general medicinal works as a handbook.

Abu Ali Husain ibn Abdullah ibn Sina is the actual name of Avicenna; (980-1037), who at the age of eighteen, had already achieved fame as a physician. At twenty-one, he composed a twenty volume encyclopedia and soon after, became visier to the Emir of Hamadan, and became involved in the affairs of the government. Eventually he limited himself to science and was regarded by many as a second Aristotle. His most important work on medicine, "The Canon of Medicine," contains sections dealing with general diseases, simple drugs, pathology, therapeutics, pharmacology and medicinal theories. This systematized work was utilized in the West from the thirteenth to seventeenth centuries and is still highly regarded in the Middle East.

The Moslem Empire was threatened by invasions of the Mongols in the thirteenth century who, in 1258, took Bagdad and the remnants of the Roman Empire crumbled when the Turks took Constantinople in 1453. Moslem rule, however, continued in many areas, especially in parts of Spain until 1492, the year Columbus sailed into the western ocean, and discovered a New World. Medieval medicine was based upon some Greek-Roman works that had survived in the West and the legacy of the Moslems who brought their translations of the Greek and Roman works and their own ideas into Europe. During the Crusades to the Holy Land, many manuscripts had been discovered which had been preserved by the Moslems and Hebrews. In the early Middle Ages, the majority of the physicians were priests or monks, and the monasteries and religious schools kept the literature of medicine alive by their translations of Greek and Arabic works into Latin, which is why Latin became the language of physicians. One of the most famous translators of these works was Constantine of Africa (1010-87), who, after traveling for many years, became a monk in the Abbey of Monte Cassino in Italy.

Medicinal beliefs of this period might best be explained by consulting a medical text of that time. In 1913, E.A. Wallis Budge published a Syriac text, edited from a rare manuscript that he had found and copied in Mosul, on the Tigris River, opposite the ruins of Ancient Nineveh.[10] Budge believed that the text was written in the twelfth century by a Nestorian monk for use in the library of a monastery. The introduction, the first two chapters and the ending of the book were missing but there remain 19 chapters on diseases and disorders plus a section on divination, forecasts, omens, and the influences of the planets and the Signs of the Zodiac on men and human affairs. There are nearly 1000 prescriptions in the text many of which are attributed to physicians such as Galen, Dioskorides, Solon and others, plus many of Egyptian, Persian and Indian origin. The following are excerpts from the translation by Budge.

"On epilepsy, which is the sickness of falling down.

> Now also the disease of those who fall down in that sickness which is called 'epilepsy' is a rigidity of all the members of the body. It is not always thus like the rigidity which cometh from behind, or like that which cometh from the front, or like the other kind of rigidity which cometh from both of these and is of the mind and is in all the body, but it lasteth for a short time only. And it is not different in this respect only from the other kinds of rigidity (or stiffening) of which we have spoken, but also in respect of injuries of the understanding and of the senses (or feelings), and from this it is known that the source of this disease is in the brain. But, inasmuch as it is speedily relieved in the cavities of the brain, it is meet to declare emphatically that it is the thick chyme which blocketh up the exits of the breath (or spirit) and causeth the disease, at the same time shaking and making to twitch the very beginnings of the nerves. Therefore thou must eject therefrom that which afflicteth it. Perhaps also each of the ends of the nerves being submerged, after the manner of those which go forth from the back, there then cometh into being the disease (or pain) of those who fall into epileptic fits and become ill."

---

10. E.A. Wallis Budge, "Syrian Anatomy, Pathology and Therapeutics" or "The Book of Medicines," edited and translated by E.A.W. Budge, Volume II, Humphrey Milford, Oxford University Press, London, 1913, pgs. 10, 14, 15, 47, 48, 531, 532, 547, 625, 685, 687.

"On the madness which ariseth from black bile.

Now therefore as no small change taketh place in the diseases which attack the head through sympathy, so also the change which taketh place in them through the peculiar property of suffering is not small. The thick chymes which are gathered together and increase in the natural matter of the brain affect it sometimes like an organic disease, and sometimes like substances made up of homogeneous particles. Now when they block up the vents (or openings) and the exits (of the brain), the disease is organic, but when they work on the brain itself the disease is (due to) a change in the substance made up of homogenous particles. The author of this observation is Hippokrates, who maketh it in the Sixth Chapter of his treatise on the Comings of Sickness."

Prescriptions for Ailments of the Head. Great Hiera-leghudhaya.

This expelleth from the body all the manifold forms of ailments which arise from the chymes without producing in it weakness, and it cureth all the sicknesses of the head, namely disease in the hemicranium, and idiocy, and dementia, and stupidity, and raving, and vertigo, and deafness, and the falling sickness, and asthma of long standing, and pains in the kidneys and in the sciatic nerve, and pains in the tendons, and gout, and those whose limbs shake and are palsied, and elephantiasis, and leprosy, and scabies, and tumours, and running sores, and pig-sores, and cancers, and all the sicknesses which are begotten of black bile, or of crude phlegm which is not distributed. And it reestablisheth the constitution which is impaired, and it healeth pains in the eyes and pains in the ears, and it bringeth on the menstrual flow, and it cureth protracted fevers, and fevers which come on for a day, and those which come on every third day.

Pith of colocynth	5	drachims	(Poisonous carthartic)[11]
Roasted sea-onion	2 1/2	drachims	
Agarikon fungus	2 1/2	drachims	(Agaric mushroom, poison)
Skamônia (convolvulus)	2 1/2	drachims	(Diuretic, laxative)
Black hellebore	2 1/2	drachims	(Poisonous cathartic)
Ammoniac	2 1/2	drachims	(Stimulant, expectorant)
Flowers of thyme	3	drachims	(Aromatic, carminative)
Bdellium	3	drachims	(*Balsamodendron* resin)
Chamadraos (chamaedrys)	3	drachims	
Aloes	3	drachims	(Stimulant, cathartic)
Thyme	2	drachims	
Malabathrum (betelnut?)	2	drachims	(*Cinnamomum tamala*)
Haprikon	2	drachims	
Parsion (horehound)	2	drachims	(For coughs, vermifuge)
Teucrium polium (germander)	2	drachims	(Treatment of abscesses)
Cassia	2	drachims	(Purge)
Peppers, of the three kinds	2	drachims	
Crocus	2	drachims	(Stimulant)
Cinnamon	2	drachims	(Carminative, astringent)
Jackal's fat	2	drachims	
Polypodium	2	drachims	(Styptic, hemostatic)

---

11. Author's notes.

Sagapenum (fennel)	2 drachims	(Stimulant, carminative)
Betonica	2 drachims	(Emetic, cathartic)
Myrrh	2 drachims	(Stimulant, astringent)
Petroselinum (parsley)	2 drachims	
Aristolochia makra (snakeroot)	2 drachims	(Poison, diuretic)
Juice of the artemisia pontica	2 drachims	(Stimulant, vermifuge)
Euphorbium	2 drachims	(Stimulant, counter-irritant)
Bearded grain	2 drachims	
Amomum gingiber	2 drachims	(Stimulant, diuretic)
Khĕmâma balsam	2 drachims	
Strychnus	1 1/2 drachims	(Poison, stimulant)
Gentian	1 1/2 drachims	(Tonic, stomachic)
Honey, as much as necessary		

Take in a draught of three drachims of warm water and honey, or in an infusion of flowers of thyme."

"Again a calculation concerning those who are sick.

First of all reckon up the (numerical values of the letters of the) name of the sick man, and of those of the name of his mother, and cast them out nine by nine (i.e., divide them by nine). If one remaineth to thee, his sickness is from God. And if two, it is caused by the Evil Eye. And if three, it is caused by sorcery (or witchcraft), but if it be a child who is sick, he is too young for the disease to be a punishment (or revenge). And if four, the sickness is caused by an evil spirit. And if five, there is a 'shidha' (i.e., a devil) in it. And if six, the sickness is from heaven. And if seven, it is due to trembling caused by fear. And if eight, the sickness is caused by a blow of Satan. And if nine, it is from his mother's womb (i.e., congenital), or is due to vengeance, or disturbing dreams."

"Auguries concerning sicknesses.

He who is smitten in the Bull. Of this man the following are the sign: His arms give him pain, and his left side, and his neck, and the soles of his feet, and he is smitten in a secret place, and his eyes are 'hard' to him. And if the sun be in the House in its going down, the pain will never move from him.

He who is smitten in the Two Images, that is to say the Twins. Of this man the following are the signs: His shoulders and bowels cause him pain, and fever will have dominion over him in the hour wherein the flux smiteth him. And if the moon be there on the day when it smiteth him, cure is nigh unto him, and the atmosphere will be changed about him, and he will be healed.

He who is smitten in the Lion. Of this man the following are the signs: His loins and his heart cause him pain, and if he be smitten in Aphrodite there will be grievous (or deep) sickness to him, and . . . will go forth to him."

"Divination by letters. That thou mayest know whether a woman hath conceived a boy or a girl.

Find out what day of the moon it is, (reckon up the numerical values of the letters in the name thereof,) and reckon up the numerical values of the letters in the name of the woman, and add to it twenty-eight, and then divide each by two. If the remainder is one, the child is a boy, and if it be two, the child is a girl."

"Miscellaneous native prescriptions.

For hiccoughs. Let him that hath them drink three mouthfuls of strong vinegar, or of very cold water, or very hot water; or shake him violently.

To prevent a man from snoring in his sleep. Put the tooth of a stallion under the head of him that snoreth in his sleep, and he will not snore.

For the man who is possessed of a devil. Tie the heart of an ass in the skin of a stag and hang it over him. Or burn the heart of a dove under him, and the devil will flee from him.

For the bite of a mad dog. Pound 'gufta' and salt, and lay upon the wound. Or take the hair of a man, and macerate it in vinegar, and apply. Hang up a dog's tooth over thee, and a mad dog will not bite thee.

Another, concerning things secret and things revealed. Take the head of a black raven, empty out its brains, and place in the cavity thereof five grains of coriander seed, and bury the head in dung. Visit it every day until the grains and then eat them, and thou shalt see whatsoever thy heart desireth to see."

the new world

Christopher Columbus undertook three voyages to the west and, until he died, believed that he had discovered a route across the ocean to India, calling the people that he had found living there, Indians. Columbus has been credited with the discovery of America, but there were already people living there who, today, are thought to be the descendents of migrants from Asia, who had crossed the ice bridge to North America about 40,000 years ago. However, recent investigations by Leakey (1970) in the Mojave desert and Fryxell (1973) near Puebla, indicate that man was in the Americas 100-250 thousand years ago. Recently[1], in Ecuador, excavations have been carried out on the Santa Elena peninsula, west of Guayaquil which have yielded artifacts that suggest that a culture, contemporary with or possibly older than those of the Fertile Crescent and Egypt, existed in South America. This is one of the oldest culture sites known in the New World, dated to about 5000-6000 years ago, and will dramatically alter perceptions of the origins of American civilizations. The diggings have unearthed clay figurines and pottery, temple foundations and evidence of corn cultivation. One figurine has only one eye, a deformed ear, a club foot, a crippled arm, skin that appears ravaged by syphilis, and lumps on the forehead, elbows and ankles typical of the disease, *verruga*, transmitted by the bite of an infected sand fly. The culture has been named "Valdivia" after the name of a nearby village. An even more dramatic find occurred in 1983[2] which reported the unearthing of ruins of 14 row houses at Monte Verde, in southern Chile by Thomas Dillehay, from the University of Kentucky and colleagues at the University of Chile. Each unit was about 6 × 10 feet and had clay-lined hearth pits. Radioactive carbon dating of charcoal and animal bones found at the site indicate that they were 12,500 to 14,000 years old.

It is believed that the first people from the Old World to visit the Americas were a group of semites from ancient Phoenicia. This is based upon rock

---

1. San Francisco Chronicle, July 30, 1978.
2. San Francisco Chronicle, March 20, 1984.

inscriptions found in Brazil in 1872 and later publications of inscriptions by Don Bernardo da Silva Ramos in 1939. Dr. Jacot L. Friend translated the 1872 inscription as follows:

> "We are Canaanites from Sidon, from the city of the trading king. We were caste on this distant shore, a land of mountains.... We embarked from Ezion-Geber into the Red Sea with ten ships and were on the sea together for two years around Africa, but we got separated through the hand of Baal and were no longer with our companions. So we have come here, ten men and three women, onto a new shore."

Dr. Friend also noted that in 1968 some copper coins, minted about 2000 years ago, were found near Louisville, Kentucky, which could indicate that explorers from the Mediterranean also visited North America in antiquity.

The Phoenicians were noted seafarers and were utilized by the Egyptian Pharaoh Necho, in about 600 B.C., for a voyage which circumnavigated Africa and which took about three years to complete. It is approximately this period when the Phoenicians were believed to have sailed to South America.

Artifacts of the Norsemen have been discovered in North America as far inland as the region of the Great Lakes where it is believed they explored in the eleventh century. The famous Nordic map depicting Europe and North America has recently proved to be a clever forgery. In 1975, an organization of professionsal and amateur scientists, the Epigraphic Scoiety, reported evidence that indicates Celtic Europeans populated New England about 2500 years ago. The findings are based on inscriptions on stone structures said to be part of an ancient language called Ogam, used by the Celtic peoples, who ranged from southwestern Germany to Spain and the British Isles. The inscriptions have been tentatively dated to 800 to 200 B.C.

Recently, the finding of stone anchors along the California coast, similar to those used by the ancient Chinese, and estimated to be 2-3000 years old by the rate of the accumulated manganese coating, have added to accumulating evidence that the Americas were visited by Chinese navigators in antiquity. The "History of Liang", written probably in about 525 A.D., tells of the country "Fu Sang" which is located about 6000 miles to the east and which abounded in grapes and the century plant, for which the country was named. Historians believe the country described is present Mexico and Central America.

The following is a legend of the Hopi Indians, abbreviated by the author, which describes their early mythology and how they came to the Americas. It is interesting that the legend indicates that they came across the Pacific Ocean in reed boats, going from island to island, until they reached the Americas.

A Legend of the Hopi Indians

The first world was *TOKPELA* (Endless space) in which there was only the Creator, Taiowa. First he created Sotuknang as an instrument to carry out his plans for the universe. After creating the universe and, finally, Earth, Sotuknang created a female who was to be his helper, Koyangwuti, Spider Woman.

Using earth and saliva, the Spider Woman created twins: Palongawhoya, who was to keep the world in order and Poqanghoya, also known as the "Echo," for all the sounds of the Creator. After completing their work, they became the poles of the Earth and were to keep the World rotating properly.

After this, the Spider Woman created from the Earth—trees, bushes, plants, flowers, birds and animals. Finally, she mixed earth of four different colors—yellow, red, white and black—and made four male figures and then four female figures. These dried in the sunlight and she said: "That is the sun. You are meeting your Father, the Creator for the first time."

Corn was created especially as a food for mankind and the people built its flesh into their own. Hence, corn became their mother also. Thus they knew their mother in two aspects—as Mother Earth and the Corn Mother.

The people of the First World eventually neglected the teaching of the Creator and the world was destroyed. Prior to its destruction, Sotuknang led some chosen people to an Ant mound and put these people underground, under the protection of the Ant-people, while above, the Earth was destroyed by fire. Food began to diminish so the Ant-people tightened their belts and ate less food which is why all ants have very narrow midsections.

When the Second World was ready, Tokpa (Dark Midnight), the people were brought out and again became wicked. Good people again were placed with the Ant-people and the Twins at the Poles allowed the Earth to teeter off balance, destroying the Second World.

The Third World was created, Kuskurza, but again the people became wicked so the world was to be destroyed by water. The Spider Woman sealed the people to be saved inside hollow reeds which then floated on the flood waters. After the flood, they made round boats from the reeds and floated from island to island until they reached the place of Emergence into the Fourth World, Tuwaqachi. When they reached the Fourth World (somewhere in Mesoamerica) and the place of Emergence, Sotuknang pointed to the West and told them he would now destroy their stepping-stones to the Fourth World, and caused the islands to sink to the bottom of the ocean.

In the Fourth World (World Complete) the people were required to migrate to the ends of the earth and back and then they could settle permanently. This they did. The spiritual and magnetic center of their migrations is what is now the Hopi country in the southwestern part of the United States.

In 1519, Cortez entered Tenochtitlan, the city of the Aztecs, now surrounded and covered by Mexico City, and met Moctezuma II, ruler of about half of present day Mexico. The name "Mexico" was given to the country by the Spaniards who derived it from a group of people who called themselves "Mexica" and who, in general, are known as the "Aztecs." Other cultures existed in Mesoamerica at that time and others had existed before the Aztecs, who arrived in the valley of Mexico about 1168 A.D., having traveled there from northwestern Mexico. Their migrations have been traced to Tula, the ancient capital of the Toltecs, from which they then migrated towards the valley of Mexico and eventually settled on islands in Lake Texcoco. The founding of the city of Tenochtitlan is generally given as 1325 A.D.

If there is a common heritage among the early cultures of Mesoamerica it was derived from the Olmecs. They gradually appeared in the primitive agricul-

158   *Magic, Myths and Medicine*

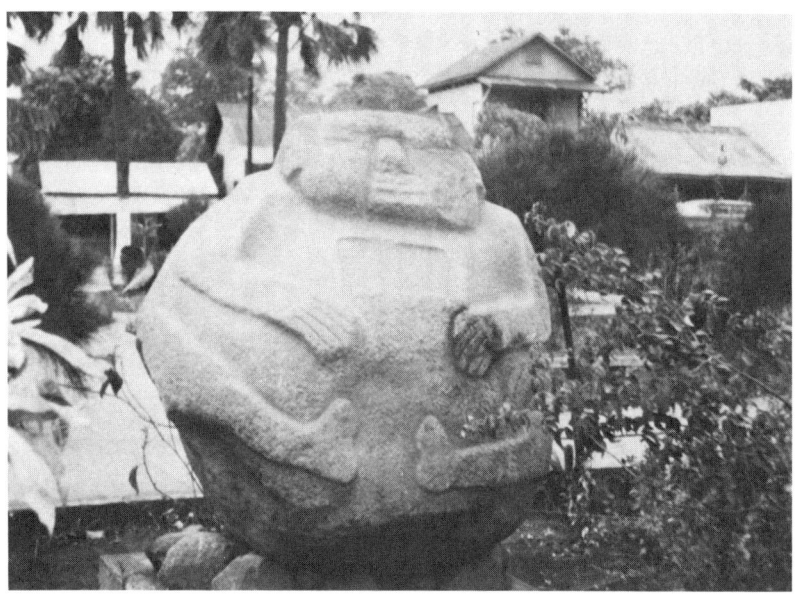

Pre-Olmec boulder carving displayed in the Archeological Park, La Democracia, Guatemala.

tural cultures and grouped together in small towns. The Pre-Olmecs were shamanistic and are frequently referred to as Magicians. These people carved rock and shaped clay figures of deformed or abnormal individuals, perhaps for some ritual; worshipped various gods who controlled the elements; utilized cotton, jade, rubber, tobacco; and farmed to support their settlements. The Olmecs may be dated to as early as 1000 B.C., in the Isthmus of Tehuantepec, but their main sites were in the hotlands of Tabasco and Vera Cruz. One such site, La Venta, was, according to carbon dating, occupied between 800 and 400 B.C. Gigantic stone heads cut from single pieces of rock and stone altars were found in the area, along with other artifacts and can be seen today in the museum in Villa Hermosa. The single pieces of rock were quarried about sixty miles away and were brought to the sites. The rocks are up to ten feet in height and weigh about twenty tons. Some of the rocks are carved into huge heads with smiling faces, thick noses and lips, and are topped with helmets which resemble present day football protective helmets. In the Museo Arqueologico of La Democracia, Escuintla, Guatemala, are similar carved boulders, though much smaller, which are termed Pre-Olmec. On these rounded boulders are carved human figures with large round heads and bodies and small thin arms and legs.

Mayan ruins and artifacts have been discovered over Mesoamerica from southern Mexico to Costa Rica and while the culture has been dated from as early as 2000 B.C., and lasting until 1697 A.D., the Classical Age is usually dated from 300 to 900 A.D. Architectural ruins of the Mayans can be seen in various areas from Guatemala to Yucatan, the best known to being Tikal, Palenque, Uxmal, and Chichen Itza. The Mayans are noted for the perfection of their calendar, glyph writing, stone carvings and their fantastic temple complexes. At Palenque was found a secret chamber within one of the temples that was the tomb of an important personage and contained carvings, offerings and jewelry. The archaeologist Ruz, investigating the Temple of the Inscriptions which stood on the top of a seventy foot pyramid, noted a stone in the floor which had three holes in it which were fitted with stone plugs. When this was lifted, a passageway was found beneath which led to the depths of the temple. After clearing rubble and rock and concrete barriers, a chest containing six sacrificial human victims was discovered. Nearby was found the burial chamber which contained a huge stone sarcophagus whose cover stone weighed about five tons. Inside the inner red-painted stone coffin were the remains of a man with a jade death mask and many articles of jade such as collars, rings, bracelets and figurines. The stone pieces involved in the tomb were too large to have been brought down the passage from above, so the tomb and sarcophagus must have been planned from the beginning and incorporated into the base of the pyramid. A replica of this tomb can be seen in the National Museum in Mexico City.

To the north of Mexico City is Teotihuacan and near Puebla is Cholula. These two sites contain huge mounds or pyramids of clay and rock. The mound at Cholula has a greater volume than the Great Pyramid of Khufu (Cheops). All were ruined and distorted by the removal of the surface stones which were used in modern buildings and the clay cores slid during rains. Later reconstructions to prevent deterioration resulted in the structures as seen today. Both sites were begun in about 200 B.C. Teotihuacan was probably destroyed about 800-900 A.D., by the Toltecs, who then moved into the area. Cholula was still in use at the time of Cortez.

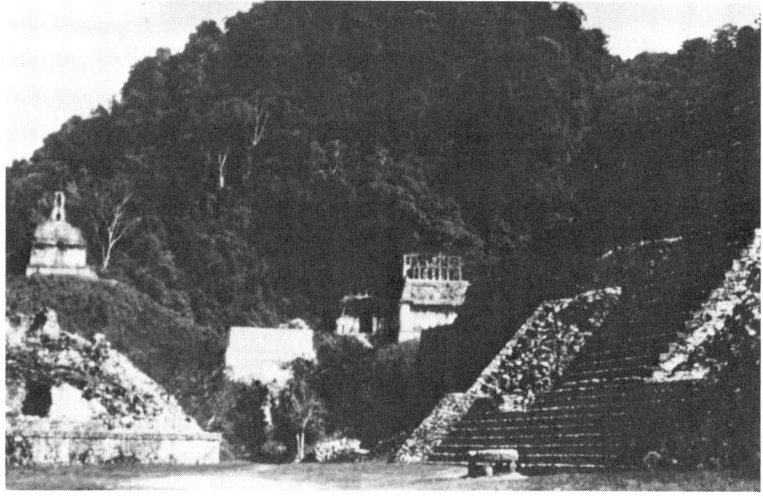

The ruins of Palenque, Chiapas, Mexico, cover approximately 15 square miles and was at its height about 700 A.D. The tomb of an important personage was found in the base of the large pyramid.

160 *Magic, Myths and Medicine*

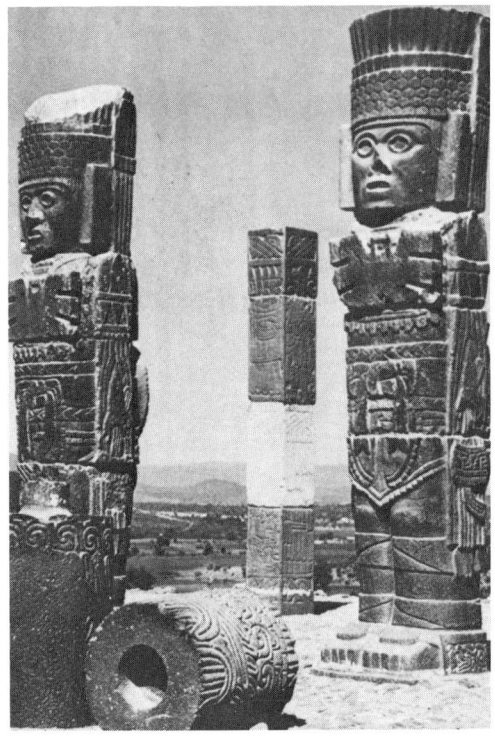

The ruins of Tula, Hidalgo, Mexico, believed to have been the capital of the Toltecs in about 900 A.D.

The Toltecs entered the valley of Mexico sometime before 900 A.D., sacked and destroyed Teotihuacan and later established their capital at Tula. Eventually they ruled a large part of Mexico and extended their influences as far away as Chichen Itza, in Yucatan. Their rule ended in 1168 A.D., and were supplanted by the Chichimecs, and other small groups.

The Aztecs, after settling on their islands in Lake Texcoco in about 1325 A.D., fought for the surrounding strong rulers until they became strong enough to stand by themselves, and Tenochtitlan grew in size and strength. About 1450, wars and famines led Moctezuma I of the Aztecs, to increase attacks on other groups as far away as Vera Cruz. His successors continued attacks near Guatemala and the Atlantic coast. One of these rulers, Ahuizotl, in ceremonies dedicating a temple to Huitzilopochtli, the Hummingbird Wizard, the Sun, sacrificed four lines of prisoners, each line being three miles long to the God of the Aztecs. This ruler died in about 1502, during a great famine, of a disease that caused him to become shrivelled and skeletonlike.

The son of Ahuizotl, Moctezuma II was elected to the throne after the death of his brother and although he had been a priest, he completed many successful military campaigns before Cortez changed the wheel of destiny. To understand how Cortez and his 550 men could take over a country, one must now examine some of the myths and religion of the Aztecs and other peoples of Mesoamerica.

There were many gods in the religions of ancient Mesoamerica which, as in other primitive cultures, can be generally divided into two groups; those who were concerned with agriculture and those who were part of the official religion of the priests and probably meant little to the average person. In general, each town and culture had a special deity as a specific patron and frequently, the deity was the same as that of another group but with a different name. Many of the gods had overlapping functions and fluidity which adds to the confusion surrounding their religions.

According to the mythology of the Aztecs, the world was created on the back of a crocodilelike monster by Tonacatecuhtli and his wife, Tonacacihuatl, the Lord and Lady of Sustenance. They produced four other creator-gods with the same name, Tezcatlipoca, but distinguished among them by color and direction as follows: blue, south or west; red, east; white, west; black, north. Later, other gods became important and were assigned these positions with frequent overlappings: Huitzilopochtli (sun, war, Aztec patron) and Tlaloc (rain) were associated with the blue color; Xipe Totec with the red; and Quetzalcoatl with the white.

Quetzalcoatl, represented as the Plumed Serpent, and called Kukulcan by the Maya, was one of the favorite gods of the peoples of Mesoamerica. Quetzalcoatl brought the bones of previous creations from the Underworld which, when mixed with the blood of the gods, became men. This seed of blood which started mankind was harvested as nourishment for the gods in human sacrifices just as mankind harvested crops in the field. He was also the god of the wind

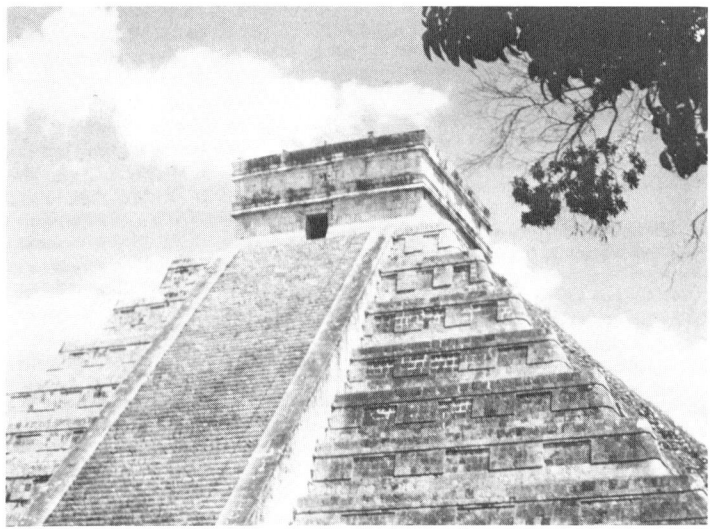

The Temple of Kukulkan (Quetzalcoatl) at Chichen Itza is 75 feet high. Each of the four stairways have 91 steps, totalling 364, and the platform on top makes 365. Each side contains 52 panels, the number of weeks in a year, and each side has 18 terraces, the number of months in the Mayan year.

and was responsible for diseases of the respiratory tract, god of life and fertility, the originator of the calendar, priestly rituals, and agricultural processes. Disguised as an ant, Quetzalcoatl stole corn from the ants and gave it to mankind for cultivation. It is interesting that the Hopi Indians, in their mythology, were saved when the First World was destroyed by fire by living underground with the Ant-people, who cared for them until the Second World was suitable for habitation. They worshipped the Earth and Corn Mother as a duality as did the Aztecs who called the deity, Tonantzin or Toci, (Our Mother). Quetzalcoatl was the main god of Cholula, where the largest temple in the world was dedicated to him. As Lord of the White Direction, he was pictured as wearing a beard, and was thought to be manifested in Cortez when he arrived in Mexico. This belief was founded upon a historical and religious legend which involved the god, Quetzalcoatl and a leader of the Toltecs, Ce Acatl Topiltzin (Our Prince) Quetzalcoatl.

The Toltecs were led into the valley of Mexico by Mixcoatl, who married Chimalma and had a child who was born on the day, Ce Acatl, named Topiltzin. The child was sent to a school for priests and later, due to his piety, was made a high priest of Quetzalcoatl. Thus his name was Ce Acatl Topiltzin Quetzalcoatl. Topiltzin eventually took over the leadership of the Toltecs and established their capital at Tula, where he attempted to convert the people from the worship of Tezcatlipoca to Quetzalcoatl. Tezcatlipoca (Smoking Mirror) was the most important god of the priests and was black, in color, and could assume any shape. He was portrayed as the night sky and the jaguar. One of his legs had been bitten off by a monster and was replaced by a mirror in which he could see anything in the world. He also represented the sacrificial knife and sacrificial blood. Topiltzin Quetzalcoatl was opposed to human sacrifices and attempted to change the religion of the Toltecs. He introduced new agricultural methods, new strains of corn and cotton, and the working of precious metals. In about 968 A.D., Topiltzin Quetzalcoatl left Tula, perhaps because of a lack of rain, or, according to legend, he had committed incest with his sister while drunk on pulque, and went to Cholula (Puebla). Here the history of the man and the religious legends of the god become confused; the two personalities merge as one; and shall be called Quetzalcoatl by the author. Quetzalcoatl remained for many years in Cholula and then, with some followers, went to the region of Vera Cruz. From here, he sent several messengers back to Cholula with the message that he would return from the direction of the rising sun on the date, Ce Acatl. Then Quetzalcoatl traveled to the south and arrived in the land of the Mayans in about 1000 A.D. There are many legends that tell of what then happened to Quetzalcoatl: he turned into the planet Venus; he threw himself onto a funeral pyre, the smoke of which turned into beautifully plumed birds; he sailed eastward into the ocean on a raft composed of intertwined serpents. However, the important story is that he would return on the date, Ce Acatl, and that was the approaching year of the calendar when Cortez arrived in Mexico. Archeology has proven the arrival of

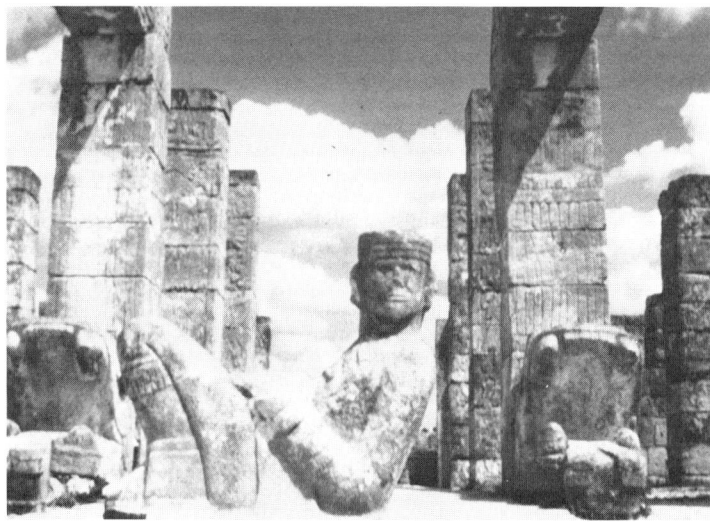

An altar of the water deity, Chac Mool, in the Temple of the Warriors, Chichen Itza, Yucatan, Mexico. The Toltecs, arriving about 1000 A.D., brought about a change in the architectural style of the Mayans. The city was abandoned in about 1200 A.D. A Steam bath and oven, with a drainage system are also included in this structure.

the Toltec influence in Mayan Yucatan at about 1000 A.D. It is also interesting that Moctezuma II had been a priest before his election to the throne and therefore was well aware of the legend of Quetzalcoatl and his promised return in Ce Acatl.

It is interesting how Moctezuma addressed Cortez at the time of their first meeting:

> "Long time have we been informed by the writings of our ancestors that neither myself nor any of those who inhabit this land are natives of it, but rather strangers who have come to it from foreign parts. We likewise know that from those parts our nation was led by a certain lord, to whom all were subject, and who then went back to his native land, where he remained so long delaying his return, that at his coming, those whom he had left married the women of the land and had had many children by them and had built themselves cities in which they lived, so that they would in no wise return to their own land nor acknowledge him as lord; upon which he left them. And we have always believed that among his descendants, one would surely come to subject this land and us as rightful vassals. Now, seeing the regions from which you say you come, which is from where the sun rises, and the news you tell of this great king and ruler who sent you hither, we believe and hold it certain that he is our natural lord: especially in that you say he has long had knowledge of us. Wherefore be certain that we will obey you and hold you as lord in place of that great lord of whom you speak, in which service there shall be neither slackness nor deceit: and throughout all the land, that is to say all that I rule, you may command anything you desire, and it shall be obeyed and done, and all that we have is at your will and pleasure."[1]

---

1. "The Letters of Hernando Cortez," translated by F. Bayard Morris, edited by Sir E. Denison Ross and Eileen Power, Robert M. McBride and Co., New York, 1929.

Cortez and his followers entered Tenochtitlan on November 8, 1519, and by August 13, 1521, had succeeded in the complete destruction of that city, and others. During the period of conquest and subjugation of the native population of Mesoamerica, Cortez and his Indian allies burned many towns, including their libraries. A systematic destruction of non-Christian buildings and books was instituted with the arrival of missionaries and members of the Inquisition, so that today, of the thousands of books or codices that were known to have existed, only seventeen remain from pre-Spanish Mexico. The first Archbishop of Mexico City, Zumarraga, reported the destruction of 500 temples, 20,000 statues and the library of Texcoco. In 1562, the second Bishop of Yucatan, de Landa reported the destruction of the library of the Mayan city of Mani. Only three Mayan codices have escaped destruction. Many of the Indians probably burned their books in order to escape the members of the Inquisition, who could enter any house or building in search of heretics or heretic materials.

The following quotations are from letters written by Cortez to the Emperor, Charles V, of Spain.[2]

"The great city of Tenochtitlan is built in the midst of this salt lake, and it is two leagues from the heart of the city to any point on the mainland. Four causeways lead to it, all made by hand and some twelve feet wide. The city itself is as large as Seville or Cordova. The principal streets are very broad and straight, the majority of them being of beaten earth, but a few and at least half the smaller thoroughfares are waterways along which they pass in their canoes. Moreover, even the principal streets have openings at regular distances so that the water can freely pass from one to another, and these openings which are very broad, are spanned by great bridges of huge beams, very stoutly put together, so firm indeed that over many of them, ten horsemen can ride at once.

"The city has many open squares in which markets are continuously held and the general business of buying and selling proceeds. One square in particular is twice as big as that of Salamanca and completely surrounded by arcades where there are daily more than sixty thousand folk buying and selling. Every kind of merchandise such as may be met with in every land is for sale there, whether of food and victuals, or ornaments of gold and silver, or lead, brass, copper, tin, precious stones, bones, shells, snails and feathers; limestone for building is likewise sold there, stone both rough and polished, bricks burnt and unburnt, wood of all kinds and in all stages of "preparation." There is a street of game where they sell all manner of birds that are to be found in their country, including hens, partridges, quails, wild duck, fly-catchers, widgeon, turtle doves, pigeons, little birds in round nests made of grass, parrots, owls, eagles, vulcans, sparrowhawks and kestrels; and of some of these birds of prey they sell the skins complete with feathers, head, bill and claws. They also sell rabbits, hares, deer and small dogs which they breed especially for eating.

"There is a street of herb-sellers where there are all manner of roots and medicinal plants that are found in the land. There are houses as it were of

---

2. "The Letters of Hernando Cortez," translated by F. Bayard Morris, edited by Sir E. Denison Ross and Eileen Power, Robert M. McBride and Co., New York, 1929.

apothecaries where they sell medicines made from these herbs, both for drinking and for use as ointments and salves. There are barber shops where you may have your hair washed and cut. There are other shops where you may obtain food and drink.

"All kinds of vegetables may be found there, in particular onions, leeks, garlic, cresses, watercress, borage, sorrel, artichokes, and golden thistles. There are many different sorts of fruits including cherries and plums very similar to those found in Spain. They sell honey obtained from bees, as also the honeycomb and that obtained from maize plants which are as sweet as sugar canes; they also obtain honey from plants which are known both here and in other parts as 'maguey,' which is preferable to grape juice; from 'maguey,' in addition, they make both sugar and a kind of wine, which are sold in their markets.

"There are a very large number of mosques or dwelling places for their idols throughout the various districts of this great city, all fine buildings, in the chief of which their priests live continuously, so that in addition to the actual temples containing idols there are sumptuous lodgings. These pagan priests are all dressed in black and go habitually with their hair uncut; they do not even comb it from the day they enter the order to that on which they leave. Chief men's sons, both nobles and distinguished citizens, enter these orders at the age of six or seven and only leave when they are of an age to marry, and this occurs more frequently to the firstborn who will inherit their father's estates than to others. They are denied all access to women, and no woman is ever allowed to enter one of the religious houses. Certain foods they abstain from and more so at certain periods of the year than at others. Among these temples there is one chief one in particular whose size and magnificence no human tongue could describe. For it is so big that within the lofty wall which entirely circles it one could set a town of fifteen thousand inhabitants.

"Certain of the priests but not all are permitted to enter, and within are the great heads and figures of idols, although as I have said there are also many outside. The greatest of these idols and those in which they placed most faith and trust I ordered to be dragged from their places and flung down the stairs, which done I had the temples which they occupy cleansed, for they were full of the blood of human victims who had been sacrificed, and placed in them the image of Our Lady and other saints, all of which made no small impression upon Muteczuma and the inhabitants.

"The images of the idols in which these people believed are many times greater than the body of a large man. They are made from pulp of all the cereals and greenstuffs which they eat, mixed and pounded together. This mass they moisten with blood from the hearts of human beings which they tear from their breasts while still alive, and thus make sufficient quantity of the pulp to mould into their huge statues: and after the idols have been set up still they offer them more living hearts which they sacrifice in like manner and anoint their faces with the blood. Each department of human affairs has its particular idol after the manner of the ancients who thus honoured their gods: so that there is one idol from whom they beg success in war, another for crops, and so on for all their needs.

"Along one of the causeways connecting this great city with the mainland, two pipes are constructed of masonry, each two paces broad and about as high as a man, one of which conveys a stream of water very clear and fresh and about the thickness of a man's body right to the center of the city, which all can use for drinking and other purposes. The other pipe which is empty is used when it is desired to clean the former.

"Another palace of his (Moctezuma), not quite so fine as the one we were lodged in, had a magnificent garden with balconies overhanging it, the pillars and flagstones of which were all jasper beautifully worked. In this palace there was room to lodge two powerful princes with all their retinue. There were also ten pools of water in which were kept every kind of waterfowl known in these parts, fresh water being provided for the river birds, salt for those of the sea, and the water itself being frequently changed to keep it pure: every species of bird, moreover, was provided with its own natural food. . . . In one room of this palace he kept men, women and children, who had been white since their birth, face, body, hair, eyebrows and eyelashes. Other large rooms on the ground floor were full of cages made of stout wood very firmly put together and containing large numbers of lions, tigers, wolves, foxes and wild cats of various kinds; these were also given as many chickens as they wanted. In another palace he had men and women monsters, among them dwarfs, hunchbacks and others deformed in various ways, each manner of monster being kept in a separate apartment, and likewise with guards charged with looking after them.

"I (Cortez) myself with some twenty horse went to sleep that night at Cholula. The natives had asked me to go there, since many of their chief men had died of the smallpox which rages in these lands as it does in the Islands, and they wished me with their approval and consent to appoint other rulers in their place.

"On entering Tezcuco this time we had found the skins, hoofs and horse-shoes nailed up on the walls of some of their temples and placed there very carefully as a sign of victory, together with many clothes and other belongings of the Spaniards, which they had offered to their idols. The very blood of our companions and brothers was strewn and sacrificed all over their idol towers, which was so piteous sight that it renewed in our minds all our past troubles.

"All that I (Cortez) could think of was to burn their houses and the towers in which they kept their idols. Accordingly that day, that they might feel it the more, I ordered the large houses surrounding the square to be set on fire, those houses, namely, in which we had fortified ourselves when we were besieged in the city and which were large enough to contain the native chieftan and some six hundred of his retinue; we also burnt certain smaller ones hard by still more elaborate and finely worked, in which Muteczuma had been wont to keep all his birds. I was much grieved to do this, but since it was still more grievous to them, I determined on burning them.

"That night our native allies dined well enough, for all those that we killed they cut into pieces and took off with them to eat."

Fortunately, the missionaries also reported on the customs and practices of the Indians whom they were converting to Christianity, so many excellent reports exist on these subjects. Others regretted the destruction and gathered as much information concerning the language; writings and beliefs as possible, so some restitution was made. Hundreds of post-conquest manuscripts are known to exist, some written by Indians and some by Spaniards; some in the local language and some in Spanish. Cortez and Diaz both wrote about the conquest of Mexico and in 1570, Hernandez came to Mexico and prepared an herbal of Mexican plants. In 1931, Professor Charles Clark reported that he had discovered an Aztec herbal in the Vatican Library, America's oldest medical book, the Badianus Manuscript, which is dated to 1552.

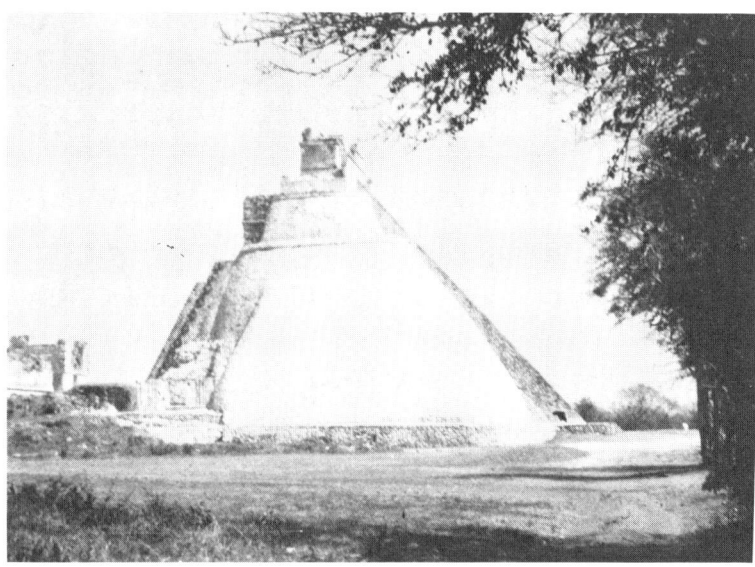

The temple of the Magician (Dwarf) at Uxmal, Yucatan, Mexico, believed to have been built by the Mayans in about 1007 A.D. The two temples at the summit are believed to have been used for astronomical observations.

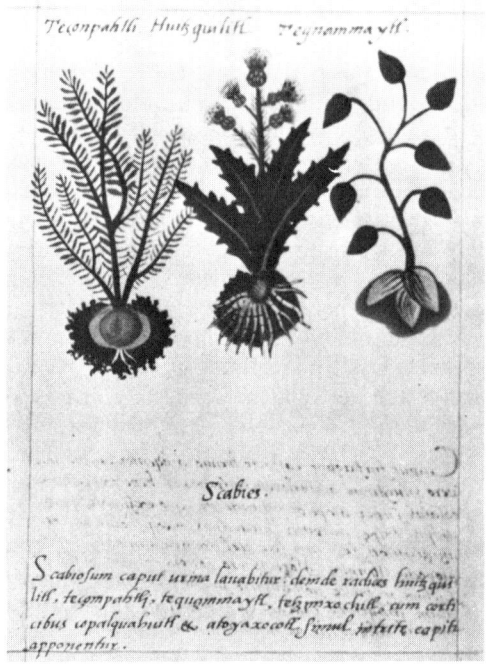

The Badianus Manuscript, an Aztec Herbal of 1552, plate 10. "The scabious head should be washed with urine;" and afterwards, ground roots and barks were applied to the head. (Photograph reproduced from "The Badianus Manuscript" by Cruz, translation and annotations by Emmart, The Johns Hopkins Press, Baltimore, Md.)

The Badianus Manuscript was first written in Aztec by Martinus de la Cruz, an Indian physician of the College of Santa Cruz, and was then translated into Latin by an associate, Juannes Badianus, in 1552. The book is mainly an herbal dealing with the pharmacological treatment of diseases with the aid of charms of various stones and parts of animals. The Christian author omitted the use of incantations to the native gods which were known to be in use prior to the conversion of the population to Christianity. This book is considered to be the only known medical text of Aztec origin that was not influenced by European medicine. The herbal is arranged into thirteen chapters, each of which deals with the afflictions of the various parts of the body, from the head to the feet. Included, are brightly colored drawings of the medicinal plants under discussion, with their Aztec names, which, after the discovery of the manuscript, greatly aided in the identification of the herbs involved.

The Indian nobility were noted for their beautiful gardens and collections of plants, many of which were utilized by physicians in the treatment of diseases. These gardens were described by Cortez and Diaz at the time of the conquest, and later by Dr. Cervantes de Salazar (1565), Friar Motolinia, Dr. Francisco Hernandez. The following quotation refers to the gardens of Moctezuma. It was written by Dr. Salazar, translated by Zelia Nuttall, and appears in a translation of the Badianus Manuscript by Emily W. Emmart.[3]

> "This great monarch had many pleasances and spacious gardens with paths and channels for irrigation. These gardens contained only medicinal and aromatic herbs, flowers, native roses, and trees with fragrant blossoms, of which there are many kinds. He ordered his physicians to make experiments with the medicinal herbs and to employ those best known and tried as remedies in healing the ills of the lords of his court. These gardens gave great pleasure to all who visited them on account of the flowers and roses they contained and of the fragrance they gave forth, especially in the mornings and evenings. It was well worth seeing with how much art and delicacy a thousand figures of persons were made by means of leaves and flowers, also the seats, chapels and other constructions which so greatly adorned these places.
>
> "In these flower gardens Montezuma did not allow any vegetables or fruit to be grown, saying that it was not kingly to cultivate plants for utility or profit in his pleasance. He said that vegetable gardens and orchards were for slaves or merchants. At the same time he owned such, but they were at a distance, and he seldom visited them."

The following diseases and treatments were selected from Emmart's translation of the Badianus Manuscript. The Aztec names of the plants are utilized in the translation but, unfortunately, many have not been properly identified. Whenever possible, the author has identified the plant and its medicinal uses, as known today.

---

3. "The Badianus Manuscript," (Introduction, Translations and Annotations by Emily Walcott Emmart, The Johns Hopkins Press, Baltimore, Md., 1940.

"Boils: Leaves of the herb 'tlantlanquaye,' the root 'tlalhaueuetl' (*Acalypha*-euphorbic, purgative, emetic, antiarthritic), 'tlayapaloni' and 'chipahuacxihuitl' (*Dioscorea*—wild yam, diaphoretic, emetic), well ground with yolk of eggs without water, are applied daily, in the morning of course, and at evening too, to boils of the head which have been carefully cleansed of the pus; when this has been done the head is to be well covered. But if only in some one part of the head festers, then it is to be washed with urine and the same medicine is to be applied."[4]

"Glaucoma (an incorrect title for a fleshy growth): Pierce with a needle a fleshy growth in the eye, loosen it and draw it out, and sprinkle the white of the eye with burnt human excrement and salt, a little at a time. Then, next day apply to it sundried and ground roots of native acid herbs." (Probably refers to *Begonia*)[5]

"For Cough: One troubled with cough is to drink frequently the juice of the root of 'tlacoxiloxochitl' (stalky cornsilk flower, *Calliandra,* antiperiodic, antifever) peeled and ground in water, with part of which, mixed with honey, the 'hroat is to be smeared. But if he spits blood, he is to take this same drink before the midday meal. And it would be somewhat useful if he would merely nibble the same root in honey and chew it. The root of the herb called 'tzopelicacococ' (*Lippia*-Yerba dulce, contains camphor, expectorant, demulcent) ground in tempid water is also useful to one who has a cough. He is to drink the juice or nibble on the root."[6]

"For Glands or Spongy Swellings: Glands are to be cut with lancet or razor, and when they are cut all the sanies (discharge) is to be very carefully removed, and a plaster is to be put on the cut place. And it is to consist of the leaves of the small herb 'tonatiuhyxiuh, which springs up in the summer, and 'tolohua' (*Datura*—jimson weed, narcotic, antispasmodic, contains hyoscyamine and atropine), ground in yolk of egg."[7]

"Bladderwort or Halicacabus (stoppage of the urinary passage): When the urinary meatus is closed up, to open it the stalk of the herbs 'mamaxtla' and 'cohuanenepilli' (*Dahlia*), 'tlatlauhqui amoxtli,' the very white blossom of 'yolloxochitl' (*Talauma*), and the tail of the animal 'tlahquatl' (opossum) are ground in bitter-tasting water, with which is to be mixed the well-known 'chian' (*Saliva*) seed, which is also to be macerated in the same."

"The abdomen is to be washed with the juice, infused with a clyster, of the stalk of the herb 'ohuaxocoyolin' ground in hot water. If this medicine does no good, it is necessary that the pith of a very slender palm made up with a little piece of cotton and smeared with honey and with the root of the ground herb 'huihuitzmallotic,' be taken and very cautiously put into the well of virility; for thus the stoppage of the urine will be opened."[8]

4, 5, 6, 7, 8. *op. cit.*, pgs. 211, 221, 240, 246, 263, 306.

"How One Who Has Been Affected by a Whirlwind or Bad Wind is to Be Treated: Let one who has been caught in a whirlwind drink the wholesome juice of the herb 'quauhyayaual,' 'acxoyatl' (fir tree), branches of pine and laurel, ground in water. The juice is to be boiled. Let him drink the decoction; for if drunk it drives out the bad air invading the inside. Secondly, he is to drink the juice of stones ground in water, a red crystal, a white pearl, whitish earth, and leaves of the herb 'tlatlanquaye' (*Capsicum*—red pepper), which you are to boil together with incense. Anoint him with the carefully prepared liquid of the cones of cypress and cedar, and of the leaves of the 'quauhyyauhtli' tree, as well as the leaves of the herb 'xiuhecapahtli,' crushed in water with incense."[9]

"Phthiriasis (lice infestation) of the Head: A medicament made of the root of the shrub 'zohzoyatic' (*Agave,* or *Yucca* or *Veratrum*—hellebore, antipruritic, parasiticide) crushed in water of acrid taste, the herb 'yztauhyatl,' the fat or suet of a goose, the head of a mouse burned to ashes, the straw taken from a swallow's nest, which you are to crush also; this medicament you are to pour on the head."[10]

"The wise physician foretells from the very eyes and nostrils of the sick man whether he is going to die or live. And so according to his probable opinion, if the eyes still have the redness of blood, they are an indutable indication of life, if they are pale and bloodless, of uncertain recovery. The signs of death are: a certain sooty color found in the middle of the eyes, the top of the head becoming cold or contracting into a certain depression, the eyes becoming black and having little sparkle, the nose becoming thin and pointed, as it were, like a rod, the jaws becoming rigid, the tongue cold, the teeth disintegrating and covered with much tartar and no longer able to move and separate. The very gritting of the teeth and when a vein is lanced a flow of blood that is either pale or black are heralds of coming death. Furthermore: the face becoming pale, black and putting on and assuming now one expression, now another, and finally, if he, like parrots, rolls, pours out and repeats unintelligible words in no order.

"But in a woman one especial prognostic has been observed, namely, if her buttocks, calves and sides feel pricked as it were by a very sharp thorn.

"Yet when we have despaired of and given up all hope of recovery, even then you can drop into the dying man's eyes a medicine carefully made of the precious stones tlahcalhuatzin' (bird stone), 'eztetl' (bloodstone-jasper), a pearl and a white pearl, whitish earth ground together in water.

"You shall anoint the breast with a liquid made of pine crushed in water, laurel and the herb 'tonatiuhyxiuh' (Sun god's dew plant), which you are to pluck in the summer and save for this time. You are to prick the breast with a sharpened bone of a wolf, that of an eagle or of a white lion or of the lion whose skin is variegated, distinguished and sprinkled with black color. On the buttocks you shall suspend an eagle's heart concealed and wrapped in a stagskin.

9, 10. *op. cit.*, pgs. 246, 263, 306, 313.

"Finally you shall give him to drink a potion of precious stones, a white pearl, a very green pearl, an emerald, whitish earth, the moss of stones found in the forest and 'tlahcalhuatzin' (bird stone), all of which you are to grind together. Likewise of the cones of the cypress, the leaves of the laurel, the herbs 'tlanextiaxihuitl,' 'tonatiuhyxiuh,' which has an excellent golden gleam, the 'quetzalaylin' tree, and the stones which you are to seek in the stomach of the birds: eagle, quail, swallow, rooster, diver, wryneck, 'quecholtototl,' 'tlapaltototl,' 'nochtototl,' 'huitlatotl,' and dove, all of which you are to grind. But when the fatal necessity is close and we are near to dying, an abundant flow of blood pours over the heart, with the passing of which into all the members we finish our mortality." [11]

The previous quotations indicate that the medicinal beliefs of the Aztecs were basically the same as those of Europe at that time. Various herbs were utilized by physicians in an attempt to cure diseases, some of which proved to be effective. In addition, charms such as precious stones, pearls and animal-stones (bezoars) were utilized in the New World just as they were in the Old World. However, missing from these examples are those concerned with the religious beliefs of the peoples of Mesoamerica.

Before the Spanish conquest, the medicinal beliefs were, as in other ancient civilizations, closely associated with religious beliefs. The gods of the elements and seasons caused natural disasters which were frequently accompanied by certain diseases, and which could be prevented or cured by appeals and sacrifices to the god associated with the disaster or sickness. Since different areas and cultures had different gods, virtually all the gods of ancient Mexico had a dual role in which they dispensed diseases and healed the sick.

Xipe Totec, the Flayed One, was regarded by the Aztecs as the god of spring planting, harvesting and pulque. He had been a god of the Zapotecs, Xipe, the goddess of fire and vengeance, who caused diseases of the eyes, itching and abscesses. The Zapotecs had a goddess of medicine, Tzapotlatenan. The Aztecs converted the goddess of the Zapotecs, Xipe, into the god, Xipe Totec, and considered him the teacher of medicine and also one who could cause diseases, especially of the skin. Each year a great feast was held in his honor at which victims were sacrificed and then flayed, and the priests then drew the human skins over their bodies for further religious rituals. It was believed that diseases of the skin could be transferred to the skin of the sacrificed victim.

Toci (Tonantzin, Centeotl), Our Grandmother, was a harvest goddess who was also associated with the moon, childbirth and medicinal herbs. Doctors, midwives and shamans regarded her as the guardian of medicine and medicinal herbs. Sacrificial victims, in her honor, were thrown from a great height onto a pile of rocks and then had the heart removed as an offering.

---

11. *op. cit.*, pgs. 323, 324.

At the time of the conquest, medicine was practiced by physicians, surgeons, midwives, herbalists and shamans. Theoretical instruction was given to physicians by the priests but the practical teaching of medicine was generally passed from father to son, or to an apprentice. The chief therapeutic measures were venesection, baths, scarification, enemas, suppositories, urethral injections, snuffs, perfumes, inhalations, purgatives, diaphoretics, sedatives, narcotics, diuretics, aphrodisiacs, poisons, antidotes and medicinal herbs. Religion, magic, and astronomy and astrology were also utilized. Broken bones were set and immobilized with a caste made of gums, resins, feathers and eggs that hardened and was further strengthened with splints. Cuts or wounds were sewn together with hair, were washed with liquids, and dressed with honey, salt and various herbs. Embryotomy was practiced but the permission of the female's parents was required prior to the performance of the surgery.

Fray Bernardino de Sahagun of the College of Santa Cruz at Tlaltelulco, between 1529-1590, recorded many observations of Mexico and the people. The following is concerned with women doctors.

> "The woman doctor is well versed in the knowledge and preparation of herbs, trees and stones; in the knowledge of those things in which she has experience and she does not ignore the many secrets of medicine. She who is a good doctor knows how to cure sickness and always brings them back from death to life, and with the cures which she composes makes them better and convalescent. She knows how to bleed, give physic, administer medicaments, rub the body to soften up hardened parts, to set bones, to clean and cure ulcers, the gout, diseases of the eyes, and to cut out fleshy growths of them.
>
> "The one who is a bad doctor uses witchery, is superstitious in her trade and has made a pact with a demon. She knows how to give drinks which kill men. She does not know the cures; instead of curing she sickens and still worse, puts in danger the life of those who are ill and finally kills them. And so she fools the people with her witchery by blowing upon the painful part, by tying and untying strings, gazing on water and throwing grains of corn which she uses in her divinations, saying that by them she is able to know and understand the kind of illness. In order to emphasize her superstitious practices, she pretends to extract worms from teeth and paper and flint from other parts of the body. In extracting all this she, being false and superstitious, says that she destroys the illness." [12]

Hygiene was at a fairly high level, at least in Tenochtitlan, where aqueducts or pipes brought fresh water to the city; the streets were cleaned and swept. Garbage was collected and taken to the mainland, as was the material removed from the public toilets. Hot, cold and mineral baths were available, as were pharmacies and barbershops.

Moctezuma not only had a large botanical and zoological collection in his palace, he also had a collection of deformed, dwarfed and crippled people, perhaps just as curiosities, but it is not certain. The extent of the Aztec knowledge of anatomy is unknown.

---

12. Sahagun, pg. 36, Vol. 3, Bustamente, 1830. Cited in the Badianus Manuscript, Emily Walcott Emmart, The Johns Hopkins Press, Baltimore, Md., 1940, pg. 48.

The contributions of Mesoamerica to Europe at this time were mainly cheap labor, precious metals and stones, and a variety of plant or plant derivatives. Sarsaparilla, obtained from the root of *Smilax mexicana,* contains the glucoside parillin, a diuretic, which later would be administered by the Europeans with iodides and mercurials in the treatment of syphilis. The seeds of *Theobroma cacao* were used to make cacao, chocolate and cacao butter. Chocolate was considered an aphrodisiac when it was introduced into Europe and was especially used then and now as a flavoring in drinks and desserts. Cacao butter is still used in various suppositories. The Mexican cactus, *Anhalonium,* produced peyotl (peyote) a drug that produces a state of intoxication and ecstasy and was used by the priests and shamans in order to predict the future and the outcome of diseases and treatments. The night-blooming cereus, *Cactus grandiflorus,* contains compounds which act as spinal, cardiac and vasomotor stimulants. The century plant, *Agave mexicana* was, and still is, cultivated for its fibers, as roofing material, as a food, as a sweetener and for its juices, which, when fermented, are called aquamiel or pulque. The juice may also be used as a laxative and diuretic. The tobacco plant, *Nicotiana,* was sacred to the Aztecs, and was used as a medicine and in religious rituals. Tobacco contains several compounds of medicinal importance, especially nicotine, an alkaloid which is exceedingly poisonous, but which has been used as an antitetanic agent and in treating strychnine poisoning. The *Guaiacum* tree yielded a resin which was highly valued by the Europeans and was sent to Europe in vast quantities where it was regarded as a cure for many diseases, especially syphilis. It was used as an expectorant and diaphoretic, as an empyreumatic, as a stimulant, as an eye anesthetic, as an antiseptic and in the treatment of tuberculosis and rheumatism. Ipecac, or ipecacuanha, is derived from a variety of rubiaceous *Cephaelis* plants and is still used today as a local irritant, emetic, expectorant, diaphoretic and stimulant. It is frequently used as an emetic because it is unaffected by gastric juices in the stomach and remains inactive until reaching the small intestine and can be administered in large doses without causing nausea or vomiting.

Strychnine is a bitter, poisonous alkaloid derived from the seeds of *Strychnos nux vomica,* which was extracted by Indians, especially in South America, and used as an arrow poison. It acts as a powerful stimulant to the central nervous system. Curare, used in a like manner, was prepared from several species of *Strychnos* and *Chondodendron* plants. An extract of *Chondodendron tomentosum* paralyses the skeletal muscles.

Other contributions include corn, a wide variety of beans, chilli (chili) peppers, pumpkins, squash, calabash, tomatoes, popcorn, peanuts, chewing gum from the chicle of the sapodilla tree, sweet potatoes, a variety of nuts, egg plant, pineapples, many berries, avocado, papaya, vanilla, coriander, sage, cascara, sassafras, dyes such as indigo, cochineal, from the insect *Coccus cacti,* was used as a red dye and in the treatment of nervous affections, and royal purple from the Pacific coast *Molluksko,* rubber, sisal and others.

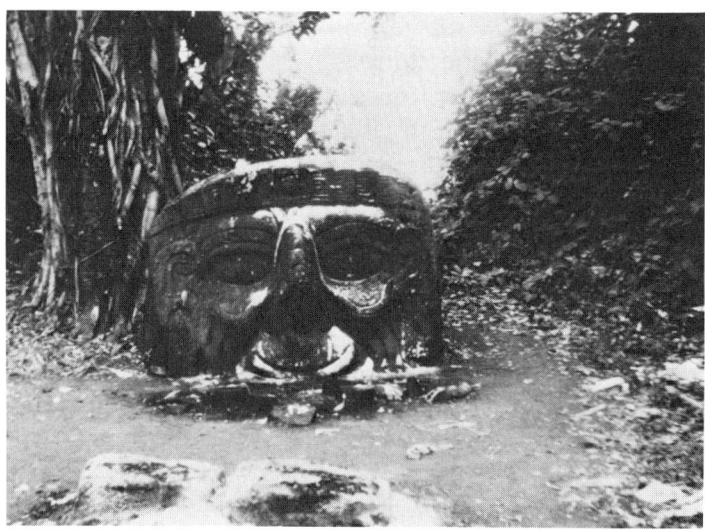

An unexcavated site at El Baul, Guatemala situated on a large mound in an agricultural area. The half-buried head was surrounded with corn-husks, flowers, wax from candles and the ashes of fires which indicate that the site is still used for some religious ceremonies.

Indians of North America

At the time of the conquest of Mexico, to the north, were many Indian tribes which never adopted large scale urban living and architectural achievements as did their neighbors to the south. These widespread peoples had more than 50 unrelated linguistic stocks and over 700 dialects, with no common vocabulary or grammatical structure and no phonetic writing, although pictographs were used.

One of the most important members of these separated groups was the medicine man. Socially, the medicine man ranked next to the Chief and he was greatly respected by members of the tribe, since he acted as a healer, or seer, or both. A healer described what caused an ailment; attempted to cure the sick; treated battle wounds caused by clubs, knives and arrows; and later, bullet wounds. A seer could look into the future and foretell what would happen to a person, the tribe or the hunting party. The medicine man had "supernatural powers" which he received from a "dream person" who instructed him concerning the various herbs and remedies to be used in the treatment of diseases or wounds. These visions or meetings were usually brought about by fasting and meditation. Medicinal teas were made from herbs, tree bark and leaves, which when ground, could also be mixed with fat or honey and applied to the body as salves. Charms and talismans were also utilized to ward off diseases and death. The medicine man usually wore a distinct costume which set him apart from the other members of the tribe and carried a medicine bag filled with charms, medicines, and paints, with which he carried out his profession. These bags were highly valued and were passed from father to son. Successors were selected from the members of the tribe who had frequent visions and seemed to qualify for the position. The pupil lived with the medicine man until he had learned all the medicinal rituals and songs; then he was allowed to perform alone and work as an additional medicine man. Frequently, they would work together on important cases or events.

Among the Sioux, it was believed that, before birth, their medicine men lived among the Thunders. Some medicine men specialized in visions; healings; wounds; snakebites; and intestinal ailments. Magic was used in some treatments, especially the procedure of sucking at various parts of the patient's body until a splinter or stone, which had been previously hidden in the mouth of the medicine man, was found, and was supposed to have been the reason for the pain or illness. Some of the medicine men could carry burning cornhusks or put their hands into boiling water, with no apparent signs of burning or pain. Boiling water rituals are still carried out in Hindu and Shinto rituals and the firewalkers of Asia are still well-known. It has been documented by some British investigators that the firewalkers could walk on a surface where the heat reached 1550°F., without burns, as long as they had to take no more than two steps on each foot. If more than two steps were taken, the foot was burned. However, not all treatments were magical and the medicine men utilized massage, bleedings, herbs, fumigations, sweat lodges, the sewing of wounds and the setting of broken bones.

The Iroquois believed that the "Great Maker," after he created the first man, caused him to strike his face against a mountain, which distorted his face so that he was called "Crooked Face." Crooked Face was directed to protect man against all causes of diseases and became known as the "Helper" or "Our Grandfather." He instructed the people on the methods used to conduct medicinal ceremonies and carved a false-face for them, in his likeness, for use in the ceremonies. The power of the mask grew as his instructions spread through the land and gradually, replicas were made and the False-face Society, which still exists today, was formed. Contrary to most cultures, the leader of the False-face Society was a woman who represented the Earth-Mother. During ceremonies she carried a miniature false-face, a corn husk mask and a turtle shell rattle, which was the symbol for a long life. All the masks were carved from living trees and represented terrifying characters so as to frighten away evil spirits that were causing the disease being treated. A red mask with a ridged forehead was the "Doctor" or Medicine Mask which had the power to drive away diseases. The Iroquois relied more upon their magic than actual medicines.

Apache medicine men, like those of many other cultures, were magicians and clairvoyants. Frequently they were called upon to find lost or stolen articles and sometimes could name the thief. They were especially important during times of war, when they were responsible for the preparations and ceremonies, and of course, during times of sickness. Chantings and the methodical beating of a drum were used to hypnotize a patient into a deep sleep and, possibly, a cure. Of special importance to the people was the pollen of the "tule" plant, a cattail. The pollen was ground into a powder and was carried around the neck in a small pouch. The powder, called "Hoddentin," was blown from the fingers toward the rising sun, and also to the moon, the stars and special animals. It was believed to represent the Milky Way which was caused by the Great Spirit spilling the powder through the heavens. The powder was applied in various ways to the bodies of people who were ill.

Medicine men of the Navaho obtained their medicine or magic by collecting herbs, seeds and grasses and burying them in the ground in a newly fashioned medicine mound. Prayer sticks were stuck into the mound and the medicine man would spend five days and nights, fasting and sleeping by the mound. He would pray to the Ancient Ones for their assistance and hoped that the medicine, and himself, would grow stronger and stronger. Ceremonies for the making of medicine might last from one to nine days, the longer the time spent, the more important the medicine. The Mountain Chant lasted for nine days and was carried out to heal the sick and to bring all those involved into close contact with the Gods. Patients were cleansed and purified by washing with yucca suds, sweat baths and emetics. Many of the ceremonies involved the use of sand paintings. The War Eagle God originally drew pictures on the clouds and later, taught the Indians how to draw them on the ground, using colored sands. The sand paintings had to be started at dawn and destroyed before sunset so that they could not be used during the night by evil spirits. During the ceremony, the patient was seated in the center of the sand painting so that the power of the Gods could be transmitted to him.

The Totem Indians of the American Northwest, like many other cultures, believed that each person had a spiritual helper who, if contacted, could help the person to achieve great wealth, power and fame. It was believed that the greatest gift that a person could receive was the power to cause or cure illness. A person who claimed to have this power was called a shaman, which is a Siberian word meaning medicine man. The shaman could be a male or female and they generally worked their charms and magic in "spirit houses," which were constructed with double walls, trap doors, hollow tubes of kelp and other constructions in order that they could magically appear and disappear and cause voices to apparently come out of the air.

The Indians of North America were not known for their great knowledge of medicines or surgery but they apparently were able to combat the endemic diseases with various herbal remedies and many of the early European settlers in this country had to utilize Indian remedies, since there were no physicians here with medicines. Some of the simple remedies used were sassafras, oil of wintergreen and birch oil, which in the hands of Europeans became root beer. Capsicum, sarsaparilla, ginger, vanilla and allspice were converted into cream soda, ginger ale and other refreshing beverages.

Teas were made from a large number of plants and were used as stimulants, emetics and diuretics. Most frequently used were the *Ceanothus;* the *Ledum;* the holly, *Ilex;* the goldenrod, *Solidago;* the fern, *Monarda;* the wintergreen, *Gualtheria;* the cathartic may-apple root; *Podophyllum;* the purgative jalap root, *Ipomoea;* the emetic, white hellebore, *Helleborus;* and *Cascara.*

Fevers were treated with a variety of barks that acted as quinine but of much less strength: dogwood bark, *Cornus florida;* cherry bark, *Prunus;* poplar bark, *Populus;* centaury plants, *Erythraea, Centaurea* and *Sabbatia;* and boneset, *Eupatorium perfoliatum.*

The most widely used vermifuge in North America was the pinkroot, *Spigelia marilandica.* Others included the Jerusalem oak, *Chenopodium ambrosioides;* roots of the wild plum, *Prunus americana;* roots of the wild cherry, *P. serotina;* the horsemint, *Monarda mollis;* and the turkey pea, *Tephrosia virginiana.*

A variety of poisonous plants were known and were utilized as poisons to kill, commit suicide or to bring about sleep. Commonly used were the may-apple root, *Podophyllum peltatum;* the black nightshade, *Solanum nigrum.*

Many of the previously discussed plant materials contain substances which are useful in the treatment of certain conditions. When they were utilized by the early settlers of the United States, Indian medicine and medicine men were frequently credited with great curative powers. Consequently, "medicine" shows traveled throughout the country, selling medicines that were supposed to cure virtually everything, and were based upon secret Indian remedies. Actually, all they usually contained were alcohol and colorings. Approximately 170 drugs were, and some still are, in the "Pharmacopeia of the United States of America," which were known to have been utilized by Indian medicine men. There are still medicine men in the remaining Indian tribes in North America and frequently they take their patients to physicians and hospitals for professional treatment in conjunction with their own methods of healing.

It is believed that the Indians were free of the disease tuberculosis until they came in contact with the European migrants. Then, and now, they have a high incidence of infection. The causative agents are bacteria, *Mycobacterium tuberculosis, M. bovis,* and other members of this *Genus,* which cause a wide variety of symptoms and lesions in man and animals. Laennec, in 1819, described tuberculosis lesions and Villemin, in 1865, transmitted tuberculosis among man, cattle and rabbits. However, it was not until 1882 that Koch discovered the microorganism, *M. tuberculosis*, that is usually the cause of infections in pulmonary cases, whereas *M. bovis* s usually involved in tuberculosis of the bones, joints, and cervical lymphadentitis. After infection, the bacteria multiply unopposed in the body due to their production of a toxic effect on phagocytic white blood cells, but later, multiplication is restricted due to the development of resistance, and the bacteria become contained within lesions or tubercles. Some bacteria remain alive within the contained lesions or tubercles and when the resistance of the host decreases, the disease may develop again. In the United States, the primary infection is usually in the lungs, but in countries where milk is consumed without being pasteurized (Louis Pasteur, 1822-95), the primary infection is usually in the intestines and cervical lymph nodes. In about 1900, tuberculosis was one of the leading causes of death in the United States but now, due to Public Health measures and drug therapy, the disease has disappeared from the list of the ten most frequent causes of death in the United States. However, the disease is still present in the population. San Francisco, California, a city with a mixed population of about 750,000 whites, blacks, Indians, Chinese, Japanese and others, has a case rate of approximately 300 new cases per year, with the highest incidence in the Indians and the least in the whites. Throughout the world, the disease causes more deaths between the ages of 15 and 45 than any other disease, and may be the cause of more deaths today than any other disease. The disease can be controlled by finding, isolating and treating the infected person and destroying diseased animals. The drugs commonly used in the United States are Streptomycin, PAS (paraminosalicylic acid) and INH (isoniazid), which are administered together in order to destroy drug resistant organisms that frequently develop when Streptomycin is used alone. In various countries of the world, people have been immunized with killed or attenuated mycobacteria which can confer some protection against naturally acquired infections. The attenuated strain of *M. bovis,* BCG (Bacille Calmette-Guerin) is usually utilized in these immunization procedures. Many countries, such as the United States, do not have an active immunization program because of a low infection rate and the fact that once immunized, the person would have a positive skin test or Tuberculin test, which is one of the tests utilized in determining tuberculosis in the population.

However, a disease somewhat similar to tuberculosis, is found in arid regions of the Americas which may cause an acute respiratory disease. The causative agent is a mold, *Coccidiodies immitis,* which produces spores that are inhaled and which cause lesions in the lungs. Dissemination of the infection results in symptoms similar to those of tuberculosis. In whites, the disease is usually self-limiting, the infection resembling a cold or the flu, but in the darker-skinned peoples the infection frequently disseminates and death results. The infection was first described in Argentina in 1892 by Posadas and Wernicke and in 1894, in California, by Rixford, who named the mold. It occurs in the San Joaquin Valley of California where it is called Valley Fever, and other desert areas where it is called Desert Rheumatism. The mild form of the infection requires no treatment since it is usually not diagnosed until the patient has recovered. The disseminated infection has been treated with Dihydroxystilbamidine and Amphotericin B with some successes.

The Indians of North, Meso, and South America had a variety of common diseases and some that were unknown to the European conquerers who ventured there. The Europeans brought with them diseases that were unknown to the Indians and which caused many deaths in the population. Epidemics of smallpox, chicken pox, measles (little leprosy) decimated the natives of the Americas. Likewise, in Europe at this time, a disease called "the pox" came into prominence. The pox became epidemic in Western Europe at about the time of the voyages of Columbus to the New World and many believe that the disease was carried back to the Old World, from the New, by the travelers on these voyages. Others believe that syphilis was endemic in Europe and Africa for centuries prior to 1492 and became epidemic due to the movement of armies and peoples in the fifteenth and sixteenth centuries. However, if this were true, why did not the disease appear in about 300 A.D., when the Germanic tribes invaded the Roman Empire or when the Moslems, conquering from India to Europe, were halted at Tours, France, in 732, or during the Crusades? Others have speculated that Neanderthal man was simply *Homo sapiens,* distorted by infection with syphilis, since the bone changes which have been noted resemble those of congenital syphilis or rickets. Also, if syphilis were endemic in Europe and Africa prior to 1492, one would expect many examples to then be found in the numerous mummies of ancient Egypt. Examination of many Egyptian mummies has taken place and, to the knowledge of the author, no definite case of syphilis has been reported. There are too few examples of skeletons of man in North and Mesoamerica prior to 1492 to state whether or not syphilis was present in the population but, there are numerous mummified remains of Indians of South America which indicate endemic syphilis.

There are two diseases of man which are caused by microorganisms similar to the spirochete causing syphilis and which are morphologically indistinguishable from one another. These diseases are yaws and pinta.

Pinta is a disease found in tropical America and other parts of the world, the causative agent of which is *Treponema carateum,* a bacterial spirochete. The disease is characterized by the presence of colored spots on the skin from which the name is derived. It was originally thought to be a fungous infection until the spirochete was identified in 1938 by Saenz, Triana and Alfonso. This is not a venereal disease but is believed to be transmitted from person to person by direct contact or by flies. The infection is usually restricted to the skin but cardiac and central nervous system involvement has been reported. The infection is today treated with antibiotics, such as penicillin, as are yaws and syphilis. Prior to the introduction of antibiotics, arsenicals and mercurials were utilized in their treatments.

Treponema pertenue is the causative agent of Yaws, a disease of the skin and bones in which frambesial sores develop which gradually increase in size, erode and ulcerate. After the "mother yaw" heals, secondary lesions may develop and eventually may result in mutilation and incapacitation. Cardiac and involvement of the central nervous system have been reported. The disease is mainly restricted to tropical areas of the world with a high humidity. It is not a venereal disease and it is thought that flies and mosquitos, feeding on the ulcerative lesions, pick up the spirochete and may then infect the next host when biting. The organism cannot penetrate the intact skin, so there must be a mechanical breaking of the skin to bring about infection. There is a yawlike treponemal disease found in monkeys. Other local names for yaws are bejel, siti and njovera, pian and framboesia.

The Pox received the name Syphilis as the result of a medical poem published in 1530 by the Veronese physician, Fracastorius (Fracastoro), entitled, "Syphilis sive Morbus Gallicus," and which concerned a young man named Syphilis, who contracted the infection then called the pox. At that time, the spirochete was extremely virulent and many people died of the infection in the early stages of the disease. Today, the mild course of the infection is regarded as being due to a decrease in virulency, a change in the organism, or perhaps the gradual development of resistance in man. If the latter were ture, then isolated tribes, such as those recently found in the Philippines, New Guinea and South America, would develop, if infected, the old, rapidly fatal, form of the disease. A new parasite, when introduced to a new host, if it survives in the host, frequently causes the rapid death of the host, if the host has no resistance to the parasite. Examples of this were the introduction of smallpox, measles, and chicken pox into the Americas and the islands of the Pacific Ocean, notably, the Hawaiian Islands. Recently, in the United States, a mosquito-borne virus which causes encephalitis in horses and man, has proven to be extremely virulent, causing many deaths.

Treponema pallidum is the causative agent of Syphilis which, in nature, is limited to man, but has been clinically transmitted to monkeys and rabbits. The human infection is generally transmitted by sexual contact. It is thought that the microorganism cannot penetrate the intact skin, requiring a small cut in order to enter the body, but they can penetrate mucosal membranes, or so it is believed. In general, a primary lesion, or chancre, develops at the site of penetration within two months. This is called the Primary Stage. Within three months of the Primary Stage, the Secondary Stage develops in which the host is covered by a skin rash, or pox. In the Third Stage of the infection, the spirochetes may attack the cardiovascular system or the central nervous system, causing death. At the present time, the disease is treated with antibiotics, such as pencillin, but formerly, many unusual treatments were utilized.

In China, the "Materia Medica" of Li Shih-chen (1518-93) mentioned syphilis, which appeared in China in about 1505, and was treated with mercurial compounds and China root. China root is ginseng, *Panax (Aralia) ginseng,* which appears to have no medicinal value, but became very popular in the treatment of syphilis. It was shipped from China to the Portuguese colony in India, Goa, from which it was shipped into the Middle East and Europe. Vesalius even included China root in his writings. Fracastorius rejected the use of fumigations and steambaths and recommended sarsaparilla, China root, sassafras and guiacum. Mercurial and arsenical compounds were found to be effective and Paul Ehrlich, in 1909, combined an arsenical, arsphenamine with copper, and produced Salvarsan, the "silver bullet" that was used in the treatment of syphilis and protozoan infections. The spirochete is susceptible to increased body temperature and some of the first attempts at treatment used methods which attempted to raise the body temperature such as fumigations and baths and sweating agents. Infection with malaria or some other disease in which the body's temperature is elevated for long periods of time, may effect a cure of syphilis, if the temperature reaches 42°C.

The most infectious stages of syphilis are the Primary and Secondary although some people remain infective after the disappearance of the rash for years. The infection can be transmitted to the fetus if the mother is infected and may result in congenital syphilis, with distortion of the brow, Parrot's nodes, a thinning and pitting of the occipital and parietal areas, depression of the bridge of the nose, the lack of incisors, mulberry molars, a shortening of the long bones of the body and syphilitic meningitis. If the child lives, the bone changes persist into adult life. Strangely, reconstructions of Neanderthal man, as seen in a variety of museums, do resemble the expected results of congenital syphilis, which again brings us to the question, where did syphilis come from?

The three voyages of Columbus stimulated other explorers to set out for the New World and to find a route through it, or around it, to the Orient. In 1513, Balboa and his companions, one of whom was Pizarro, crossed the isthmus of Panama and reached the Pacific Ocean which, along with all lands surrounding it, was claimed for the Spanish throne. In 1516, Solis explored the Rio de la Plata and later Magellan found his way around South America. In 1498, Vasco da Gama sailed around Africa, reached India, and the Portuguese established their trading colony of Goa there which controlled the trade of the Orient. Scurvy had broken out on the Portuguese ships and had caused many deaths as it had on others, including the voyage of Magellan. The most unfortunate voyage was that of Lord Anson in 1740, on which 626 of 961 crew members, died of scurvy and associated maladies. Captain James Cook prevented the disease by providing his men with a beverage made from dried sprouted barley and later, many English ships provided limes in the diet. The Chinese had utilized sprouted seeds in antiquity and today, many people include bean sprouts in their regular diet.

With these explorations into tropical areas of the world, other diseases were encountered, one of which was Yellow Fever, which became extremely important to the United States when the Panama Canal was being built. Many of the early writings of this time mention fevers, but the first epidemic of

Yellow Fever which can be definitely identified occurred in Yucatan in 1648. Early investigations of the disease were made by Walter Reed in Havana in 1901, who showed, through the use of human volunteers, that the causative agent was a virus that passed through bacterial filters and was transmitted by mosquitos, *Aedes aegypti* and others. Man is not the only host of this virus since all monkeys of South America and Africa have been found to be susceptible. Following infection, man becomes suddenly ill with fever, headache and body ache. Nausea and vomiting are common and the gums become spongy and bleed easily. Black vomit may result from this bleeding. Jaundice may appear. The mortality rate is about five percent with degeneration of the liver, kidney and the heart, accompanied by hemorrhages. There is no treatment since this is a viral infection. The disease is prevented today by vaccination.

Francisco Pizarro had been with Balboa during the expedition that had discovered the Pacific Ocean and had remained in Panama, attracted by stories of fabulous cities and treasures to the south. In 1527, he and a small group of followers made contact with the fringes of the Inca Empire and in 1528, he went to Spain and was appointed Governor and Captain-General of Peru, by Charles V. An expedition was organized, consisting of approximately 180 men and 27 horses, which left Panama in 1530 and sailed southward. In 1532, Pizarro succeeded in capturing the Inca, Atahualpa, who had been involved in a civil war, and was in Cajamarca, in the northern part of the Empire. In order to obtain his release, Atahualpa offered to fill a room with gold, the offer of which, Pizarro accepted. In 1533, reinforcements arrived from Panama which made it possible for Pizarro to plan a further advance into the Inca Empire. The gold was melted down; Atahualpa was baptized and strangled; and Pizarro and his men began their march to the capital city of Cuzco.

Pedro Pizarro, a cousin of Francisco Pizarro reported:

"Then Atabalipa wept, and he besought them not to kill him, for there was not an Indian in the land who would stir without his command, (and he asked) what had they to fear, holding him, as they did, a prisoner? (And he said) that if they were doing this thing for gold or silver, he would give them twice as much as had already been ordered. I saw the Marquis weep with sorrow at not being able to grant him his life, for he certainly feared the exactions (of the officials) and the risk which there was in the land should he (Atabalipa) be set free. This Atabalipa had given his wives and Indians to understand that, if they (the Spaniards) did not burn his body, he would return to them, for the Sun his father would resuscitate him. Then, when they took him out into the plaza to give him the garrote, padre fray Vicente de Valverde, already mentioned, preached to him, bidding him become a Christian. And he asked if they would burn him should he become a Christian, and they told him no, and he said that if they would not burn him, he would be baptized, and so Fray Vicente baptized him, and they gave him the garrote, and on another day they interred him in the church which we Spaniards have in Caxamalca."[13]

13. "Relation of the Discovery and Conquest of the Kingdoms of Peru," Pedro Pizarro, translated by Philip A. Means, The Cortes Society, New York, 1921, pgs. 218, 219.

Cuzco was easily taken in the same year, but its location in a mountain valley of the Andes, at an elevation of approximately 11,000 feet, was unfavorable to the Spaniards, so Pizarro established Lima as his base, close to the ocean, where he was assassinated in 1541. The Indians of the Inca Empire, accustomed to the organized state of the Inca, accepted the organized government of the Spanish conquerors headed by a puppet Inca on the throne; were converted to Christianity; and were subject to the King of Spain. Missionaries were very tolerant of the converted Indians and even established their church on the foundations of the sun temple in Cuzco. However, the Indians were exploited, many being forced into labor, especially in the mines, and in some areas, it still exists today.

The most puzzling thing about the cultures of South America is that very little is known about them and the first date, of certainty, is that of Pizarro, in 1527. The cultures in South America apparently did not use any form of writing, but utilized knotted strings, "quipus" and, "rememberers," who could read the strings and related the messages. Unfortunately, they are all dead.

One legend states that in the past they had writings but were visited by a great plague which caused many deaths. The priests blamed the disease on the use of writing, so it was abandoned. The plague ended and writing was never used again.

According to mythology, the Sun God, Tici Viracocha, created the first Inca, Manco Capac, on the Island of the Sun, in Lake Titicaca. Manco Capac and his sister, Mamma Ocllo, were instructed to teach the arts of civilization to

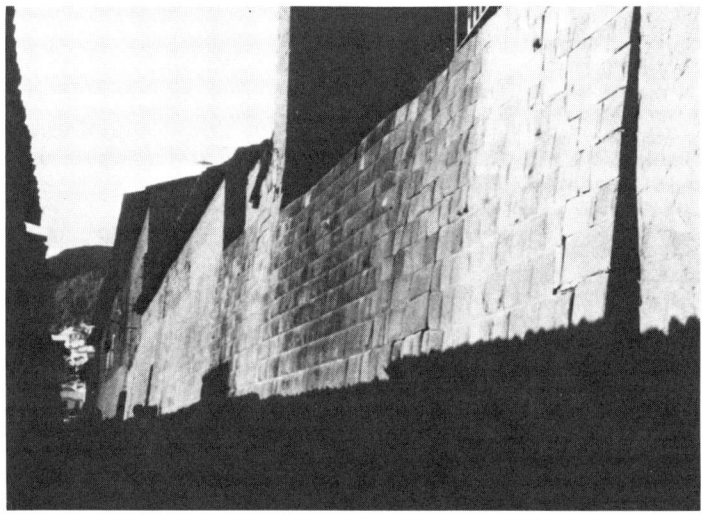

The stoneworkers of ancient Cuzco were extremely skilled in building foundations which still support more modern structures despite numerous earthquakes.

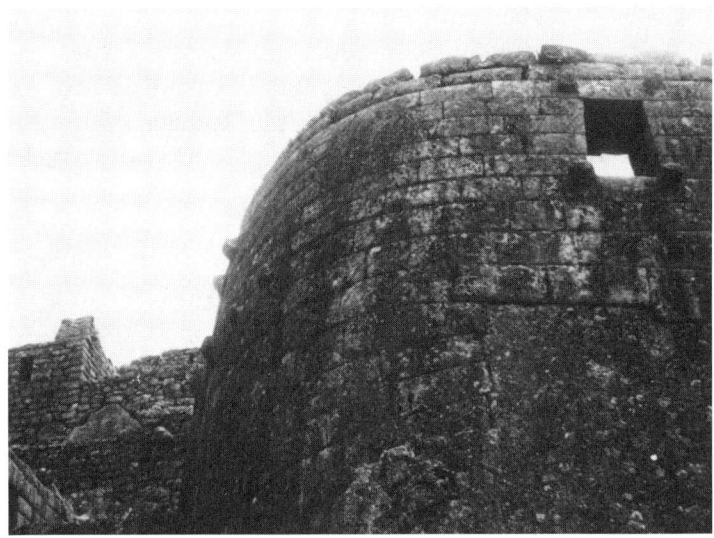

The royal palace at Macchu Picchu believed by some historians to have been erected on the orders of the Inca Manco I, in about 1000 A.D., at the place of his birth. Others believe that the first Inca came from the region of Lake Titicaca.

mankind and left the island to establish their city, which led to the founding of Cuzco and the Inca Empire. It is believed that this event occurred in 1200 A.D. and that by about 1430, the Inca Empire had been extended from what is now Argentina and Chile in the south, to Colombia, in the north. The Empire adopted the Quechua language and the history of previous cultures was eliminated by the official "Rememberers."

Pedro Pizarro described the ceremonies and the temple of the Sun in Cuzco, which was later destroyed, except for the foundation, on which a church was built, and may still be seen today:

> "This Sun had many guardians and servitors who were like priests. One among them was the chief, for he was like a bishop, and to him all the others yielded obedience, and without the permission of these (priests) they did nothing, and he (the chief priest) was called Vila.... He was Lord of ... of the Lords of the kingdom. They had for this sun certain very large houses, all of very well made masonry, in the manner of that near ... very high and well worked. On the right of it there was a band consisting of plates of gold a palm wide, fastened upon the stones (of the wall). And above all this, on the entire front of the enclosure, which was not larger than a small patio, there was a ... like a bench with the casing of gold which, as I have said, covered it, and which they carried to Caxamalca. Here they seated the Sun when he did not go out into the plaza by day. At night they placed him in a small but very well made room, likewise adorned with golden plates in every part. Here lived many women who said that they were the wives of the Sun, and they pretended to keep their virginity and to live chastely, and they lied, for they involved themselves with the male servants and guardians of the Sun, who were many.

"Away from the room where the Sun was wont to sleep, they made a small field, which was much like a large one, where, at the proper season, they sowed maize. They sprinkled it by hand with water brought on purpose for the Sun. And at the time when they celebrated their festivals, which was three times a year, that is: when they sowed the crops, when they harvested them, and when they made orejones (large ears), they filled this garden with cornstalks made of gold, having their ears and leaves very much like natural maize, all made of very fine gold, which they had kept in order to place them here at these times. In this house where, as I say, the Sun was, more than two hundred women were wont to sleep daily, all of them being the daughters of important Indians. They slept on the floor, and they placed the bundle of the Sun upon a high bench, very rich with much trimming of turnsoles, and they pretended to sleep there and that the Sun had connexion with them." [14]

Remnants of early man have been found in the coastal valleys which date to, perhaps, 3000 B.C. By 1500 B.C., man was cultivating the earth, erecting structures, weaving cloth and using pottery. The cultures were given names, mainly by their location, since it is not known what the people called themselves. In the north, the Chavin, Mochica and Chimu cultures developed, the latter being conquered by the Inca in about 1466 A.D. The Paracas and Ica-Nazca cultures were to the west of Cuzco, on the Pacific coast, the latter being

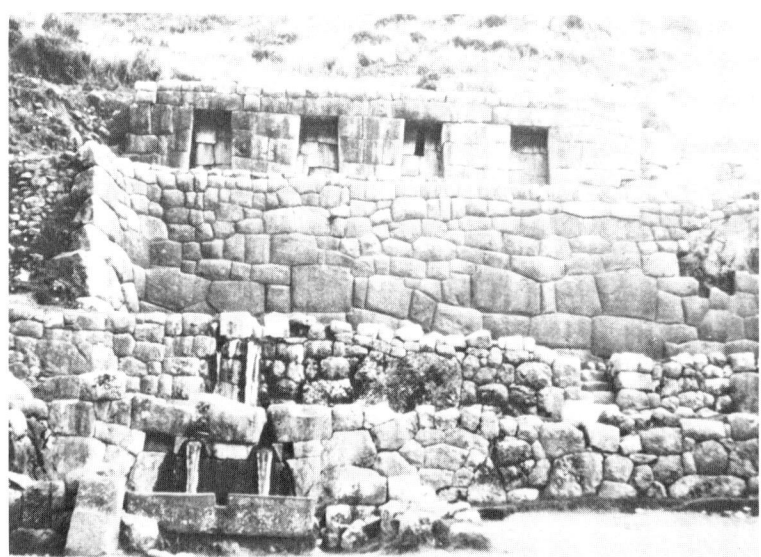

An Inca bath near the ruins of Sacsayhuaman still in an excellent state of preservation.

---

14. "Relation of the Discovery and Conquest of the Kingdoms of Peru," Pedro Pizarro, translated by Philip A. Means, The Cortes Society, New York, 1921, pgs. 254-256.

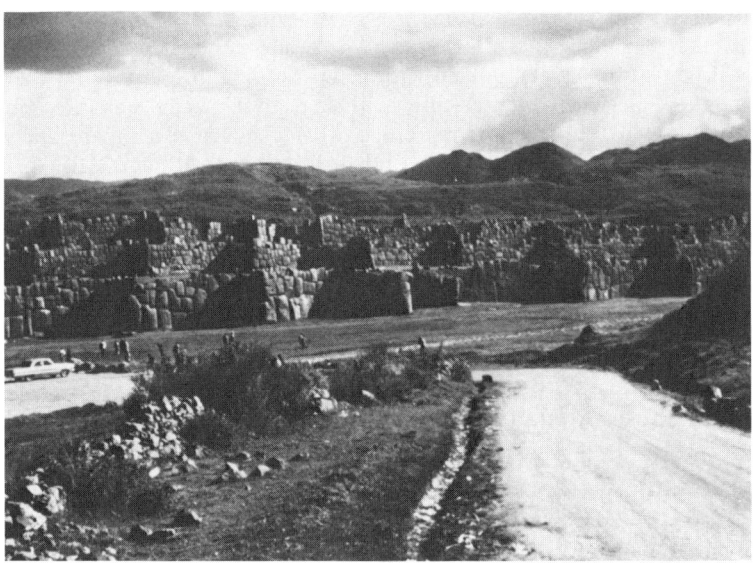

Huge stones were carefully fitted together to form the walls of the fortress of Sacsayhuaman which overlooks Cuzco.

conquered about 1436 A.D. the Ica-Nazca left the puzzling lines, diagrams and figures dug into the desert sands which are still a matter of great controversy. In about 900 A.D., a culture centered around Lake Titicaca invaded the coastal areas and became the dominant culture in southern Peru and Bolivia, the Empire of Tiahuanaco, from about 1000 to 1300 A.D. Their culture is noted for their building and stonework and, like the others, was forgotten by the Inca "rememberers." It is probably a tribe from this culture which migrated to what is now Cuzco, and began the Inca Empire. The term "Inca" referred to the ruler of these people of the Inca Empire, not to the people, whose name we do not know. Whoever these "late" conquerors were, they built on the cultures of former peoples and eventually established a great, organized Empire in South America.

All the land in the Empire belonged to the Inca and was allocated to family groups who kept one portion of their produce for themselves; gave one portion to the upkeep of their religion; and one portion to the Inca and the government. In order to keep control over the Empire, a secondary capital was established at Quito (Ecuador) and a system of roads and bridges was extended throughout the land over which runners carried governmental messages. Like their northern neighbors, the Indians of South America had no draft animals but they did have the llama, alpaca, vicuña and guanaco, all related to the camel. The llama and alpaca appear to have been developed by crossbreeding the latter two animals. These animals were used as beasts of burden and provided wool for various purposes. At one time it was believed that man acquired syphilis as the result of sexual intercourse with llamas, but the animals have not been found to harbor the spirochete, which ruined another legend concerning the origin of that disease.

The people believed in life-after-death and, in many instances, attempted to mummify the body of the deceased, so that the soul could return. A natural mummification of the body occurred in the desert regions, but in the mountainous regions, with high humidity, little has survived. The viscera were removed and the cavity filled with cloths; beyond that, little is known. The body was placed in a sitting position with the head resting on the knees, and was wrapped in bindings and protective coverings. The mummies of deceased Incas were especially venerated and were kept in their houses as if they still lived. They sat on their thrones and were "fed" and cared for as if they were still living. The royal mummies were noted by the Spaniards when they entered Cuzco. Several were carried off into the wilderness capital of Vilcapampa by the Inca, Manco Capac II, in 1536. Three mummies were reported to have been moved from Cuzco to Lima, and were later buried in the courtyard of the San Andrés Hospital in 1562. It was also reported that on warm, sunny days, the mummies were brought outside to enjoy the sunlight. This would help to keep them dry and would prevent deterioration of the tissues.

> Pedro Pizarro reported: "These Lords had the law and custom of taking that one of their Lords who died and embalming him, wrapping him up in many fine clothes, and to these Lords they allotted all the service which they had had in life, in order that these bundles (mummies) might be served in death as well as they had been in life. Their service of gold and silver was not touched, nor was anything else which they had, nor were those who served them (removed from) the house without being replaced, and provinces were set aside to give them support. The Lord who entered upon a new reign had to take new servants. His vessels had to be of wood and pottery until there was time to make them of gold and silver, and always those who began to reign carried out all this, and it was for this reason that there was so much treasure in this land, because, as I have said, he who succeeded to the kingdom always hastened to make better vessels and houses (than his predecessors). And as the greater part of the people, treasure, expenses and vices were under the control of the dead, each dead man had allotted to him an important Indian, and likewise an Indian woman, and whatever these wanted they declared it to be the will of the dead one. Whenever they wished to eat, to drink, they said that the dead ones wished to do that same thing. If they wished to go and divert themselves in the houses of other dead folk, they said the same, for it was customary for the dead to visit one another, and they held great dances and orgies, and sometimes they went to the houses of the living, and sometimes the living came to theirs." [15]
>
> "It was the sight of the soldiery who were in this city of Cuzco that caused wonderment ... most of who served these dead folk whom I have mentioned, for each day they took them all out into the plaza and sat them down in a row, each one according to his antiquity, and there the men and women servitors ate

---

15. "Relation of the Discovery and Conquest of the Kingdoms of Peru," Pedro Pizarro, translated by Philip A. Means, The Cortes Society, New York, 1921, pgs. 202, 203.

and drank. And for the dead they made fires before them with a piece of very dry wood which they had worked into a very even shape. Having set this piece of wood on fire, they burned here everything which they had placed before the dead in order that he might eat of the things which they eat, and here in this fire they consumed it. Likewise before these dead people they had certain large pitchers, which they call 'verquis,' made of gold, silver or pottery, each one according to his wish, and into (these vessels) they poured the chicha which they gave to the dead man with much display, and the dead pledged one another as well as the living, and the living pledged the dead." [16]

Thousands of skulls from burial sites of pre-Inca and Inca cultures reveal that trepanning was widespread and frequently performed, with regrowth of bone indicating that the surgery was successful. The surgical procedure was known in antiquity and was highly developed by the Inca culture. It is believed that one of the battle weapons of South America, a club with projections, frequently caused head injuries that resulted in a portion of the skull pressing against the brain. In order to relieve the pressure, a portion of the skull was removed, which relieved the paralysis. In addition to trepanning, it is believed that amputations were carried out which are represented by numerous pottery figurines. It is not known whether the "surgeons" used anesthetics or narcotics on their patients, but several were available, including the coca plant, which yields cocaine.

The coca plant, *Erythroxylon coca,* was, at the time of the Inca, grown and distributed by government control. The leaves of the plant were utilized mainly by the shamans, priests, runners, the aged and the royal family. However, after the Spanish conquest, coca came into widespread cultivation and use, and eventually became a state monopoly. The leaves act as a nervine and stimulant when chewed, and also as a mild anesthetic. A crystalline alkaloid, methyl benzoyl ecgonine, can be extracted from the leaves and is known as cocaine. Although the coca leaves may stimulate the user, its continued use causes addiction; prolonged use of the stimulant may lead to degeneration of the central nervous system, glandular disorders, a general physical breakdown and death. Cocaine was once widely used throughout the world as a local anesthetic and nerve tonic, but its use has been regulated in most countries since about 1900.

In 1885, John Pemberton, a pharmacist from Atlanta, Georgia, copyrighted "French wine of Cola," prepared from coca leaves and later combined coca leaves and the African cola nut, to make Coca Cola. Years later when the drink became world famous, the coca leaves were omitted from the preparation.

Spanish missionaries mentioned the presence of physicians, or healers, in the population who were skilled in the use of herbs, powders and waters, and also others who were skilled in medicine and surgery. Their local names were

---

16. *op. cit.,* page 251.

"hampi-camayoc" (remedy keepers), "sircac" (possessors of medicine and surgery) and "oquetlupuc" (doctors). Frequently, if the patient died, the family could claim malpractice, and the physician was buried with the patient.

The Spaniards brought the diseases of Europe to South America, such as smallpox, chickenpox, measles and others; and contracted various endemic diseases such as Uta, Verruga and South American Trypanosomiasis.

Uta, American Leishmaniasis, is similar to the Leishmaniasis previously discussed in Plague VI, during the Exodus of the Hebrews from Egypt. The causative agent is *Leishmania braziliensis,* which was first observed in ulcerative lesions in man in 1909, by Carini, Paranhos and Lindenberg, and was named in 1911. The infection is distributed from Mexico to Chile, where it is transmitted by sandflies of the Genus *Phlebotomus.* The disease was pictured in Mochica pottery, as were most of the endemic diseases of the area, and showed a disease which caused facial disfigurement. Uta is a destructive, ulcerative infection which generally begins on the face, especially on the nose or lips, destroying the tissue and gradually extending into nearby areas, causing great deformity. The Indian physicians treated the infection with sulphide of arsenic, the death-medicine, and today, infections are treated with antimony derivatives and antibiotics, which prevent bacterial infections. Immunity to infection can be brought about by vaccination and the disease can be controlled by the treatment and isolation of infected individuals and animals, and the destruction of sandflies. There is an incidence of 10 to 20 percent in endemic areas, but it varies with the location and the occupation of the people and the density of the sandflies.

Verruga was so named because of the development of warty, red-colored pimples all over the body, which bled and resulted in an anemia which caused death. It only occurs in the mountainous regions of Ecuador, Colombia and Peru, and occurs in two forms; a febrile anemia, Oroya fever, and a benign eruption of the skin, Verruga peruana. The death rate in the former is 40 percent and in the latter, about 5 percent. The causative agent is a bacterium, *Bartonella bacilliformis,* which was reported by Barton, in 1909. The bacterium is transmitted to man by *Phlebotomus,* sandflies, which may be controlled with insecticides. Since the infective agent is a bacterium, it will respond to the use of antibiotics.

Pedro Pizarro, in his "Relation of the Discovery and Conquest of the Kingdoms of Peru," described this disease:

> "In this Coaque they found many mattresses of wool from the ceyua, which is a tree they grow there and thus name. And it befell then that some Spaniards who threw themselves down upon the mattresses got up crippled, for if the arm or the leg was doubled up during sleep it could not be straightened out again except with very great difficulty. This was the lot of some people, and it was understood to be the origin of a disease called berrugas, a disease so bad and tormenting that it caused many men to be wearied and worn by pain just as if they had tumors, and even great sores came out all over the body, and some

were as big as eggs, and they corrupted the skin, and much pus and blood ran out of them so that it was necessary to cut them out and to throw strong things (herbs?) into the wound to kill the root. There were other sores as small as measles, because of which the whole body swelled up. Few were those who escaped having them, though they attacked some men more than they did others. Some wished to claim that the cause of this infirmity was some fish which they ate in the provinces of Puerto Viejo, and which the Indians maliciously gave to the Spaniards."[17]

South American Trypanosomiasis was discovered in Brazil in 1907 by Chagas and has been reported from southwestern United States throughout South America. The causative agent, *Trypanosoma cruzi*, is a protozoan which is transmitted to man by a large number of species of reduviid, or kissing bugs. After a cyclic reproduction in the intestine of the kissing bug, the protozoan is deposited on the skin of the host, in the feces of the bug, while it is taking a blood-meal. The bite wound is easily infected. The trypanosomes enter various tissue cells and reproduce. If the heart and brain are infected, death may occur rapidly. In chronic infections, the disease may go unnoticed for years, with no symptoms. The trypanosomes can usually be found in blood smears only during the first two months of infection, after which time it may be located in biopsied lymph node material. Dogs and cats are the most important reservoir hosts, especially since they are so closely associated with man. A quinoline derivative, Bayer 7602, has been used to successfully clear the trypanosomes from the blood, but not from the tissues, where arsenical compounds have sometimes proven useful. Some experimental immunity has been shown in the innoculation of animals, but has not been utilized in endemic areas. Preventative measures include the destruction of the vectors with insecticides and measures to prevent the insects from biting man.

One of the greatest contributions of South America to the medicine of the world was quinine. Although malarial fevers, and other fevers, were described in antiquity, the parasite which caused malaria was not discovered until 1880, by Alphonse Lavaran. The ancient Chinese used the plant "Ch'ang Shan," *Dichroa fibrifuga,* which contains alkaloids, and was effective in the treatment of malaria, but Europe had not yet found a drug which was successful in the treatment of the infection. In 1633, Padre Calancha of Lima, Peru, described the native treatment of fevers with the powdered bark of the "Fever tree," now called *Chinchona ledgeriana.* Although the Europeans had readily adopted the use of coca leaves, sarsaparilla and others, they did not readily take to the Peruvian bark. It was introduced into Europe in about 1645, and in 1649, Cardinal de Lugo, cured of malaria by taking the bark, began distributing the bark with instructions for its use. Protestants were reluctant to use the bark, or powder, since it was a Catholic preparation, and others discovered that its use

---

17. "Relation of the Discovery and Conquest of the Kingdoms of Peru," Pedro Pizarro, translated by Philip A. Means, The Cortes Society, New York, 1921, pgs. 150, 151.

did not always cure the fever. This was probably due to the disease causing the fever, not being malaria, or the bark being used, not being from the correct tree. The demand for the bark became so great that the suppliers in South America were sending any bark that was brought to them that resembled the *Chinchona* bark. In 1711, the Italian physician Torti gave the disease the name "Malaria" (bad airs) and showed that quinine was useless in the treatment of other than malarial fevers. However, quinine has other effects on the body: it is a stimulant to the CNS and may cause congestion of the brain, vertigo and deafness; it is a depressant to the heart, circulation and respiration; it increases the number of white blood cells, but arrests their migration; it acts as an antiseptic and reduces fevers. In overdoses, it causes destruction of red blood cells, a rash, deafness, blindness and death from respiratory failure. Today, quinine is rarely used, except when combined with primaquine, in treatment of relapsing malaria. Primaquine is the least toxic and the most effective of the aminoquinolines used in malarial prophylaxis throughout the world.

The countries of South America eventually had a monopoly on the production of quinine bark and forbade the exportation of any portion of the tree except the dead bark. In 1853, Hasskarl, of the Java Botanical Gardens, disguised as the tourist, Muller, with some gold, bribed some people and managed to get some plants and seeds. He was knighted by the Netherlands and was placed in charge of a plantation for the raising of the trees. Unfortunately, all the trees died and he was relieved of his position. However, by 1860, Dutch plantations in the Malabar mountains had succeeded in raising almost one million trees which, when the bark was assayed, produced little or no quinine. The trees may not have been the *Chinchona* tree, or ones that produced little quinine.

In 1863, a dealer in quinine bark, Ledger, succeeded in getting a bark collector, Manuel, to bring him some of the seeds from the trees, which he sent to his brother in England. Manuel was captured, tortured and died in jail. The British government declined the seeds, but the Netherlands bought some for about twenty dollars. These seeds produced the tree, *Chinchona ledgeriana*, which yielded a high quantity of quinine, and was the start of the Dutch monopoly: 9/10ths of the world's supply of quinine bark. However, in 1930, German chemists synthesized Atabrine, which led to the synthesis of other antimalarial compounds such as Chloroquine, Pentaquine, Primaquine, and others, and the decline in the use of quinine. The widespread use of antimalarial compounds, although successful in the control of malaria in many areas of the world, has also led to the development of *Plasmodium* strains that are resistant to some of the compounds, and quinine is frequently used in treatment of these drug resistant infections.

Other trees utilized by the Indians were the Ratantici tree, which contained tannic acid, and was used in the treatment of diarrhea; the Pepper tree, whose resin was used to expell intestinal parasites; and the "huilca" tree, which was used as a purgative and in enemas. The seeds of the tree were powdered and inhaled, which caused an intoxication, and was used by the shamans and priests, who used the hypnotic state to discover the causes of sickness.

The Indians also were aware that certain plants were poisonous and could be used to kill other people. Pedro Pizarro reported:

> "This man (Tubalipa, a brother of Guascar, Inca at Cuzco) had come to see Atabalipa when he was in prison, and he pretended to be very friendly (to the Spaniards), and he feigned illness throughout the time when Atabalipa was not leaving his room. He did this in fear lest Atabalipa order him siain, as he had the rest of his brothers. Then, having been raised up as Lord, in conformity with (the laws of) the natives, and while he was eating one day, Challicuchima (an army captain) being with him, Challicuchima pledged him with a cup of chica, for they had this custom of pledging thus, and Challicuchima put poison in the chica of Tubalipa, in such a way that he consumed it, and he came to die at Xauxa at the end of seven or eight months. These Indians knew herbs by means of which they can kill at the end of as many months or years as they desired." [18]

Strangely, when the Inca, Manco Capac II, fled from the Spaniards in Cuzco, he went to a wilderness area called Vilcapampa or Uilcapampa. This is believed to actually be "Huilcapampa," the pampa where the "huilca" tree grows. In 1911, Hiram Bingham was searching for the lost capital of the last Incas, and found the city now known as Macchu Picchu, which is believed by many to be the origin, and last capital, of the Inca. The majority of the burials in the area were of women, so it is believed that Macchu Picchu was a hiding place for the "Virgins of the Sun" and the wives of the Inca. Following the defeat of the Inca forces and the introduction of Christianity, the old religion gradually died away, the priestesses died, and the city was abandoned. Bingham reported the finding of the burial place of the High Priestess and reported that, "Pathological examination of the skeleton of this delicately formed woman shows that unfortunately she suffered from syphilis." [19] Paleopathologists, who have examined the skeletal remains of Peruvian Indians, have reported lesions of syphilis and physicians have noted that the Indian, who contracted syphilis, did not suffer the effect that the European did, which might indicate a resistance to the infection due to a period of long, endemic infection in the population.

---

18. "Relation of the Discovery and Conquest of the Kingdoms of Peru," Pedro Pizarro, translated by Philip A. Means, The Cortes Society, New York, 1921, pg. 228.
19. Hiram Bingham, "Lost City of the Incas," Duell, Sloan and Pearce, New York, 1948, pg. 207.

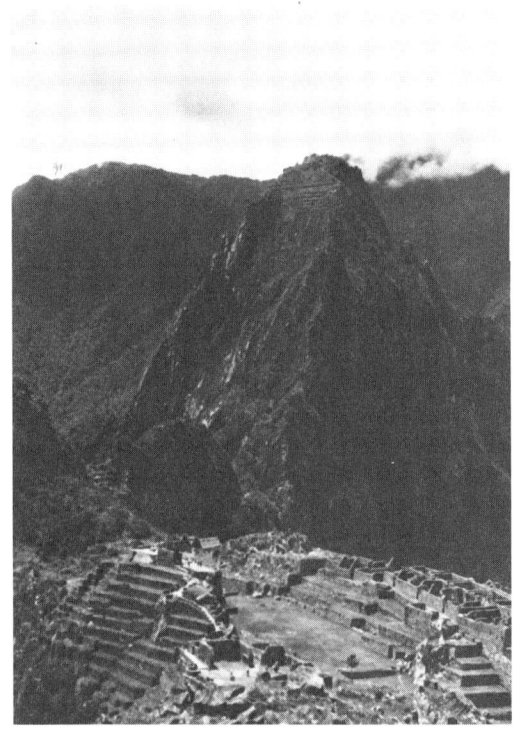

Macchu Picchu.

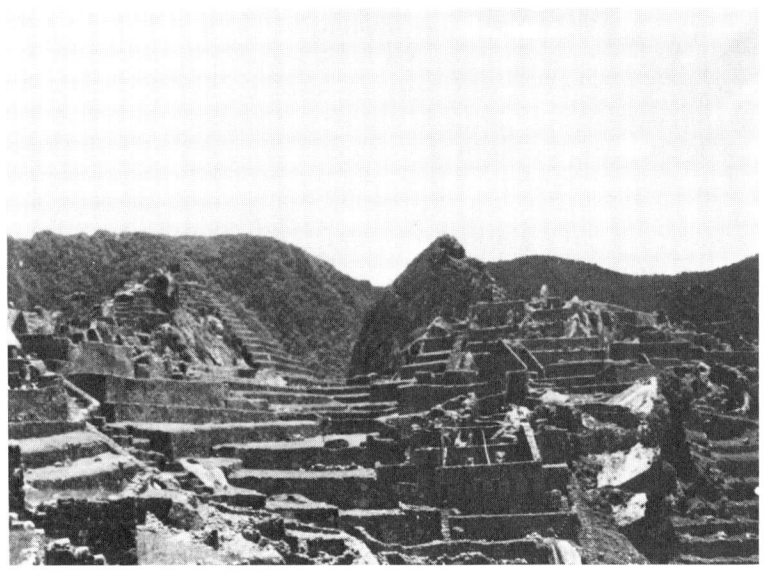

Macchu Picchu.

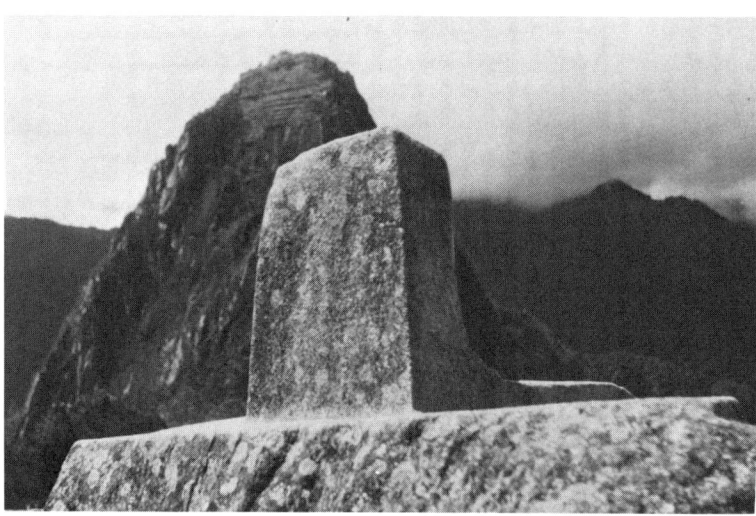

The sun dial at Macchu Picchu was probably utilized by the priests for celestial observations.

1500~present explorations and discoveries

The period of time that followed the discovery of the New World by Columbus is frequently referred to as the "Age of Exploration," during which time many explorers visited lands that were unknown to people living in Europe. Previously, writers such as Herodotus, Pliny, St. Augustine, Prester John and others, had written of strange countries, animals and men; which were very different from those found in their normal surroundings. Especially noted by the travelers and explorers were strange men. Columbus had described the Indians that he had met as being intelligent and handsome, but also mentioned people who were hairless, tailed or had the heads of dogs. Other explorers returned to Europe with sightings of other monsters which finally led to the declaration, by Pope Paul II, in 1537, that the Indians of the Americas were human and possessed souls. The celebrated scientist, Carl von Linhe (Linnaeus), in 1735, in "System of Nature," classified man as a quadruped and, in the tenth edition of the same work, in 1758, along with man, *Homo sapiens,* classified another species, *Homo monstrous,* into which animal-like men were placed. The pupil of Linnaeus, Hoppius, continued the classification of these monsters and produced *Homo troglodytus, H. luciferus, H. satyrus* and *H. pygmaeus.* Strangely, today there are still being circulated stories concerning the sightings of creatures such as the "abominable snowman" of the Himalayas and "big foot" of the western United States. The author has seen a short film of "big foot" which would be convincing except that the creature filmed looks like someone wearing a badly fitted fur suit, that moved around a great deal when he ran. Of course, both creatures could actually have been someone with hypertrichosis. The pictures of these monsters were obtained from "Homo monstrous," by Annemarie de Waal Malefijt, Scientific American, October, 1968, pgs. 112-118.

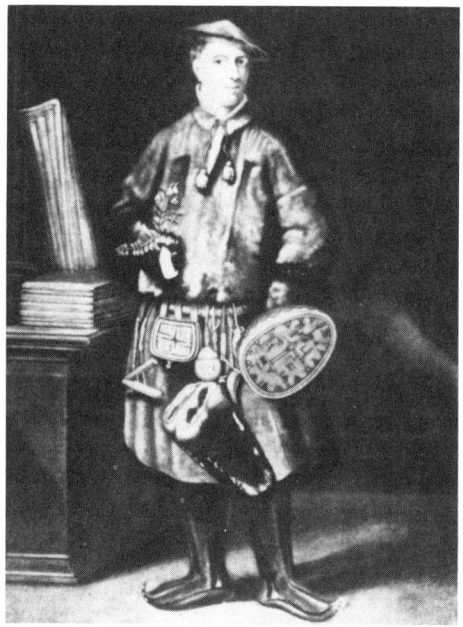

Carolus Linnaeus. Mezzotint by Robert Dunkarton after Hoffman, from Thornton's "Temple of Flora," London, 1805. From *Medicine and the Artist* by Carl Zigrosser, Dover Publications, Inc., New York, 1970. Reprinted through the permission of the publisher and the Philadelphia Museum of Art.

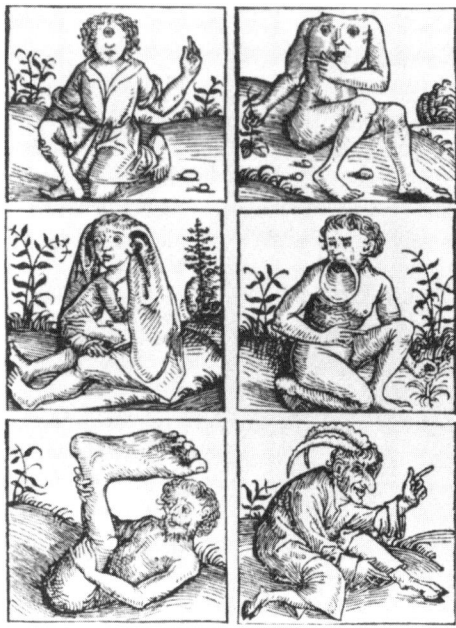

Monstrous people described by Herodotus and other early writers were pictured in Hartmann Schedel's "Liber Chronicarum," 1493. (Courtesy of Picture Collection, The Branch Libraries, The New York Public Library.)

This same period of time is found to contain the beginnings of scientific investigations into medicine which had for centuries, from the fifth to thirteenth, been hindered by the Church which controlled the Universities. Medical schools appeared in several Universities during the thirteenth century, but the teaching had very little to do with medicine except for the writings of Galen. Surgery was not taught and was considered a degrading craft, so the dissection of the human body was seldom carried out. In 1299, Pope Boniface issued a Bull which forbade the boiling and stripping of flesh from cadavers, which hindered the study of anatomy. By 1315, a few dissections were being performed in the University of Bologna, but these were rare and ceremonial, rather than instructive. A noted physician would lecture to the students from the writings of Galen while a barber-surgeon dissected the cadaver and displayed the organs under discussion. In 1407, the University of Notre Dame, in Paris, was given the official sanction for the dissection of three human cadavers. These early physicians were required to have a priest to aid and advise them during the treatment of a patient, which was mainly diet, bleedings, leechings, the use of certain herbs and religious prayers. Women were not admitted into the Universities, but many were involved in the study of medicine as midwives and healers. It was these healers, or witches, who developed an understanding of anatomy, herbs and drugs while physicians were using religion, Galen, astrology and alchemy in the treatment of diseases. In 1527, Paracelsus, the "Father of Pharmaceutical Chemistry," burned some of his medical books claiming that all that he knew about medicine he had learned from a sorceress. The partnership among the physicians, the Church and the government reached its height during the witch trials.

The Inquisition began in 1179, when the Third Lateran Council passed strict decrees against heretics and reached its height in 1542, with the beginning of the Roman Inquisition under Pope Paul III. The two most famous examples of the Inquisition were the heretic theories of Copernicus, who believed that the earth rotated daily on its axis and that the planets revolved in orbits around the sun; and Galileo, in 1632, for his investigations in physics and astronomy. The female healers, or witches, were also attacked and thousands were arrested, tortured and burned at the stake for heresy. So thoroughly were women discredited that by the seventeenth and eighteenth centuries, men, mainly barber-surgeons, began undertaking the delivery of babies by using obstetrical forceps which, being classified as medical instruments, could not be used by midwives. The physicians entered this lucrative business in the eighteenth century. From the confessions of many of the witches, it can be observed that many of them believed that they had flown through the air, attended "witches sabbaths" and other unusual things. Strangely, if one examines the ingredients of many of

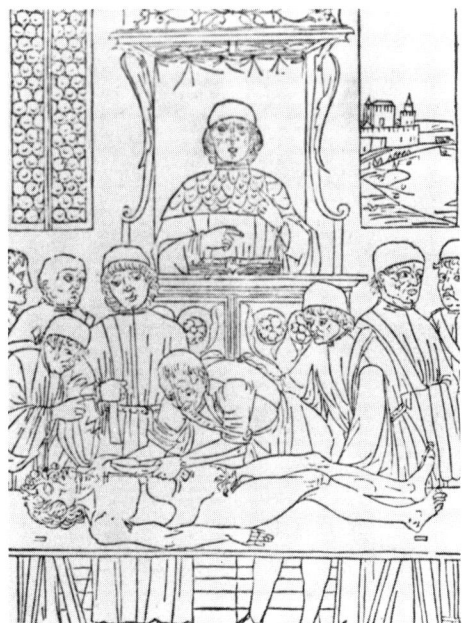

Lesson in Dissection. Woodcut from Ketham's "Fasciculus Medicinae," Venice, 1522. From *Medicine and the Artist* by Carl Zigrosser, Dover Publications, Inc., New York, 1970. Reprinted through the permission of the publisher and the Philadelphia Museum of Art.

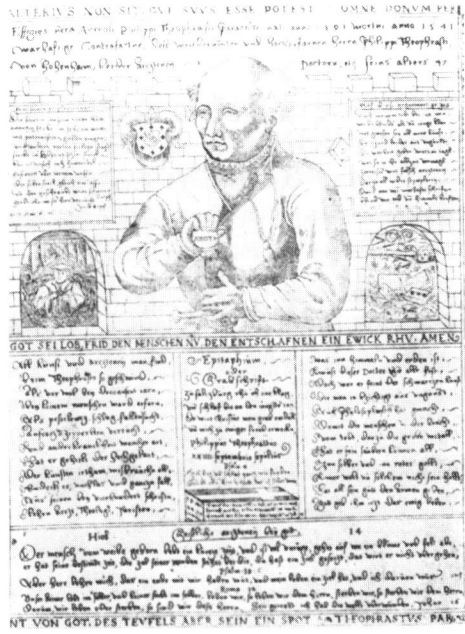

Paracelsus. An etching by B. Jenichen (German, 1520-1600), ca. 1550. From *Medicine and the Artist* by Carl Zigrosser, Dover Publications, Inc., New York, 1970. Reprinted through the permission of the publisher and the Philadelphia Museum of Art.

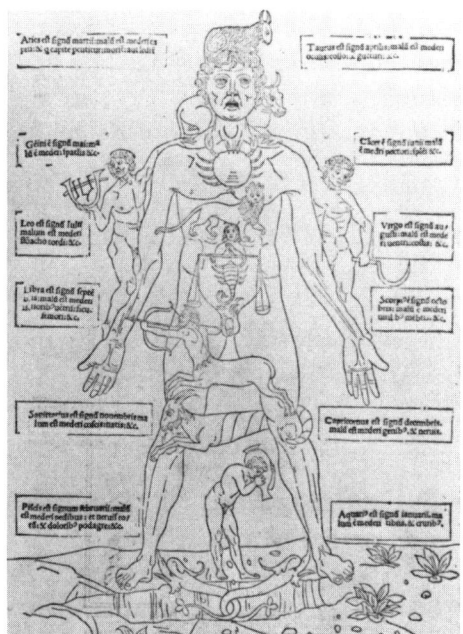

The Zodiac Man. The woodcut from Ketham's "Fasciculus Medicinae," Venice, 1493, is the oldest known blood-letting chart.

their potions, one can find many substances which have a hallucinogenic effect when consumed. The skin of toads contains bufonin, a poison also found in certain lizards; various mushrooms contain toxic alkaloids; ergot, *Claviceps purpurea,* a fungus infection of various grains, was used to stop bleeding following childbirth, but also can act as a hallucinogen; others are monk's-hood, belladonna, nightshade and the mandrake. Witchcraft is currently enjoying a renewed interest by so many people that several religious groups, such as the Episcopalian Church, in England, have introduced witchcraft and exorcism into their curriculum.

Despite the rather rigid control of the Universities by the Church, several important discoveries were made by their graduates. One of the classmates of Copernicus at the University of Padua in the early 1500s was Girolamo Fracastoro (1478-1553). The art of printing with movable type had recently been invented and books were being used more frequently than manuscripts. Fracastoro studied medicine and the classics, and following completion of his studies, investigated and wrote about infectious diseases. He studied the "love-pestilence," or "pox," and published three books, in 1530, entitled "Syphilidis sive de morbo gallico," which described the disease and methods of treatment. Included, was a poem concerning a man, Syphilidis, which was thereafter adopted as the name of the disease known today as syphilis. In 1546, he produced "De contagionibus" in which he explained how infectious diseases were spread from person to person by contact, fomites or through the air. In spite of his theory, it was over 300 years before Pasteur demonstrated that microorganisms caused diseases. Fracastoro described and distinguished among a variety of fevers and discovered the disease now called typhus fever, which is described in this book in the section dealing with India.

Philipp Theophrastus Bombastus von Hohenheim (1493-1541) studied in the University of Ferrara, Italy and Latinised his name to Paracelsus (above Celsus, a Roman physician of 25 A.D.) After graduation he traveled about studying diseases and learning of the remedies used by healers, midwives, barbers and barber-surgeons, which he had never been introduced to in the university.

In 1527, utilizing his acquired knowledge, he cured the famous book printer, Frobenius, after other physicians had advised amputation of his foot; and shortly after, Erasmus of Rotterdam. His fame as a physician spread and in 1527 he went to Basle as the town physician and professor at the university. There, he distributed a pamphlet which stated that he did not believe in the old doctrines of complexions and humours as the causes of all diseases, and invited students to come and reform medicine. The faculty of the medical school was shocked and attempted to forbid his teaching at the University of Basle, but the town council allowed him to do so. He lectured in German, rather than Latin, which further alienated him from the University members, who were joined by many of the students. He lost a court case in 1528 concerning a fee, and left the city. Using his lecture notes as a guide he wrote "Paragranum," a book concerning philosophy, astronomy, chemistry and virtue. In chemistry, he taught the use of antimony, mercury, copper, iron, lead and sulphur, and stated that chemists should be seeking effective drugs and investigating biological processes, rather than attempting to change lead into gold and making the Philosopher's stone.

> "In the dark interior of an old laboratory cluttered with furnaces, crucibles, alembics, stills and bellows, bends an old man (Trevisan) in the act of hardening two thousand hens' eggs in huge pots of boiling water. Carefully he removes the shells and gathers them into a heap. These he heats in a gentle flame until they are white as snow, while his co-laborer separates the whites from the yolks and putrifies them all in the manure of white horses. For eight long years the strange products are distilled and redistilled for the extraction of a mysterious white liquid and a red oil. With these potent universal solvents the two alchemists hope to fashion the 'philosopher's stone.' At last the day of final testing comes. Again the breath-taking suspense, again—failure!—their stone will not turn a single one of the base metals into the elusive gold."[1]

He had a great deal of trouble getting anyone to publish his books but he continued to write concerning syphilis, the plague, surgery and his medicinal beliefs. He was summoned to Salzburg by Prince Ernest of Bavaria, a patron of the sciences, but he died shortly after in 1541. Paracelsus is frequently referred to as the "Father of Pharmaceutical Chemistry."

---

1. "Crucibles, The Story of Chemistry," Bernard Jaffe, Fawcette Publishing Co., Greenwich, Ct., 1975. (Refers to Bernard Trevisan, 1406-1490.)

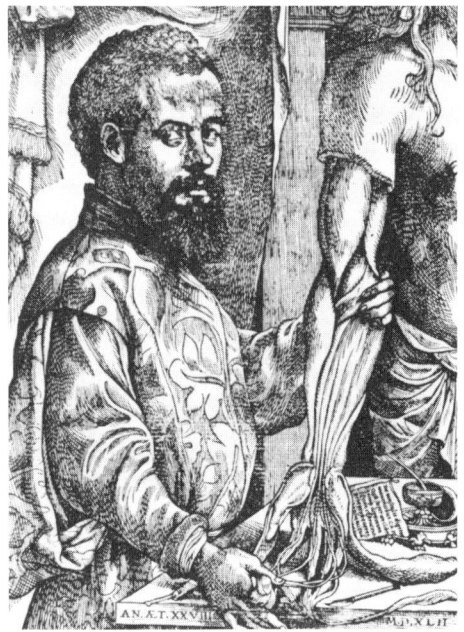

Andreas Vesalius. Woodcut by J. S. von Calcar from A. Vesalius' "De Humani Corporis Fabrica," Basle, 1543. From *Medicine and the Artist* by Carl Zigrosser, Dover Publications, Inc., New York, 1970. Reprinted through the permission of the publisher and the Philadelphia Museum of Art.

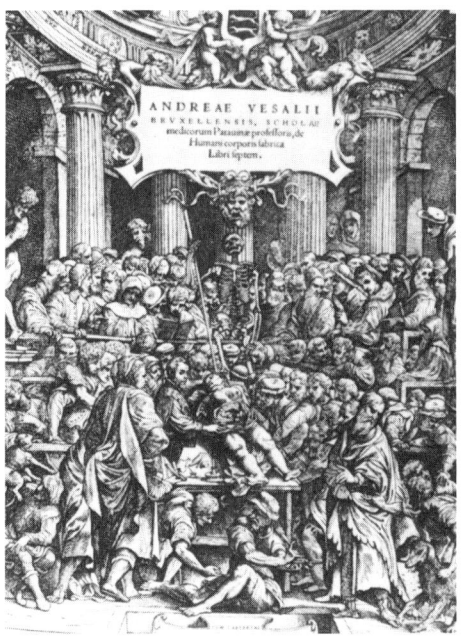

Vesalius Teaching Anatomy. Woodcut by J. S. von Calcar, title page of Vesalius' "De Humani Corporis Fabrica," Basle, 1543.

Living during the same time as Paracelsus and Fracastoro was Andreas Vesalius (1514-1564), who studied anatomy and dissection at universities in Paris, Louvain, Brussels and Padua. He obtained a complete human skeleton by stealing a corpse from a gallows. He compared Galen's works with his own observations and found many errors so he wrote a textbook on human anatomy, "De humani corporis fabrica libri septem," which was published in 1543 and contained over 300 illustrations of the human body. This was the first complete text on human anatomy. He was attacked by defenders of Galen so he left university life and became physician to the Emperor Charles V and, later, to Philip II of Spain. He died in 1564 while on a trip to Jerusalem. According to one story, Vesalius, unknowingly, dissected a living body and was brought before the Inquisition. He was rescued by the Emperor but had to leave the country. This story has not been verified.

The first attempts by man to describe the circulatory system are found in the Egyptian medical papyri, Smith and Ebers, and the Sashruta Samhita of India. For centuries, Galen had been the authority on circulation, but gradually, investigators such as Servetus (1553), Vesalius (1564), Colombo (1560), Falloppio (1565) and d'Acquapendente (1537-1619) made more scientific studies of the circulation of the blood. In 1602, William Harvey received the degree of Doctor of Medicine, at Padua, having studied under d'Acquapendente, and returned to England, later being appointed physician at St. Bartholomew's Hospital. He practiced as a physician and investigated the heart and circulatory system, eventually being appointed physician to King James I, and later, to Charles I. In 1628, he published "Exercitatio anatomica de motu cordis et sanguinis in animalibus," in which he described the action of the heart and the circulation of the blood through the body. He omitted the capillaries, by which the blood passes from the arteries to the veins, believing that the blood made its way through gaps in the tissues. Harvey also was interested in embryology, and investigated developing eggs and embryos which led to publication of "De generatione animalium." This was the most advanced work of its time on embryology. In 1661, the Italian anatomist, Malpighi, using a microscope, reported the finding of capillaries and in them, red globes, which he believed to be fat droplets, but were actually erythrocytes. He also investigated plant structure and like Harvey, embryology and then glands of the body.

Fracastoro, Paracelsus, Vesalius and Harvey are excellent examples of physicians who broke away from the Galenic system of medicine, but the medical schools of Europe changed very slowly and advancement was not rapid. In England, medicine was controlled by dogma and the guilds. In the Americas, medical education consisted mainly of an apprentice system in which the aspiring physician studied with an established physician who himself, may have had no formal education. These physicians, unlike their European relatives, were not bothered with professional or legal regulations and acted as physicians, pharmacists and surgeons. The medical practice was actually open

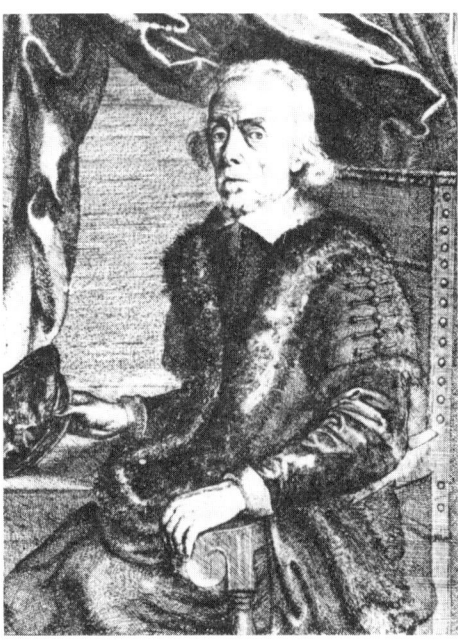

William Harvey. Etching by Richard Gaywood, London, ca. 1649. From *Medicine and the Artist* by Carl Zigrosser, Dover Publications, Inc., New York, 1970. Reprinted through the permission of the publisher and the Philadelphia Museum of Art.

202 *Magic, Myths and Medicine*

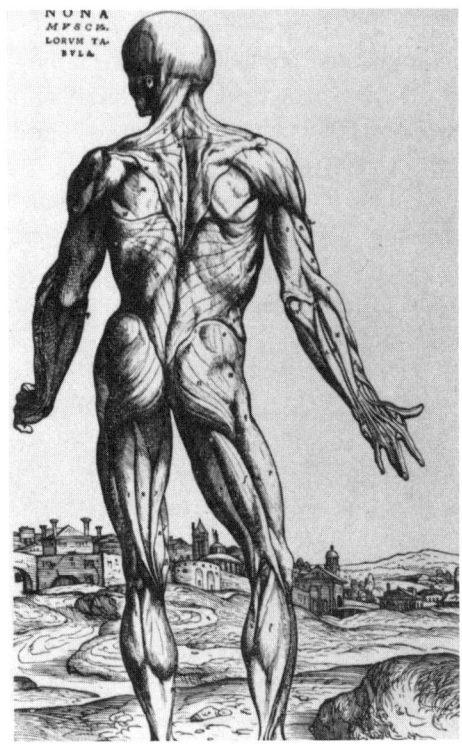

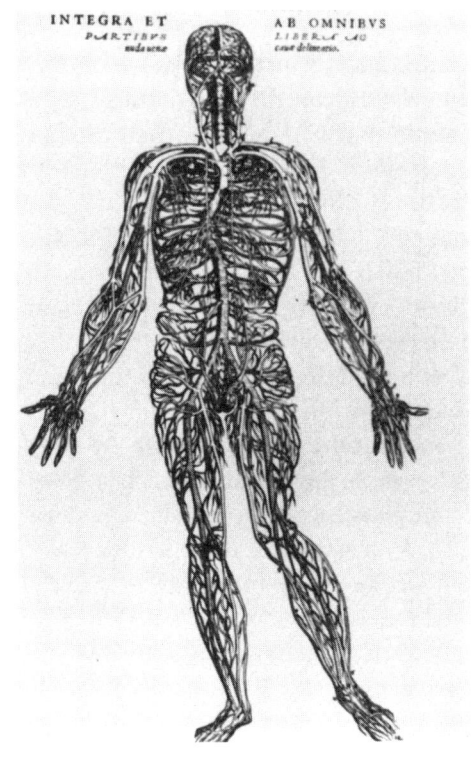

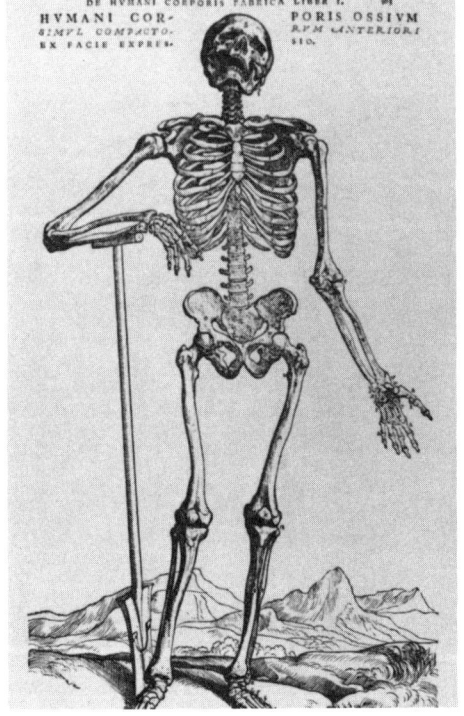

Top Left The Ninth Plate of Muscles. Woodcut from Vesalius' "De Humani Corporis Fabrica," Basle, 1543. Workshop of Titan. From *Medicine and the Artist* by Carl Zigrosser, Dover Publications, Inc., New York, 1970. Reprinted through the permission of the publisher and the Philadelphia Museum of Art.

Top Right A Chart of the Veins. Woodcut from Vesalius' "De Humani Corporus Fabrica," Basle, 1543. Workshop of Titan. From *Medicine and the Artist* by Carl Zigrosser, Dover Publications, Inc., New York, 1970. Reprinted through the permission of the publisher and the Philadelphia Museum of Art.

Left Skeleton Leaning on a Spade. Woodcut from Vesalius' "De Humani Corporis Fabrica," Basle, 1543. Workshop of Titan. From *Medicine and the Artist* by Carl Zigrosser, Dover Publications, Inc., New York, 1970. Reprinted through the permission of the publisher and the Philadelphia Museum of Art.

to anyone with healing skills, so physicians who had been formally trained were very careful to distinguish themselves from the many lay practitioners. Eventually, medical departments were established in American universities such as the College of Philadelphia, in 1765; King's College in 1768; and Harvard College in 1783; but the majority of American physicians were not educated in these universities. Proprietary medical schools arose in the United States and Canada at the beginning of the nineteenth century with the only entry requirements being the ability to read, write and to pay the fees. These schools fit in well with the apprentice system, and since there was little science in medicine at this time, and very little that the physician could actually do for the patient with the medicines available, the lack of a university education had little effect on the practice of medicine. Medical philosophies such as Homeopathy, Grahamism and Eclecticism sprang up and established their own medical schools and produced physicians who entered the competition for patients. In 1848, the national organization of physicians, the American Medical Association, AMA, was formed, and began attacking sectarian and lay physicians. During the late 1800s several American physicians began studying medicine in Europe, especially in Germany, where the germ theory of diseases was being taught, and when they returned, they brought new ideas with them that resulted in the formation of an American medical school, based upon the German system. Johns Hopkins Medical School, which also introduced the present educational system of four years of college followed by four years of medical school, was such an institution. In 1904, the AMA established the "Council on Medical Education and Hospital," which became a force for reform in the field of medical education. The Carnegie Foundation was responsible for the report of Abraham Flexner, in 1910, "Medical Education in the United States and Canada," in which he visited 155 medical schools. The report recommended the closing of all proprietary medical schools and criticized those schools associated with the colleges and universities. Only John Hopkins Medical School, of which Flexner was a graduate, escaped criticism. It was described as a suitable model for other medical schools to follow. Within a short time, laws were established that defined the requirements for admission into medical schools and the subject matter that would be included in the curriculum, so the proprietary schools were forced to adopt or close. This was the basis that launched American medicine to assume a dominant role in medical education and medicinal sciences. In 1937, the National Institutes of Health were established, which aided research and medical advances, and the practice of specializations in medicine which we have today. Family physicians are becoming a rarity, are poorly distributed, and appear to be in short supply, due to the limitation of the medical schools in the United States to graduate more students. Many students who cannot enter American medical schools are now going to foreign medical schools and then are returning to the United States to be licensed. According to the California Medical Association, only 37 foreign doctors were licensed in 1968 but 432 foreign doctors were licensed in 1973. In contrast, foreign coun-

204 *Magic, Myths and Medicine*

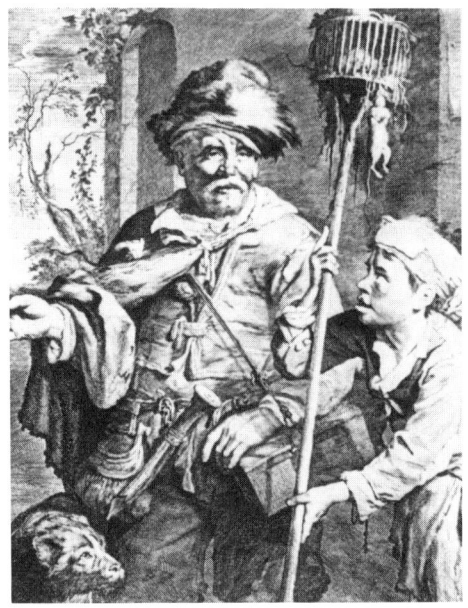

The Rat Catcher. Engraving by C. Visscher, 1655. From *Medicine and the Artist* by Carl Zigrosser, Dover Publications, Inc., New York, 1970. Reprinted through the permission of the publisher and the Philadelphia Museum of Art.

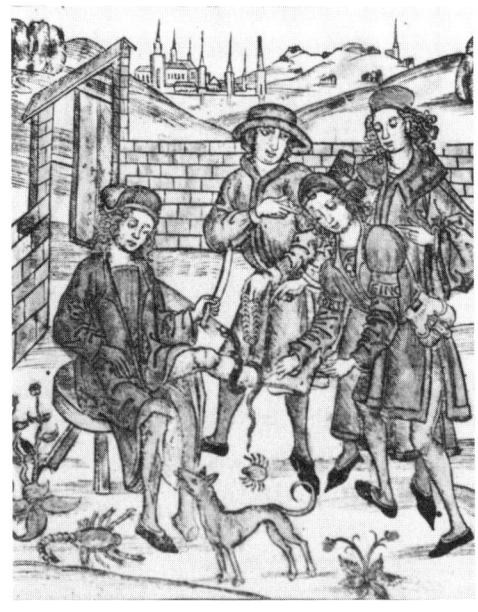

The Physician and his attendants have various methods of treatment which include surgery, herbs and astrology as pictured in H. Brunschwig's *Buch der Cirurgia*, 1497. (Photograph from Medicina Rara Ltd., New York.)

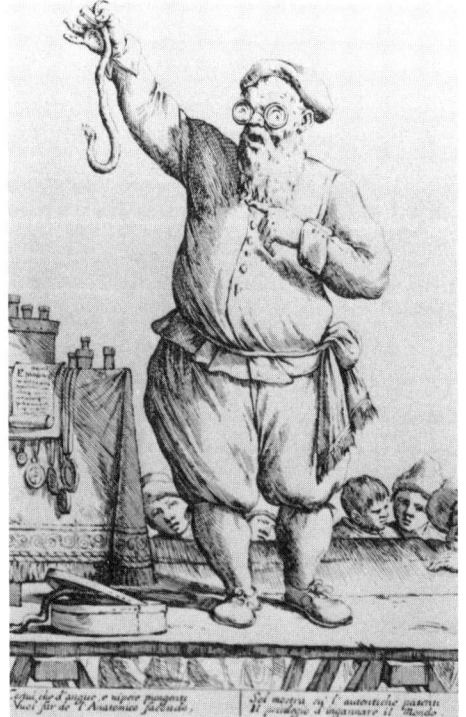

The Quack. Etching by G. M. Mitelli after the design by A. Carracci. From *Medicine and the Artist* by Carl Zigrosser, Dover Publications, Inc., New York, 1970. Reprinted through the permission of the publisher and the Philadelphia Museum of Art.

tries are sending students here for medical training and the AMA reported in 1972 the following foreign students in training: India—3229; the Phillipines—2440; Korea—1171; Taiwan—889; Thailand—789; Iran—769; Pakistan—615; Spain—492; Mexico—458; Italy—454; Argentina—393; and the UAR—386. Are the medical institutions of the United States, by training these foreign students, depriving citizens of this country of medical care in the near future?

Today, if one visits a physician or a hospital, one usually can observe a nurse or nurses in attendance, assisting the physician or caring for a patient. This was not always so. Nursing, as a paid occupation, was invented in the nineteenth century.

Since antiquity, women had cared, nursed and treated sick members of their families, using physicians only when necessary. When hospitals became established for surgery and the treatment of diseases, someone had to care for the patients, and it was usually one of their relatives. Some hospitals did employ people to clean the rooms and give token care to the patients, but they were usually not the type of persons that we see in hospitals today. Frequently, persons arrested for drunkenness, prostitution and thievery were used in the hospitals in these positions. Although armies had physicians and surgeons, once the patients were treated, their care was usually left to the orderlies and camp followers. The hospitals were also not the cleanest places in which to practice medicine, since the idea of asepsis was not really accepted until after the time of Lister (1912). Someone had to initiate reforms in hospitals and nursing care. Miss Florence Nightingale got the chance to do so during the Crimean War, in 1855.

Miss Nightingale and her assistants were trained to be obedient to physicians, devoted to the patients and firm with other hospital employees. They

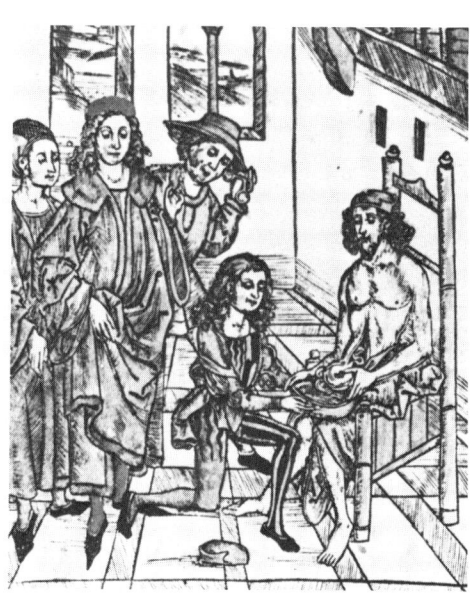

Abdominal surgery as pictured in H. Brunschwig's *Buch der Cirurgia,* 1497. (Photograph from Medicina Rara Ltd., New York.)

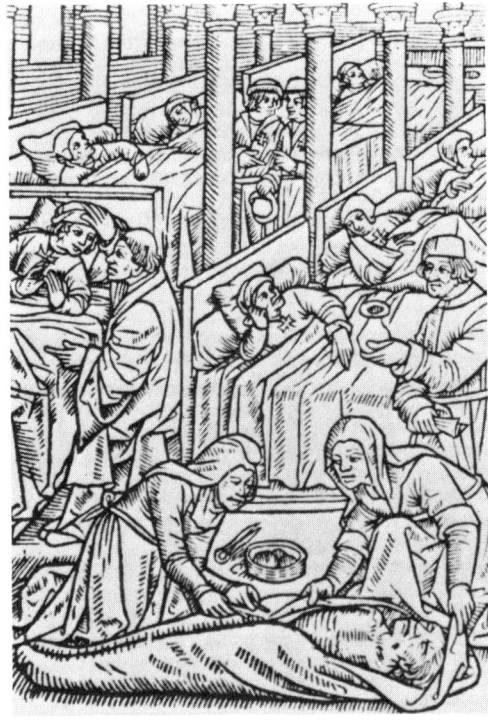

Hospital Interior. Woodcut from Saint-Gelais, "Le Vergier d'Honneur," Paris, J. Petit. ca. 1500. From *Medicine and the Artist* by Carl Zigrosser, Dover Publications, Inc., New York, 1970. Reprinted through the permission of the publisher and the Philadelphia Museum of Art.

actually transferred the image of a Victorian lady; the obedient wife, the devoted mother and the manager of the household to the hospital.

When Miss Nightingale and her nurses arrived in the Crimea, they were ignored by the physicians. Nightingale refused to allow her nurses to help any of the thousands of sick and wounded until ordered to do so by the physicians. The physicians finally allowed them to clean up the rooms and, realizing what competent workers they now had for virtually any task, allowed them to care for the patients after they had been treated.

The image of "the lady with the lamp" making her rounds and caring for the sick and wounded caught the attention of the public and soon after the war, nursing schools appeared in England and a little later, in the United States. The number of hospitals began to increase, as it was recognized that physicians needed training, and good hospitals required someone to run them, so, nursing schools were established to fulfill this need. Dorothy Dix and Louisa Schuyler were the leading forces behind the establishment of Nightingale-type nursing schools in the United States. At first, their training emphasized character rather than skills, but now, nursing curricula are requiring college education and many skills that were formerly relegated to the physician. A movement is currently underway to expand the position of nurses in health maintenance. We soon may see the image of the physician "curing" and the nurse "caring" undergo a change due to the Women's Liberation Movement and the entrance of many men into the occupation of nursing. Recently, a new position has appeared in

1500–Present. Explorations and Discoveries 207

the field of medicine; this is the "Medical Assistant," whose role is not clearly defined, but lies somewhere between that of the nurse and the physician.

Surgery had been practiced by many civilizations in antiquity and has been discussed in those sections, but due to the influence of religion over medicine, physicians had been expected to refrain from all surgical practices which left surgery to the barbers and surgeons. The barbers and surgeons were generally not very well educated and therefore, were deprived of the teachings of the Greeks and were forced to rely upon their own observations of human anatomy, wounds, cuts and methods of healing. People who wanted to become barber-surgeons became an apprentice to an established barber and learned the trade by observations, instruction and practice. Cuts, wounds and amputations were cauterized with boiling oil or hot metallic implements, and the opening was sutured together in the hope that there would be no poisoning. The introduction of guns into general use by European armies led to horrible wounds that generally became infected and resulted in amputation and death, unless the surgeon was extremely lucky. One surgeon of this period was very successful, Ambrose Pare (1510-90).

Pare had been a barber's apprentice in France until he learned his craft and then went to Paris and worked as a surgeon in the hospital, Hotel-Dieu and as a regimental surgeon with the army. While in the field treating the wounded by cauterization, he ran out of oil and so substituted plugs of lint smeared with a salve which he placed in the wounds. The next day he noted that those patients who had been cauterized had pain and fevers, while those treated with the salve had little pain and were comfortable. He declined to continue cauter-

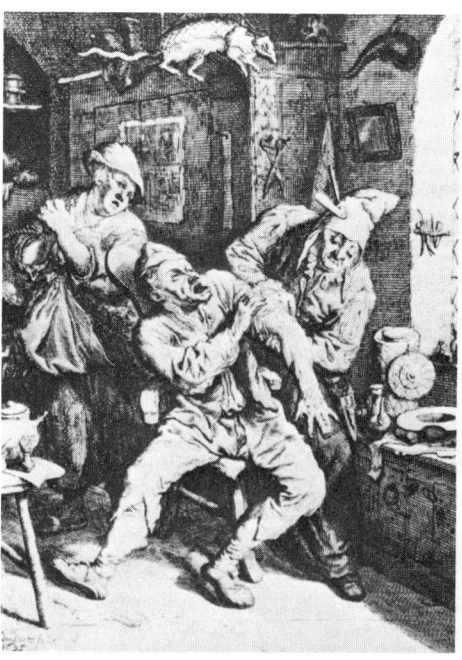

Village Surgeon. Etching by C. Dusart, Haarlem, 1695. From *Medicine and the Artist* by Carl Zigrosser, Dover Publications, Inc., New York, 1970. Reprinted through the permission of the publisher and the Philadelphia Museum of Art.

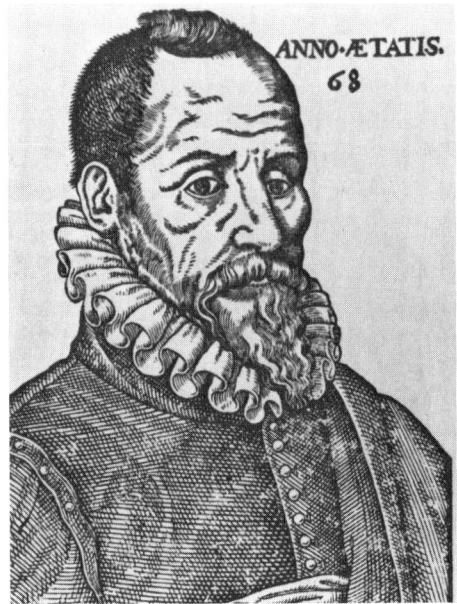

Ambrose Pare. Woodcut from the Latin edition of A. Pare's "Opera Chirurgica," Frankfort, 1594. From *Medicine and the Artist* by Carl Zigrosser, Dover Publications, Inc., New York, 1970. Reprinted through the permission of the publisher and the Philadelphia Museum of Art.

ization and utilized his new method of treating wounds, so that he soon became widely known due to his many successes. In 1544, Jacques Dubois, one of the teachers of Vesalius, met with Pare and persuaded him, under his auspices, to publish his findings concerning the treatment of gunshot wounds, which appeared in 1545. Pare studied and accepted the anatomy of Vesalius and practiced dissection which led to the production of several books on anatomy, as practical guides for the surgeon. In 1552 he rediscovered that ligature was preferable to cauterization for stopping bleeding, following an amputation. Many of the operations that Pare utilized were not new discoveries, but had merely been forgotten until he publicized them and for many years, France was the leader in the field of surgery. During his life, this former barber's apprentice, who knew no Latin, was appointed head surgeon at the College of Saint-Come; and was appointed the surgeon of Henry II, Francis II and Charles IX.

In Italy, at the University of Bologna, Professore Gasparo Taglicozzi (1546-99) rediscovered the method of restoring a damaged nose, rhinoplasty, which had been performed in India in antiquity, and is frequently called the "Father of Autoplastic Surgery."

In spite of these investigations into surgery and the healing of wounds, operative surgery was extremely limited because of the prevalence of infections and the lack of a general anaesthesia. In universities, physicians received some instruction in surgery, generally in the study of anatomy, but the practicing surgeon was, in general, a poorly educated craftsman. The person who is frequently noted as the one who opened the field of surgery to the study of medicinal practioners is John Hunter (1728-93).

1500–Present. Explorations and Discoveries   209

John Hunter started his career as an assistant in his brother's surgery in London, where he cleaned the dissecting room and secured cadavers, eventually becoming a skilled dissector. He became an apprentice surgeon at Chelsea, and several other hospitals, until he had mastered his techniques and became interested in comparative anatomy. After serving as an army and naval surgeon, he settled in the country and collected many rare and unusual animals for his studies, including the Irish giant, O'Bryan, whose body was purchased from his friends for 500 pounds, although they had promised O'Bryan that they would put his corpse in a leaden coffin and sink it in the sea to prevent Hunter from dissecting it. The skeleton is in the museum of the Royal College of Surgeons. He was appointed surgeon to St. George's Hospital, and shortly after began lecturing on the theories and practice of surgery which included general surgery, pathology, physiology and anatomy. He was especially interested in inflammations and recognized three types; alterative, secretive and regenerative; and also that inflammation was frequently the mode of cure. His best work, "A Treatise on the Blood, Inflammation and Gunshot Wounds," is considered a great advance in the study of general pathology.

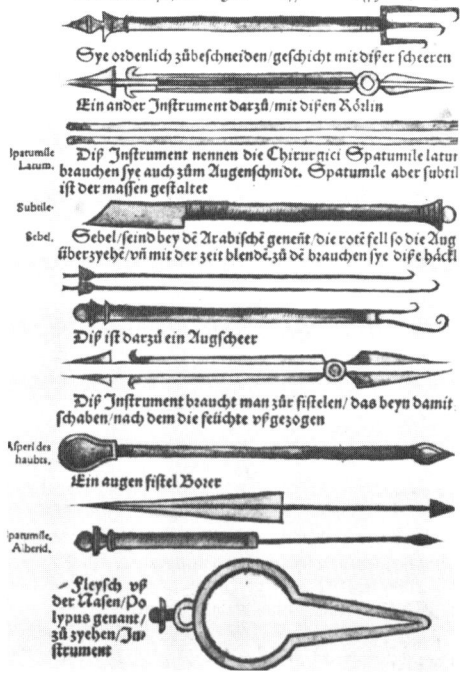

Surgical Instruments. Colored woodcut from H. von Gersdorff's "Feldtbuch der Wundartzney," Strassburg, 1540. From *Medicine and the Artist* by Carl Zigrosser, Dover Publications, Inc., New York, 1970. Reprinted through the permission of the publisher and the Philadelphia Museum of Art.

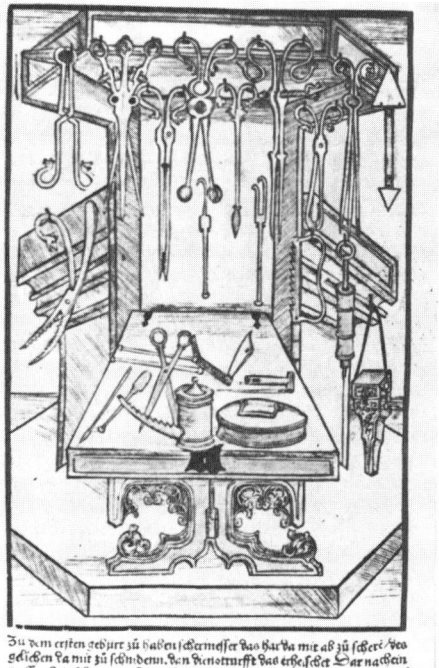

The surgeon's instruments as pictured in Hieronymus Brunschwig's *Buch der Cirurgia,* 1497. (Photograph from Medicina Rara Ltd., New York.)

The next great advances in surgery were the discovery, between 1844 and 1847, of "laughing gas," nitrous oxide, by an American dentist, Horace Wells; ether, by another American dentist, William Morton; and chloroform, by Dr. Simpson of Edinburgh. Physicians, surgeons, and dentists now had the means to render a patient partially or totally unconscious during surgery, extractions, or childbirth. However, wounds still became infected and patients died. Joseph Lister, (1827-1912), was to discover methods for the prevention of surgical infections.

Joseph Lister studied surgery in London and then took the post of house-surgeon at Edinburgh Hospital, where he conducted a variety of research projects which led to his appointment as professor of surgery in Glasgow. His father had been a wine-merchant who had spent much of his leisure time in microscopial investigations, and Lister was well aware of the microbial world and the work of Pasteur and Koch. In surgical procedures, the wounds generally became infected and, if Pasteur were correct concerning fermentation and putrefaction, these microorganisms could also enter wounds and cause putrefaction. The boiling procedures used by Pasteur could not be applied to the patient, so Lister began experimenting with chemicals that would destroy the microorganisms, finding carbolic acid to be the most successful. Lister operated in a carbolic acid mist and, when surgery was completed, covered the wound with a thick bandage soaked in carbolic acid. Wound infections and gangrene virtually disappeared from his wards. The mortality rate in major amputations

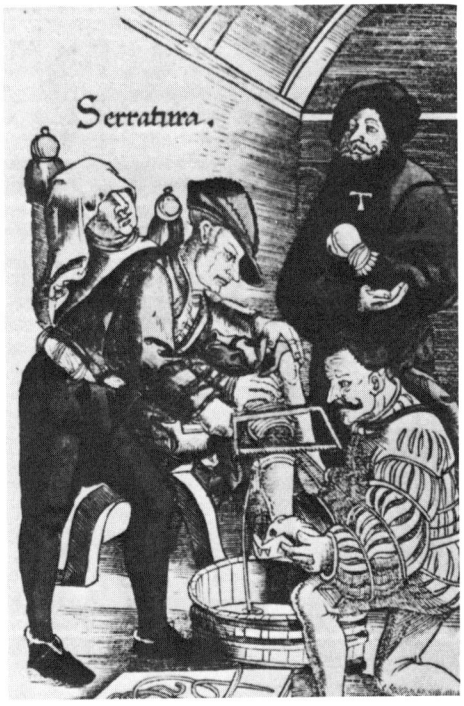

Amputation. Colored woodcut by J. Wechtlin from H. von Gersdorff's "Feldtbuch der Wundartzney," Strassburg, 1540. From *Medicine and the Artist* by Carl Zigrosser, Dover Publications, Inc., New York, 1970. Reprinted through the permission of the publisher and the Philadelphia Museum of Art.

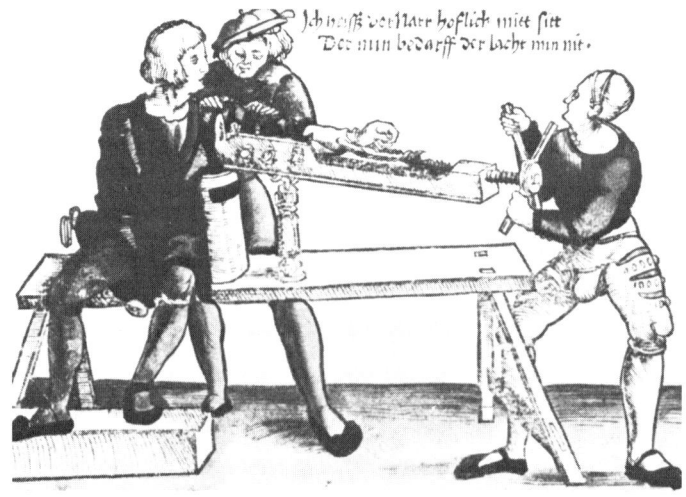

Extension Apparatus for Fractured Arm. Colored woodcut by J. Wechtlin from H. von Gersdorff's "Feldtbuch der Wundartzney," Strassburg, 1540. From *Medicine and the Artist* by Carl Zigrosser, Dover Publications, Inc., New York, 1970. Reprinted through the permission of the publisher and the Philadelphia Museum of Art.

carried out with his procedure dropped from about 46% to 15%. Lister began publication of his results in 1867, but they received little recognition until the Franco-German War, when many of the army surgeons who practiced "Listerism," reported very favorable results. Gradually, antisepsis received general acceptance and instruments and dressings were sterilized. In Germany, Bergmann and Schimmelbusch formulated the aseptic procedures that are utilized today in every surgery. Lister also introduced the use of absorbable sterilized catgut in sutures and ligatures.

In the early civilizations of the world, diseases were thought to have been caused by evil spirits, spells or the Gods. The Chinese used the imbalance of Yin and Yang to explain disorders of the body, while the Greeks introduced the four humors and associated tetrads in an attempt to explain diseases. In the first century B.C., Varro, in "De re rustica," explained that tiny creatures which were too small to be seen, grew in damp places and entered the body through the nose and mouth, causing illness. In 1546, Fracastoro wrote that infectious diseases were spread from person to person by contact, fomites or through the air. In 1658, the Jesuit, Father Kircher, using the microscope, examined pus and blood obtained from plague victims, and reported that he saw tiny worms which he believed were the cause of the disease. These he named "contagium animatim" or "contagium vivum," but today it is known that he was describing erythrocytes. The Dutch microscopist, Antony van Leeuwenhoek, in 1676, observed and described bacteria and, although he observed them in pus, physicians did not associate his finding with diseases. Many wealthy people had microscopes made for them with which to view the new

212   *Magic, Myths and Medicine*

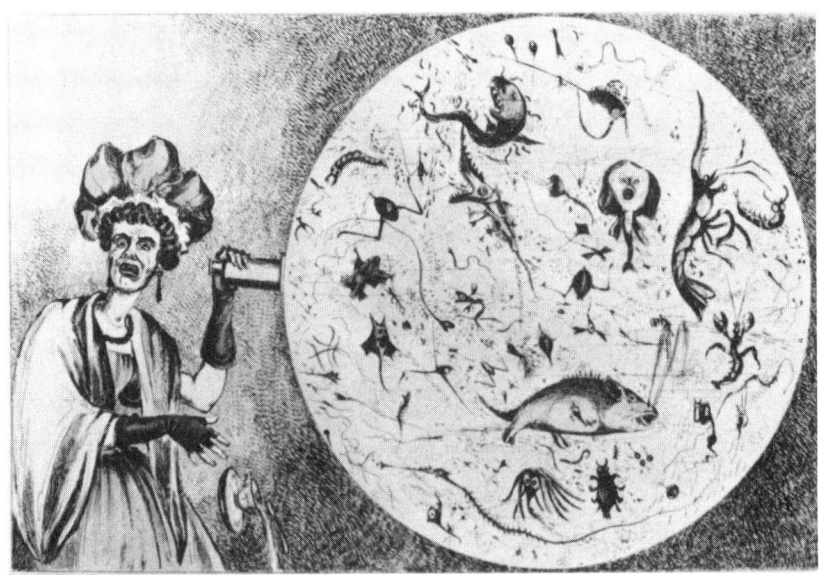

Thames Water. Colored etching by William Heath, ca. 1828. From *Medicine and the Artist* by Carl Zigrosser, Dover Publications, Inc., New York, 1970. Reprinted through the permission of the publisher and the Philadelphia Museum of Art.

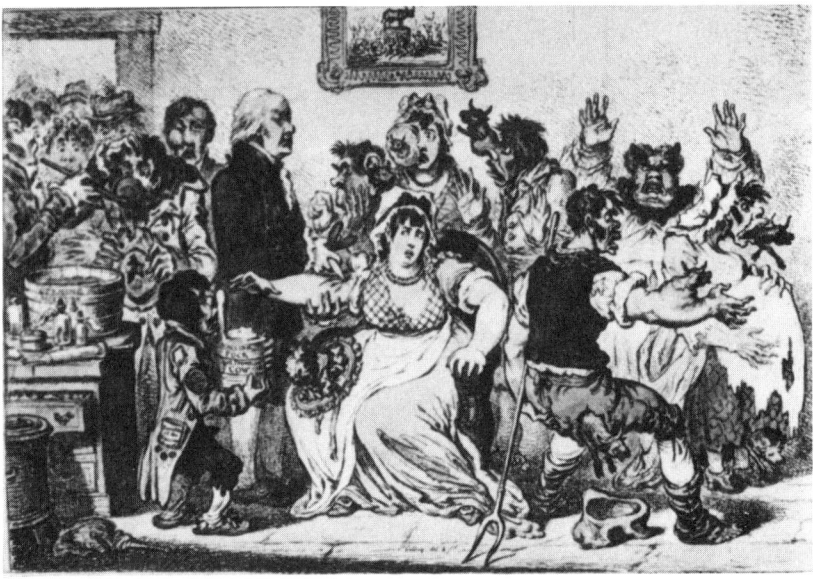

Cow Pock. Colored etching by J. Gillray, London, 1802. The administering physician is Jenner. From *Medicine and the Artist* by Carl Zigrosser, Dover Publications, Inc., New York, 1970. Reprinted through the permission of the publisher and the Philadelphia Museum of Art.

microbial world. Louis XV of France gave Madame de Pompadour a bronze microscope which was recently sold, at auction, for $74,000. Since antiquity, variolation had been practiced by many people in an attempt to obtain protection from an infection with smallpox. John Hunter, in 1767, had inoculated himself with gonorrheal pus and confused the study of venereal disease when he developed syphilis, probably because the donor had syphilis, as well as gonorrhea. The Italian anatomist, Lazarro Spallanzani (1729-99) also was interested in microorganisms and succeeded in growing bacteria on sterilized media, under aerobic and anaerobic conditions, and discovered "germs" or spores which were heat resistant. Unfortunately, the significance of his investigations was not understood by himself or the scientific world.

Edward Jenner (1749-1823) was a physician and surgeon of Berkeley, Gloucestershire, and a former pupil of John Hunter. Frequently, he was called to variolate all the members of a household, and noticed that people who had contracted cowpox, which he called "variolae vaccinae," failed to have any reaction to the inoculation.

In May, 1796, Jenner inoculated a boy, James Phipps, with pustular material from a cowpox lesion obtained from a milkmaid. The boy developed cowpox and recovered. In July, Jenner inoculated Phipps with smallpox, but no infection resulted, so he inoculated him again several months later, with the same results. The Royal Society of London returned his manuscript, but he published articles in 1798, 1799 and 1800 concerning vaccination experiments. In 1802, Parliament awarded him 10,000 pounds and later, 20,000 pounds.

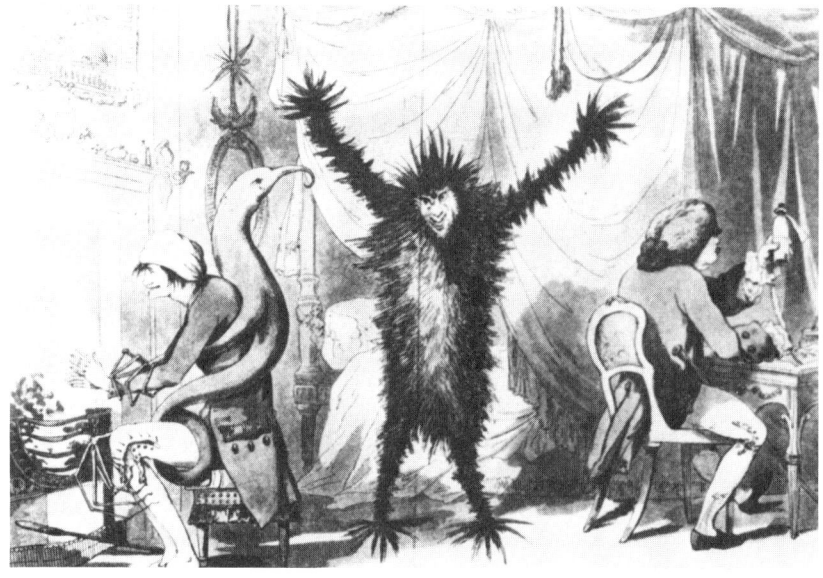

Ague and Fever. Colored etching by T. Rowlandson after a design by J. Dunthorne, London, 1792. From *Medicine and the Artist* by Carl Zigrosser, Dover Publications, Inc., New York, 1970. Reprinted through the permission of the publisher and the Philadelphia Museum of Art.

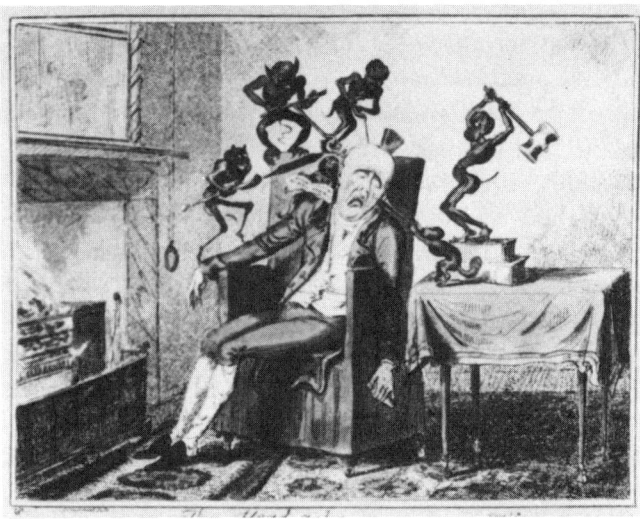

The Headache. Colored etching by G. Cruikshank after the design by Maryatt, London, 1819. From *Medicine and the Artist* by Carl Zigrosser, Dover Publications, Inc., New York, 1970. Reprinted through the permission of the publisher and the Philadelphia Museum of Art.

Vaccination, rather than variolation, spread throughout the world with the result that today, the World Health Organization has declared the disease to be extinct. However, China still requires a valid smallpox vaccination for entry.

The increased use of the microscope by investigators led to the discovery of the causative agents of many of the parasitic infections and in Sweden, Rudolphi (1771-1832), the "Father of Parasitology," organized and classified a large collection of specimens. In 1828, Peacock discovered a human infected with the worm, *Trichinella,* and in 1846, Leidy found the infection in pigs. In 1842, Gluge and Gruby discovered trypanosomes in the blood of frogs. In 1848, Gros discovered the amebic infection of man, *Endamoeba.* In 1869, Melnikov reported that the cat and dog tapeworms developed in fleas, and in the same year, Fedchenko discovered the cyclops involved in the transmission of Dracunculosis. Sir Patrick Manson, the "Father of Tropical Medicine" (1844-1922), studied the development of the filiarial worm in mosquitos and postulated a similar cycle in the mosquito for malaria. In 1880, Lavaran discovered the malarial parasite, *Plasmodium.* Nepveu, in 1890, found trypanosomes in the blood of a man with African Sleeping Sickness which was followed, in 1895, by the discovery, by Sir David Bruce, that African Trypanosomiasis was transmitted by the Tsetse fly.

The prevention of puerperal fever and blood-poisoning had been attempted by practical methods and cleanliness as early as 1773, by White. Later, advocates were Holmes (1843), Semmelweis (1847), Lister (1867), Championniere (1874) and others. Antiseptics were available for the control of infections long before physicians recognized and understood antisepsis.

The fungus that is the causative agent of favus, or ringworm of the scalp, was discovered by Schonlein, in 1839 which, in 1845, was named *Achorion schoenleinii* by Remak. Later, the Genus was changed to *Trichophyton*. Many of the fungus infections of the skin are called ringworm infections because early investigators believed that a worm was the causative agent, due to the circular raised lesions that were frequently observed. Other dermatophytes can also infect man and, in general, they are now treated with griseofulvin, akrinol, nystatin, tinactin and others. Systemic fungal infections are, in general, treated with Amphotericin B (Fungizone) which has proved effective in many cases, but which is also very toxic.

In 1835, Bassi reported that muscardine, a disease affecting silk worms was caused by a fungus and predicted, as did Henle in 1840, that microorganisms would also be found to be the causative agents of diseases of man. Also involved in diseases of silkworms was Louis Pasteur (1822-1895), a French chemist, not a physician, who was to revolutionize many biological theories by his experiments.

The son of a tanner, Louis Pasteur studied in Paris and became the assistant of the chemist Dumas. His first work, on tartaric and racemic acids laid the foundations of stereochemistry. He became Dean of the natural science school of Lille, where the investigated the fermentation theories of de la Tour and Schwann, which involved yeasts and alcoholic fermentations, confirmed them, and went on to study other fermentations. He discovered that microorganisms could convert lactose to lactic acid and that butter fat was converted to butyric acid, which made the butter rancid. He recognized that the alcoholic fermentation was carried out anaerobically, whereas the bacterial fermentations were carried out under aerobic conditions. Meanwhile, wine-producers in the area were complaining of their spoiled or "sick" wines which Pasteur now knew were due to the presence of microorganisms. He discovered that by heating the wines, the microorganisms were destroyed and the wines were preserved. This process, the application of heat for the preservation of wines, and later other foods, is called pasteurization.

While director of scientific studies at the Ecole Normale, in Paris, where he had previously been a student, Pasteur attacked the belief in spontaneous generation, or heterogenesis, by showing that sterilized substances, if sealed from the air would not decompose, but those which were sterilized and exposed to the air would decompose. The obvious deduction that he made was that the environment was teeming with microorganisms, some of which caused diseases.

In 1865, the silkworm industry of southern France suffered an epidemic of pebrine, a spotted disease of the worms, and Pasteur was sent to study the infection. He instituted procedures for breeding a healthy stock and eliminating the diseased worms, thereby saving the silk industry.

While studying chicken cholera, anthrax and swine fever, he inoculated chickens with an old culture of microorganisms which had previously caused death of other experimental birds, but at this time, did not prove fatal. Rein

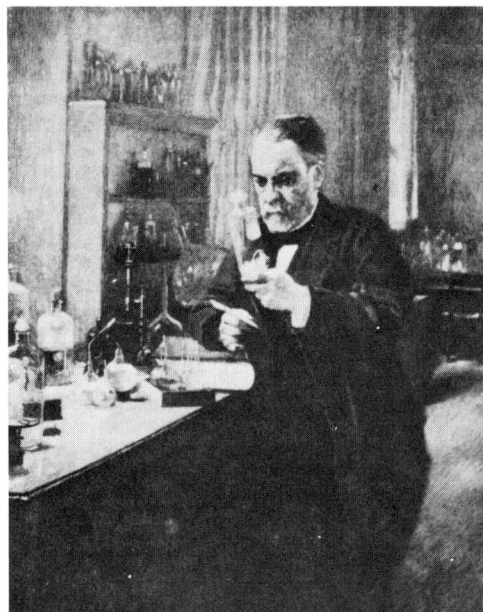

Pasteur in His Laboratory. A wood engraving by T. Cole, 1925. From *Medicine and the Artist* by Carl Zigrosser, Dover Publications, Inc., New York, 1970. Reprinted through the permission of the publisher and the Philadelphia Museum of Art.

oculation of birds with a virulent culture of the same microorganisms proved them to be immune to chicken cholera. He was able to develop inoculations against chicken cholera, anthrax and swine fever which he called "vaccines," by analogy with the cowpox inoculations of Jenner.

The development of these vaccines led Pasteur to develop the method of attenuating the virus of rabies by drying the spinal cords of animals he had infected with rabies. This material was injected into persons who had been bitten by rabid animals and usually produced immunity before the fatal attack of hydrophobia commenced. This procedure is still used today in many parts of the world, although others use the Flury egg-passed virus and an antirabies serum. Pasteur is frequently called the "Father of Bacteriology."

Although Pasteur had developed the anthrax vaccine, previous investigators had reported the presence of a bacterium in the blood of diseased animals. Pollender (1849) had observed the bacillus in the blood of animals and Davaine (1863) had transmitted the disease from animal to animal by inoculations of blood. It was also reported that blood which was free of the bacteria could also infect animals, so an impass had developed in the investigations of the infection until Robert Koch (1843-1910) completed his investigations.

Robert Koch was a physician who, after serving during the Franco-German war, settled in the country as a district medical officer. He became interested in the epidemic of anthrax that developed in his patients' animals and began his studies. Mice infected with anthrax were bled and examined, which revealed chains of bacilli which formed spores, the latter being resistant to heat and drying, and which, if transmitted to a healthy animal, could cause the disease. His results were published in 1876, when Pasteur was carrying out his own investigations on anthrax and preparing the vaccine. Koch's paper, for the first time in the history of man, proved that a microorganism was the cause of an infectious disease, by cultivating it on artificial medium and then introducing the microorganisms into a healthy animal and causing the specific disease, and none other.

In 1879, Neisser discovered the bacterium that caused gonorrhea; in 1880, Gaffky and Eberth reported the discovery of the typhoid bacillus and Hansen discovered the leproma bacillus. More were to be discovered by other researchers. In the same year, Koch was made a member of the Imperial Board of Health of Germany.

In 1865, Villemin had transmitted tuberculosis from humans to rabbits but many people still believed that tuberculosis was a nutritional disorder, until 1882, when Koch announced that he had discovered the tubercle bacillus and in the next year, the causative agent of cholera. Other diseases included in his researches were rinderpest, bubonic plague, Texas fever, malaria and investigations of the tsetse fly.

In 1890, Koch reported the discovery of "tuberculin," an extract of the tubercle bacillus, which, when injected into the bodies of infected animals or people would destroy the bacteria, heal the damaged body and would prevent and protect against tuberculosis. He wanted to keep the treatment process a secret so that Germany would have a monopoly in the treatment of the disease, but public pressure forced him to release the process of preparation of tuberculin. Soon, physicians throughout the world were injecting their patients with Koch's tuberculin and, to their horror, the patients collapsed and died.

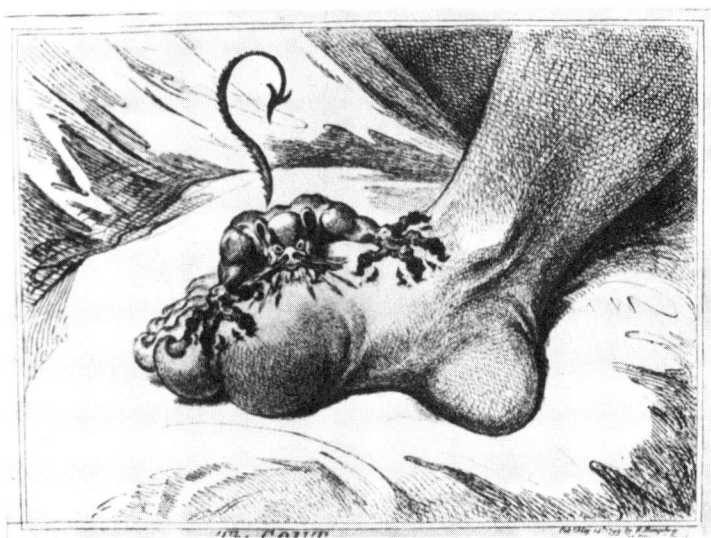

The Gout. Colored etching by J. Gillray, London, 1799. From *Medicine and the Artist* by Carl Zigrosser, Dover Publications, Inc., New York, 1970. Reprinted through the permission of the publisher and the Philadelphia Museum of Art.

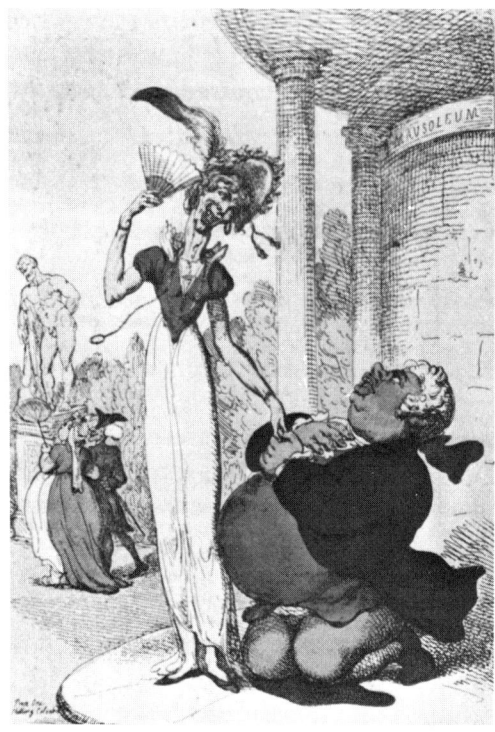

"Dropsy Courting Consumption." Colored etching by T. Rowlandson, London, 1810. (Reproduced from Medicina Rara Ltd., New York.)

It is now known that the injection of tuberculin into tuberculous people causes a swift reaction, with coma, fever, pain and death. Those patients who do not die immediately undergo a spreading of the bacteria throughout the body and death follows. The injected material destroys the tuberculous tissue by an allergenic reaction and the tissue may enter the bloodstream, causing death. Apparently, Koch had used some harmless strain in his experiments and his animals had survived.

The treatments were halted abruptly and Koch was accused of recklessness and negligence. In 1897, Koch announced a new form of the substance called tuberculin-R which he described as being perfectly safe, but few physicians would believe him. In 1901, he produced a "bacillary-emulsion," a new tuberculin which went virtually unnoticed by the medical world.

In 1896, Theobald Smith described two species of the tubercle bacillus, *Mycobacterium tuberculosis* of man, and *M. bovis* of cattle, and stated that man could be infected by both organisms. At first Koch stated that there was only one species and then said that there were two, but the bovine strain could only infect cattle. In 1907 the Royal Commission on Tuberculosis stated that Koch was in error but Koch managed to sway everyone to his belief. In 1910, Park and Krumwiede reported that one-third of the tuberculous children they had studied were infected with *M. bovis*. The thousands of children who had died between 1900 and 1910 from bovine tuberculosis could probably have been prevented from developing tuberculosis by pasteurization of milk. Koch died soon after the publication in 1910.

Koch's tuberculin and a more purified form, purified protein derivative (PPD), are still used today, but not to cure tuberculosis. Small amounts of these materials are injected into the skin to diagnose the infection.

Perhaps the greatest contribution of Koch to the study of diseases was his law, or postulates, under which the specificity of a microorganism is not demonstrated without the fulfillment of the following conditions: (1) The microorganism is present and discoverable in every case of the disease; (2) It is to be cultivated in pure culture; (3) Inoculation from the pure culture must reproduce the disease in susceptible animals; (4) It must be isolated from such animals and grown again in pure culture.

Early in the twentieth century, two French investigators, Calmette and Guerin (1908), began experiments to attenuate *M. bovis* by growing the bacteria on an artificial medium that contained ox-bile and transferring it over a period of thirteen years. Test animals were inoculated with this "Bacille Calmette-Guerin" (BCG) which did not develop tuberculosis and were found to be immune to pathogenic tubercle bacilli. They tested themselves, their associates and volunteers and finding no ill effects, in 1922 began vaccinating children with BCG. The death of 200 babies in Lubeck, Germany, stopped the vaccinations and a Commission reported that the German physicians had accidentally used a virulent culture rather than BCG. The vaccinations proceeded until scientists began reporting the isolation of pathogenic mycobacteria from the BCG cultures and many physicians refused to continue with the inoculations. The controversy over the pathogenic strains of BCG has never been settled, but BCG is today being utilized by the World Health Organization (WHO) in the immunization of children throughout the world, since tuberculosis is still one of the leading causes of death throughout the world. In the United States, the death rate has declined from about 500 per 100,000 persons in the mid-nineteenth century to about 2.8 per 100,000 persons today.

The Sloan-Kettering Cancer Center has recently reported the use of BCG in the regression of certain skin cancers.

The discoveries of Pasteur and Koch led others into the field of bacteriology, and other microorganisms, both pathogenic and nonpathogenic, were rapidly isolated or, as in the case of viruses, were discovered by filtration techniques. Interested readers should consult manuals of determinative bacteriology for a continuation of this information. Pasteur and Koch had demonstrated that animals and people could be made immune to specific diseases by the inoculation of dead or attenuated specific microorganisms into their bodies, but the mechanisms of the development of the response was unknown at that time, and is still not fully understood.

Elie Metchnikoff (1845-1916), a Russian zoologist working in Paris in the 1880s, introduced fungal spores into the water flea, *Daphnia,* and observed ameboid cells, phagocytes, surround and digest the fungal spores. He also observed that sometimes the phagocytes failed to digest the fungal spores which resulted in a fatal fungal infection. From these observations, and others, Metchnikoff proposed the theory that nonspecific resistance and acquired immunity were brought about by this phagocytic activity of the ameboid body cells. These observations shortly caused a lively controversy due to the investigations of a pupil of Koch, Emil Behring.

Emil Behring (1854-1917) studied under Koch and later worked as his associate in the Institute of Infectious Diseases, eventually becoming professor of Hygiene in Halle (1894) and in Marburg (1895). Behring experimented with the toxin produced by the diphtheria bacillus and discovered that the animals infected with diphtheria produced antitoxins which were able to combine with, and neutralize, the toxins. He was then able to demonstrate that the antitoxin could be introduced into a healthy individual which resulted in a transient immunity to diphtheria, or into an infected individual in which the progress of the infection was usually arrested. This principle of serum therapy and artificial immunization has been successfully utilized in the prevention and treatment of many diseases. Behring was awarded the Nobel Prize in 1901.

Today, it is known that the phagocytes and the antibodies are extremely important defence mechanisms of the body and that in addition to increasing the efficiency of the phagocytes, antibodies serve other purposes.

By 1900, medicine finally was established on a firm scientific basis. Human anatomy was fairly well-understood and pathologic conditions were being observed. Microorganisms were known to cause a wide variety of diseases and in some cases could be prevented by vaccination or control of the environment or vectors. Others could be treated with antisera or derivatives of mercury, arsenic or antimony. Asepsis had been introduced into surgery, childbirth and the treatment of wounds. Anaesthetics, such as ether, were available to immobilize the patient for long periods of time and pain could be controlled with opium derivatives and other drugs. Yet, something was missing for the control of infections. A substance, which, when injected into an organism, would destroy harmful microorganisms without harming the host. The alchemists had searched for the philosopher's stone for centuries but a histologist and chemist, Paul Ehrlich, was to discover one.

Paul Ehrlich (1845-1915) first studied histology and the chemical application of stains which rendered various portions of cells more readily visible due to their affinity for certain dyes or stains. In 1887, he contracted tuberculosis and went to Egypt for the cure and returned in good health, taking several posts with Koch at Moabit Hospital and the Institute for Infectious Disorders. Later he became the head of the State Institute for Serum Testing and Serological Research, which was followed by a similar appointment to the Royal Institute for Experimental Therapeutics. Working under the theory that specific chemicals had specific points of attack in organisms and microorganisms, he began studying how to destroy microorganisms without harming the host. He began investigating syphilis and its treatment with an arsenic derivative by systematically making modifications of the compound and testing them. The six hundred and sixth derivative tested, in collaboration with Benda and Bertheim, was produced in 1910 and was named "Salvarsan." It was found to have toxic properties so an improved variant "Neosalvarsan" was formulated, which proved to be effective in the treatment of syphilis, relapsing fever (*Borrelia recurrentis*), Yaws, Leishmaniasis and others. Scientists began searching for other miracle drugs. It is interesting that Ehrlich had been in Egypt for some time since, in antiquity, the Egyptians had used copper and antimony in treating a variety of infections and other cultures such as in South America had used the "death medicine," arsenic. Ehrlich's Salvarsan was composed of a derivative of arsenic and copper.

In 1908 the compound para-amino-benzene-sulfonamide (sulfanilamide) was produced in Germany, and during World War I, it was found to be effective in treating trypanosomiasis. By 1930, it had been found to be effective in the treatment of pneumonia, scarlet fever, blood-poisonings and other infections. However, the drug, Prontosil, had been patented by Farben, the Germany Trust, and could not be produced by others. At the Pasteur Institute, two chemists discovered that half of the compound was also effective and that portion, Sulfanidamide, was unpatented. In 1936 the drug was introduced into general use but continued reports of toxic side effects, such as kidney damage, led to the synthesis of less toxic compounds such as Sulfapyridine, Sulfathiazone and Sulfadiazine. These sulfa drugs were widely used by the United States during World War II to prevent wound infections.

Alexander Fleming (1881-1955) had been an assistant to Sir Almroth Wright, who had continued the vaccine research started by Pasteur. Fleming devoted many years in the search of substances which would destroy microorganisms and, in 1922, reported the discovery of lysozyme, a substance which he found in the tissues and secretions of the body which brought about the lysis of certain bacterial cells. In 1928, while working with *Staphylococcus aureus,* a bacterium frequently associated with wound infections, he noted a blue-green mold in one of his cultures around which the colonies of *S. aureus* were undergoing lysis. Further experimentation led to the isolation of the inhibitory substance which he named Penicillin, derived from the mold, *Penicillium.*

Fleming performed tests with the penicillin on animals and people with favorable, but not spectacular, results which were published in 1929, but which aroused little interest, probably due to the use of the sulfa drugs. In 1938, Chain and Florey began investigations of Fleming's mold and isolated a penicillin of greater potency, which they administered to a case of blood-poisoning, keeping the patient alive for ten days. The Rockefeller Institute and pharmaceutical manufacturers became interested in the drug and a new strain of the mold, *Penicillium chrysogenum,* isolated from a moldy cantelope, was found to yield 200 times more penicillin than the original *P. notatum.* Penicillin was found to be effective against many Gram-positive bacteria and some of the Gram-negative bacteria.

The earliest reference that the author has been able to locate in which the *Penicillium* molds were used to treat infections, dates to the 1550's, when Arabic physicians[1] used moldy green cheese[2] to treat the wounded from battles.

Since the discovery of penicillin, many other antibiotics have been discovered with which man is now able to control many microbial infections. Dubos discovered Tyrothricin; Waksman, Streptomycin; Duggar, Aureomycin; Burkholder, Chloromycetin; Pfizer and Company, Terramycin; and others.

Although the antibiotics have saved many lives, some have also caused the death of the patient. In 1968, Chloromycetin came under attack from numerous reports by physicians of patients who died while under treatment with the drug. The California State Department of Public Health estimated a fatality rate of one person per 60,000, and since approximately 40 million Americans had taken the drug, the deaths would therefore be 666. While Chloromycetin is the drug of choice in the treatment of psittacosis, typhoid and paratyphoid fevers, murine typhus, Rocky Mountain Spotted Fever, Acne and bacterial meningitis *(Hemophilus),* the number of these infections in the United States is small when compared with the sales figure of $72 million in 1966, of Chloromycetin. It is believed that physicians are prescribing it for the common cold and similar virus infections, in which it is ineffective. A fatality rate of 58% has been reported in newborn infants treated with Chloromycetin for pneumonia and diarrhea.

Recently, Dr. Paul Stolley of Johns Hopkins and Dr. Henry Simmons, deputy assistant secretary for Health, in the Department of Health, Education and Welfare, estimated the use of the miracle drugs in hospitals in the United States resulted in 50,000 to 100,000 deaths yearly. The results, of physicians who blindly treat patients with antibiotics, are the development of "resistant" bacteria which do not respond to the normal treatment. Dr. James Visconti, of Ohio State University School of Pharmacy, has estimated the cost of unnecessary prescriptions at approximately $200 million per year. Ralph Nader and the Food and Drug Administration have both reported that over one hundred Americans die daily from the result of adverse reactions to prescriptions and legal, nonprescription drugs. The benefits of the miracle drugs are currently under investigation.

At the present time, researchers are attempting to discover drugs that can be used to treat virus infections. Some drugs which have been found to be effective are: amantadine hydrochloride for the treatment of influenza; vidarabine for the treatment of herpes simplex infections; and adenine arabinoside (ara-A) for the treatment of herpes virus encephalitis.

Although there have been great advances in medicine since the time of the first recognizable physician, Imhotep of Egypt (2780 B.C.), the life expectancy of man is still about 70 years. What has changed is that more people are living

---

1. "Green Darkness," A. Seton, Houghton Mifflin Co., Boston, Mass., 1972, pg. 205.
2. Many species of the mold Genus *Penicillium* are blue-green in color. Blue cheeses are made with species of this mold.

to be 70 years of age and the diseases which are causing their deaths have changed.

In the United States, in 1900, the ten leading causes of death were: (1) all forms of pneumonia and influenza; (2) tuberculosis; (3) diarrhea, enteritis, and ulcers; (4) heart diseases; (5) intracranial lesions of vascular origin; (6) nephritis; (7) accidents; (8) cancer and other malignancies; (9) senility; (10) diphtheria.

In 1980, the ten leading causes of death in the United States were: (1) heart diseases; (2) cancer and other malignancies; (3) cerebrovascular diseases; (4) accidents; (5) all forms of pneumonia and influenza; (6) diseases of early infancy; (7) diabetes mellitis; (8) arteriosclerosis (9) cirrhosis of the liver; (10) emphysema, asthma and bronchitis.

These causes of death reveal that the majority of deaths are now those due to the process of aging, physiological disorders or viral infections which cannot be treated with drugs. When, or if, a substance is found to combat viral infections and cancers, one can expect these diseases to be removed from the list. Certain cancers, such as leukemia, are treated with drugs that suppress the immune system or with antimetabolites that interfere with cellular metabolism. With increasing frequency, viruses are being implicated with cancers so that it may be that in the near future a vaccine or vaccines will be developed for protection against this disease.

Recently, in a bold experiment, Dr. Alfonso Zavaleta, of Lima, Peru, injected himself with cancer cells taken from his half-sister. After a period of time, he bled himself and transferred antibodies and white blood cells to his half-sister. He reported, after one month, that the cancer of the uterus had disappeared, but that five years was required before the treatment could be called a cure.

For most people the word "surgery" means a necessary intervention to alter the course of a disease. At one time this was true, but today, surgery may be used in diagnostic procedures, in minor operations and for cosmetic purposes. There are now approximately one thousand classified operations listed and it has been estimated that about 50,000 major and minor surgical procedures are carried out in the United States every day.

In antiquity, the surgeon was the seer, shaman, medicine-man or priest who removed foreign objects from the patient's body, sometimes making incisions with a stone or metal knife. Trepanning, the removal of a portion of the skull, was frequently carried out in ancient cultures, especially in South America where thousands of trepanned skulls have been found dated prior to the Spanish conquest. It is believed that trepanning was carried out to relieve pressures on the brain caused by the blow of a club or mace on the skull. Others have suggested that it was also used to allow evil spirits to leave the body of the patient. Surgery was practiced in ancient Egypt and Mesopotamia and appears to have been very advanced in India at the time of Sashruta, when compared with European surgery in 1500 A.D. The understanding of human anatomy, the circulatory system, asepsis, diseases, pathology, anaesthesia and chemical interventions in the nineteenth and twentieth centuries, has led to the rapid development of surgery as it is undertaken today. In the United States, the individual States license the surgeon and the hospitals in which the surgery is performed, while "boards" specify the training required, the hospitals where the training is obtained, and examine and certify the candidates as specialists for the licenses.

The American Board of Surgery was established in 1937 to certify the general surgeon. However, not all surgeons in the United States are board-certified; it has been estimated that there are approximately 46,500 board-certified surgeons in the United States and, about 20,600 uncertified surgeons, who have designated themselves as surgeons. It might be prudent to inquire if your surgeon is board-certified prior to undertaking surgical treatment.

In 1968 the American Medical Association held a national conference on quackery in Chicago where the AMA President, Dr. Dorman, reported that if the Americans could not find the quacks they wanted in the United States that they would travel around the world to find them. He reported that 110 Americans and Canadians had, during the previous year, chartered an aeroplane and had flown to the Philippines to seek "psychic surgery" from Antonio Agpaoa, known to his friends and customers as "Dr. Tony." Agpaoa claims that he can perform brain, heart and abdominal surgery with his bare hands, without the

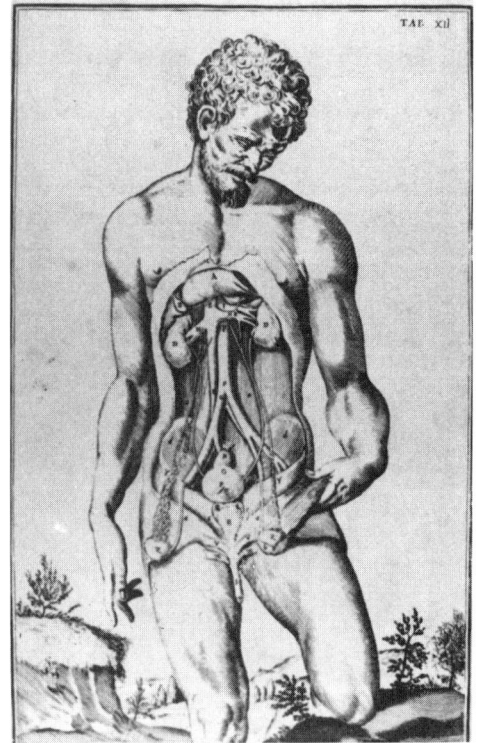

Dissection of a male. Drawings from Julius Casserius's "Tabulae Anatomicae and De Formato Foetu Tabulae" which were completed about 1616 & published in later works. (Reproduced from Medicina Rara Ltd., New York)

precautions of asepsis or anaesthesia, and can close the surgical opening without leaving a scar. He also has students training under his guidance in these procedures.

Dorman reported that in Europe there are rejuvenators who will make you young again such as Dr. Anna Aslan, who claimed to be able to restore elderly patients with injections of procaine (Novocain) and vitamins. In Switzerland, Professor Paul Niehans, a licensed physician, utilizes embryonic cells from unborn lambs which are injected into the body of the patient. Strangely, some very famous persons have undergone this treatment such as Winston Churchill, Konrad Adenauer, Somerset Maugham, Gloria Swanson, Pope Pius XII, King Ibn Saud of Arabia, and others.

Dorman also reported that Mexico has become the haven for many quacks and clinics for the treatment of diseases such as cancer and arthritis with the drugs Laetrile and Liefcort, which have been found worthless in clinical tests. It is also estimated that quackery in the United States robs victims of two billion dollars annually. Imagine what might be accomplished if that amount of money were utilized annually in research on the two diseases, arthritis and cancer.

1968 also became famous for another report and that was the report of Dr. Barnard, of Capetown, who successfully transplanted a human heart into the body of Philip Blaiberg, a 58-year-old dentist, the first long-term heart-transplant survivor. This achievement led to a flurry of heart transplants and a number of complex questions with ethical and moral overtones dealing with the establishment of a universally recognized definition of death. Legally, death became official when certified by a licensed physician that there was an irreversible cessation of respiration and circulation. A thirteen-member panel of the AMA recommended that the definition of death be based upon "brain death," although it recognized that there were such cases in which the heart continued to beat. The criteria of brain death are: unreceptivity and unresponsitivity; absence of muscular movements or breathing; the absence of reflexes such as pupil response, swallowing, yawning and others. A flat electroencephalogram was felt to be of confirmatory value.

In 1974, in Santa Rosa, California, a Sonoma County Superior Judge overruled an earlier decision by a Municipal Court Judge in which the cause of death of a girl was ruled to have been caused by the removal of her heart for transplant rather than the automobile accident in which she had suffered irreversible brain damage. Recently, State Attorney General Evelle Younger stated that he would propose legislation which would enable physicians to pronounce patients legally dead when the brain stopped functioning, even though the heart was still beating.

The history of transplantation goes back to ancient India where rhinoplasty was performed. Although the Sashruta Samhita describes a method using the patient's own tissues, another ancient description mentions the beating of the donor's buttocks with a paddle, the excision of the tissue and the securing of the donated tissue to the patient with a secret cement, the formula of which has been lost. Today, skin allografts are used mainly for temporary burn dressings, in histocompatibility tests, and in the study of the phenomenon of rejection.

During the Middle Ages there were several accounts of the transplantation of entire limbs or breasts, which were said to have been successful due to the assistance of a variety of Saints of the Church. A report by Jobus, in 1680, tells of a Russian who had a skull injury repaired with pieces of bone taken from the skull of a dog. The Russian Church heard of the operation and threatened to excommunicate the man unless the dog's bones were removed from his skull. A similar operation was carried out in ancient Egypt using an ostrich egg shell.

John Hunter, the English surgion (1728-93), successfully transplanted teeth obtained from cadavers but the development of artificial dentures made the procedure obsolete until recently, when it is again being studied more closely.

Bone allografts date to 1878, when the British surgeon MacEwen repaired the arm of a child by using bone grafts taken from patients suffering from rickets. Today, fresh and frozen allografts are used, but only when an autograft is not feasible, since xenografts are generally rejected by the recipient. Bone marrow has been transplanted primarily as therapy in the treatment of leukemias and the new tissue matching techniques may lead to more successful procedures.

The most frequently transplanted tissue is blood. Next in frequency is the cornea, which was initiated by von Hippel in 1888. The technique was improved by Elschnig, in the 1920s, which resulted in tens of thousands of corneal transplants.

At one time or another, most of the organs or glands of the body have been transplanted, as well as nerves, but with little success. In 1960, immunosuppressants were introduced into the procedures of transplantation which suppress the normal immunity reaction of the host to the donated tissue. These drugs also leave the patient virtually unable to ward off infections, other than those that can be controlled with drugs.

In 1968, Bernard Linn and colleagues at the University of Miami Medical School reported that experimental results with dogs indicate that the administration of Egyptian cobra venom extract interferred with the rejection of transplanted pig kidneys by acting on the fourth of the nine complement components in the blood serum and left the other components available for protection against infections. More recently, the drug Cyclosporin A has been found to suppress the graft-rejecting immune response, leaving the protective immune response intact to combat infections. The drug was approved for use by the FDA in November, 1983.

Kidney transplants were initiated in humans in 1950. In 1968, there were approximately 1100 surviving patients with this type of transplant. In 1971, 1610 patients received kidney transplants. Today, a cadaver kidney transplant has about a 50% chance of surviving in the patient for two years. Congress has

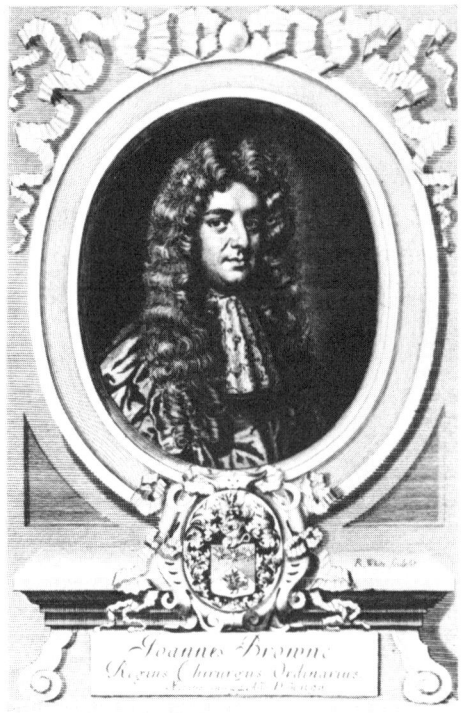 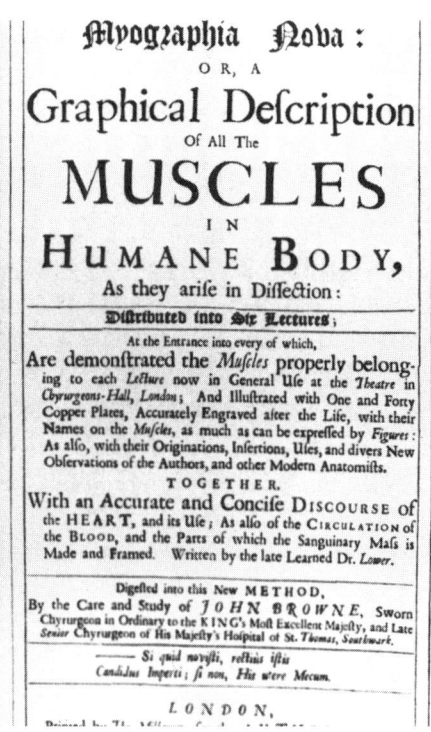

The title pages of Joannes Browne's "Myographia Nova," London, 1697. (Reproduced from Medicina Rara Ltd., New York.)

passed a law providing Medicare reimbursement for kidney transplantation or artificial kidney treatment for any patient with an end-stage kidney disease. Perhaps in the future we shall see other transplants handled in this manner so as to be available for anyone in need.

Other organs which have been transplanted in humans, such as the liver, lungs, spleen and pancreas, have not been very successful and are not, at the present, being routinely carried out.

Today everyone is a candidate for the surgeon as surgery rapidly approaches the status of a public utility. Insurance companies and the government provide the money; hospitals are the facilities; surgeons are the providers and patients are the consumers. Only the dead are immune to the knife of the surgeon unless there is an autopsy called for; or the body has been donated to a medical school; or the body is utilized in transplants, having many spare parts that can be used by the living.

Many scientists and physicians believe that the future of the replacing of portions of the human body lies with the use of artificial parts made by man, from such materials as Teflon, plastics, pyrolytic carbon, titanium and other alloys, stainless steel, Dacron and others, which are chemically inert, and therefore are not rejected by the immune systems of the body. Artificial bones have been implanted which are made of titanium and other alloys and tendons have been replaced or repaired with cords of Dacron. Ball-and-socket type joints are being replaced with artificial ones of plastic and steel, as are the joints of the knees, elbows, shoulders and knuckles. Tubes of synthetic fibers, mainly Dacron, are being used in the repairing of the blood vessels, while heart valves are being replaced with pyrolytic carbon or titanium. Patients who have undergone a laryngectomy may now have an air system installed which allows them to speak. Electronic stimulators have been installed in the ears of patients with hearing problems, and the University of Utah's researchers are experimenting with a system that could stimulate the auditory vision unit utilizing a television camera in a glass eye which stimulates electrodes in the brain. A miniaturized dialysis machine is under development for kidney patients which can be carried over the shoulder. At the Texas Heart Institute, and elsewhere, investigators are working on pumps to assist damaged hearts. A completely artificial heart was implanted in a calf which walked around for almost a month before dying from a blood clot. Perhaps in the future, hospitals will have spare parts catalogues as the auto-repair shops do today.

When one reviews the history of medicine, it can easily be noted that the majority of advances have occurred within the last one hundred years, although advances in the study of human anatomy occurred much earlier. In the early civilizations of the world priests and sorcerers were organized into various groups, one of which practiced medicine and had schools of instruction for these "physicians." Physicians and medical schools were probably established in ancient Egypt in approximately 3000 B.C., and medical papyri were probably in use, although the oldest surviving one dates to about 2000 B.C. Similar physicians and schools probably existed in Mesopotamia, although it is not certain. India and China appear to enter the field of medicine at a later time and, although by tradition, some of their works are dated to 1500 B.C. (India) or 2900 B.C. (China) the author believes that they are of a much later date.

The Egyptians appear to have made the earliest attempts in the descriptions of diseases, human anatomy, circulation of the blood and observations of the brain. These were utilized by the Greeks, along with knowledge obtained from Mesopotamia, Persia and India, who made the next advances in the descriptions of diseases, their causes and treatments, and in descriptions of human anatomy. Chinese medicine was influenced by India and later, by Persia and Greece. Few advances were made until Vesalius undertook the study of human anatomy (1543), and Louis Pasteur associated microorganisms with diseases (1860s). Vesalius and Pasteur probably did more to advance medicine than any other persons in the history of medicine.

Although chemicals had been utilized in antiquity in medicine, arsenic, antimony, copper and mercury, it was not until 1910 that Ehrlich produced Salvarsan, a copper-arsenic derivative effective in syphilis treatment. A sulfa drug had been discovered in 1908, but it took about twenty years to find out how useful the sulfa drugs could be. The sulfa drugs overshadowed the discovery of penicillin, by Fleming, in 1929 and it was not rediscovered until 1938, when its use brought about the search for other antibiotics.

The discoveries in the last one hundred years, both large and small, in medicine and associated fields are enormous and have led to specialization in many fields because there is just too much material with which to become familiar. The libraries are filled with books and journals concerned with every phase of medicine and associated sciences. Many countries of the world are now engaged in socialized medicine which guarantees the treatment of everyone. Other countries still rely on the private physician, while others have a combination of both systems. There are also cultures of the world that have no advanced medicine and still rely on their medicine men. The World Health Organization has extended modern medicine into all parts of the world with the resultant increase in life expectancy and an increase in the population of the world. The increased use of drugs and chemicals has led to an increase in the resistance of microorganisms, insects and vectors of diseases to the drugs which once were effective in their control. What will happen in the future is unknown, but warnings can be seen in cases of antibiotic-resistant bacteria, drug-resistant malarial parasites, insecticide-resistant insects and Wafarin-resistant rats. Will science and medicine learn how to control these organisms before they have a major effect on the human population of the world?

new diseases and those which have vanished

Some diseases appear and disappear with the seasons while others may disappear for centuries and then suddenly reappear, baffling epidemiologists. Other diseases may have their numbers decreased or entirely eliminated due to vaccination procedures or changes in the environment or changes in the diet or may be due to unknown causes. New diseases may appear which can be traced to changes in the diet or environment. Others may result from the transfer of a microorganism to a new host or through the mutation of the causative agent.

Chlorosis disappeared from Europe and the United States following World War I. It had commonly affected females up to the age of twenty-five, causing a greenish pallor of the skin due to an iron-deficiency anemia. The exact reason why the disease has disappeared has never been established.

Encephalitis lethargica appeared in epidemics in the United States and Europe between 1919 and 1926. During the acute stage of the disease, there was damage to the central nervous system which later, in approximately 80% of the survivors, caused a form of Parkinson's Disease, paralysis agitans. Although a pandemic of Influenza A occurred at the same time as the encephalitis lethargica, Parkinson's Disease has not been linked to other Influenza A epidemics, so the reasons for the appearance and disappearance of this disease are unknown.

Ergot epidemics, caused by the fungus *Claviceps purpurea* growing on the fruiting heads of rye grains, were widespread in Europe, especially during the Middle Ages, but are now rare. The symptoms of the disease, hallucination, black leg (vascular necrosis) and other distresses were well known before the science of mycology (study of fungi) was established. The disease was eliminated by not using infected rye grains for eating purposes. This mold, and others such as *Cladosporium cladosporides, Fusarium javanicum, Fusarium moniliforme, Aspergillus flavus* (aflatoxin), *Stachybotrys alterans, Pithomyces chartarum, Penicillium viridicatum* and *Penicillium rubrum* have all been found to produce dangerous toxins which can cause severe sickness and death in humans and animals, when foods contaminated with the mold or its toxin are consumed.

Peptic ulcers were found primarily affecting the stomachs of young women about 150 years ago. Today, this condition has become primarily, a disorder of the small intestine in middle-aged men and scientists do not know why.

Rheumatic Fever, a complication of infections with bacteria of the Genus *Streptococcus,* was very common about thirty years ago all around the world. Today, it is quite rare in advanced countries. It is believed that either the strains of streptococci which caused the Rheumatic Fever have disappeared, for unknown reasons, or that the early treatment of streptococcal infections with antibiotics prevents the complication from developing.

Smallpox, caused by the variola virus, used to appear in great epidemics, causing great numbers of deaths around the world. In 1980, the World Health Organization declared that the disease had been eradicated from the world by vaccination procedures. The virus is still maintained in a few laboratories for research purposes.

Stomach Cancer has undergone a dramatic decline in the United States which scientists cannot account for. Between 1937 and 1976, this most common type of cancer fell from second place to ninth place in its incidence rate.

English Sweating Disease occurred in several epidemics in England between 1486 and 1551. This acute, frequently fatal, infection was characterized by chills, profuse sweating and vomiting. The disease disappeared for about 200 years and then reappeared in a milder form in Europe, its last appearance being in 1907. Similar outbreaks were reported from the Soviet Union in 1932 and from Mexico in 1926. The cause of this infection is unknown.

Trembles occurred in the United States, in the Mississippi River Valley in the 1700's to 1800's. The symptoms were abdominal pain, fever, vomiting and an intense thirst. The disease first occurred in cattle which had eaten a plant, the white snakeroot, which contained a toxin which caused the disease. People who drank the milk from, or ate the meat from infected cattle developed the disease. The disease disappeared as pasture land was cultivated, eliminating the white snakeroot from the diet of the cattle.

Legionnaires' Disease was first recognized in 1976 at a convention of the American Legion in Philadelphia, Pa. The causative agent was found to be *Legionella pneumophilia,* a bacterium which caused a severe respiratory disease. The microorganism was found in contaminated aerosols from air-conditioning systems and shower units. For treatment, the drugs of choice are erythromycin and rifampin.

Toxic Shock Syndrome (TSS) was first identified in 1980 and since that time, statistics compiled by the U.S. Center for Disease Control (CDC), show that the number of reported cases have dropped by more than 70%. However, the CDC estimates that only 10% of the actual TSS cases are being reported to them. TSS is caused by the bacterium *Staphylococcus aureus* which is generally a part of the normal bacterial flora of most people, and which produces a toxin which causes TSS. Approximately 95% of the population has been exposed to the bacterium and shows antibodies to the toxin by the age of 20 years. The remaining 5% of the population is at risk to TSS. Rely tampons, used by menstruating females, were linked to 71% of the 50 TSS cases reported to the CDC during the 2 months prior to September 1980, when the tampons were removed from the market. However, TSS is still here and is still linked to the use of tampons, contraceptive sponges and childbirth. According to the CDC, in 1984, 93% of the TSS cases involved menstruating women and approximately 96% of these women were using tampons. Therefore, it would greatly reduce the incidence of TSS if females would stop using tampons or, if they insist on using tampons, to change them frequently to prevent the multiplication of the bacteria and the production of the toxin.

Cysticercosis is a parasite (tapeworm) infection which has been extremely rare in people in the United States, although the infective larval forms, cysticerci, are occasionally found in pigs. However, the U.S. Center for Disease Control has reported that the number of cases of Cysticercosis has increased 63% between 1978 and 1982, and that 62% of these cases came from states bordering Mexico. Between 1973 and 1983, approximately 500 cases were reported at four Los Angeles hospitals alone. Over 90% of the patients were Hispanic, and most were Mexicans, but 12 cases occurred in U.S. citizens who had not traveled out of the United States.

The pork tapeworm, *Taenia solium,* may be found in the intestinal tract of humans, where ova (eggs) are passed with the feces. The ova are ingested by intermediate hosts such as domesticated and wild pigs, sheep, deer, dogs and cats, and cysticerci develop in the tissues of these hosts. When the infected "measly" meat of these animals is eaten without proper cooking (50°C at ½ hour/pound of meat), the cysticerci are dissolved and the contained larvae develop into adult worms attached to the intestinal tract, producing more ova to continue the cycle.

Sometimes, people become the intermediate hosts by ingesting the ova and then, cysticerci can be found in any organ or tissue of their bodies. Since the ova from the adult tapeworms are passed in the feces, this means that people are eating or drinking foods and beverages contaminated with infected fecal material from infected people or animals. Muscle and brain tissue are the usual infected sites but the cysticerci can also be found in the eyes, heart or lungs. The symptoms depend upon the infected site.

When the brain is infected, the patient may show signs of epilepsy, encephalitis, brain atrophy and abnormal behavior. Treatments include surgery and drug therapy. In the drug therapy, the destruction of the cysticerci causes a severe immune reaction in most of the patients.

To prevent more infections, it is recommended that: adult tapeworms be removed from infected people; correct sewerage treatment and water purification be accomplished; strict sanitation procedures be used in all food and beverage handling; there be inspection of all pork products; all pork products be cooked thoroughly; people be instructed in more thorough personal hygiene.

Opportunistic fungi have been found to cause infections in many people today, whereas 20 years ago, these infections in humans were rare. A decrease in the natural immune system can allow these infections to occur or various types of chemical therapies can destroy the normal flora of the body, allowing the fungi to grow. Certain chemical therapies may also reduce the natural immune system, allowing infection.

AIDS and *AIDS Related Complex* are diseases of humans which are believed to have started as an infection in monkeys that was transmitted to people and eventually developed into an extremely lethal disease. In Senegal, Africa, African Green Monkeys carry a virus very closely related to the human AIDS virus but the monkeys do not show any signs of the disease. A similar AIDS-like virus has also been found in two research colonies of sooty mangabey and rhesus monkeys. The mangabey monkeys, like the African green monkeys, do not become sick with the infection, but the rhesus monkeys become ill and their immune systems are destroyed in much the same way humans are affected. In Africa, many of the native people have antibodies to the AIDS virus, but do not show any signs of the disease.

Apparently, when the virus was transported out of Africa, a mutation occurred and the virus became lethal. It first appeared in 1982, affecting mainly male homosexuals, prostitutes and intravenous drug users in Europe and the Americas. Some cases were also traced to blood transfusions from infected people. The causative agent is believed to be the HTLV-3 virus. Ten percent of the people who carry the virus will develop AIDS and 25% of the carriers will develop ARC. The Center for Disease Control estimated that there are already one million people infected and that by the end of 1986, 40,000 cases will have developed in the United States.

Several anti-viral drugs are being tested which inhibit viral replication or inhibit viral enzymes or break the viral envelop. These are: Suramin; Azido thymidine (AZT or S,BW A509U); AL721; HPA-23; Ribavarin (virazole); Foscarnet (phosphono-formate); and Interferon. How effective these drugs will be in controlling viral diseases is unknown at the time of this writing.

Cancer Therapy: In November 1985, the National Cancer Institute announced that a novel technique had been used on 25 advanced cancer patients which produced measurable reductions, by more than 50%, in the tumor sizes of eleven of the patients. One patient, not in the project, died during the treatment procedure. The procedure involves removing about 10 billion white blood cells from the patient and culturing the cells in a solution containing *interleukin-2*. This substance is a genetically engineered version of the protein interleukin-2 which is produced in the human body by certain immune system cells. The process apparently turns some of the white blood cells into "killer cells" which attack the abnormal cancer growths. The "killer cells" and the interleukin-2 are then injected back into the patient and, hopefully, will attack the cancer cells. The procedure must be repeated over a period of weeks and is very expensive.

Index

—A—
Abram (Abraham) 35, 38, 57, 62
Acanthocheilonema perstans 32
Achondroplastic dwarf 14
Acupuncture 117, 122-123
Adam 36
Aesculapius 4, 134-136
Agamemnon 133
Age of the Five Rulers 108, 113
Age of the Three Sovereigns 108, 113
AIDS 234
Akhenaton (Ikhnaton) 26, 27
Akkadians 64
Alexander, the Great 74, 87, 132
Amenhotep IV 26, 27
Americas, the 155-194
Amphotericin B 34
Amulet 23
Anemia 231
Ankhesenpaamon 27
Anthrax 216
Antibiotics 221, 222, 234
Antimony 19, 20, 22, 26, 44
Anti-viral drugs 234
Anubis 10
Apache (Indians) 176
Apollo 134
Arabia 35
A.R.C. 234
Ariadne 132, 133
Aristotle 146
Aryans 81, 82
Ascaris lumbricoides 77, 78
Asepsis 205, 210-211, 214
Ashoka 87
Ashurbanipol 71
Aswan 8, 14, 26
Atahualpa 182, 192
Atharna Veda 83
Athothis (zer) 13
Atlantis 4
Atreus 133
Atum 7
Avicenna 149
Ayur Veda 88
Aztecs 157, 160

—B—
Babylon 35, 62, 73
Badianus Manuscript 168, 171
Balboa 181
Ban Chiang (Thailand) 23
Beer 8
Beetles 49, 50
Behring, E. 220
Bennu (bird) 7
Bingham, H. 192

Boils 44
Brahma 85
Braidwood 61
Bubonic plague 56
Buddha 86
Budge, E. A. W. 150
Byblos 9

—C—
Cacao (chocolate) 173
Caduceus 53
Cancers 38, 234
Cancer therapy 234
Carter, H. 27
Cattle 43-45
Cauterization 24, 207
Century (*Agave*) plant 173
Chaldeans 35
Charaka Samhita 87, 97-102
Charles V 164, 182, 200
Chaulmoogra oil 94
Cheops (Khufu) 32, 47, 159
Chin Shih-huang-ti 108
China 107-129
Chlorosis 231
Cholera 95-97
Cholula 159, 162
Circulatory system 200, 201
Circumcision 38, 50
Cobra 41
Cocaine 188
Coccidioidomycosis 178-179
Columbus, C. 155, 195
Copernicus 197
Copper 19, 20, 22
Cortez 157, 159, 160, 162, 163, 164
Crete 131-134
Cryptococcus neoformens 34
Curare 173
Cuzco (Peru) 184
Cyclops 49, 52, 214
Cysticercosis 233

—D—
Daedalus 132
Darius (Persia) 15, 73, 74, 87
de Landa 164
Dentistry 14, 23, 127
Deucalion 134
Dietary laws (Hebrews) 47-50
Diphtheria 79, 80
Djoser (Zoser) 4
Dorian Greeks 132
Dracunculosis 52, 214
Dravidians 81
Dwarf 14
Dysenteries 120, 121, 214

—E—

Ebers papyrus 15, 17, 20, 200
Edwin Smith papyrus 15-17
Egypt 7-34
Ehrlich, P. 19, 220, 221
Elephantiasis 32
Embalming 10, 25, 124, 187
Embryology 201
Encephalitis 44, 231
English sweating disease 232
Epidaurus 135
Epilepsy 78, 79, 145
Ergot 198, 231
Erysipelas 143, 144
Esau (hypertrichosis) 57, 58
Etruscans 132
Evans, A. 132
Eve 12
Exodus 39-41, 46, 47
Ezekial 35

—F—

False-face society 175
Fertile crescent 61
Ficus sp. 52
Fiery serpents 52
Filarial worms 32, 52, 214
Fire walkers 175
Fleming, A. 221
Flexner, A. 203
Flood 8, 37, 108
Fly agaric mushroom 84
Fracastoro 43, 198, 211
Frogs 42
Fu Hsi 108-111
Fungi 231, 234

—G—

Galen 146-148, 196, 200
Galileo 197
Geb 7, 9
Genetic engineering 14
Germs, 213
Giants 37, 209
Gilgamesh 68
Gonorrhea 20, 51, 213, 217
Greece 134-139
Growth hormone 14

—H—

Hammurabi 69-71
Hansen (leprosy) 217
Harappa 81
Harvey, W. 200, 201
Hatshepsut 31-33
Hebrews 35-59
Helen of Troy 133
Herodotus 14, 120, 195
Herpes virus 38, 39
Hippocrates 136, 137, 151
Histoplasma capsulatum 34
History of Liang 156
Hittites 27
Homer 132-135
Hopi (Indians) 156, 157, 162
Hormones 27, 30

Horus 7
Houses of life 14, 15
Huang-Fu Mi 122
Humors (Four) 145, 211
Hunter, J. 208, 209, 213
Hygeia 135
Hypertrichosis 57, 195

—I—

I-Ching 112, 113
Icarus 132
Ikhnaton (Akhenaton) 26, 27
Imhotep 4, 13, 135
Inca(s) 182-194
Incest 27
India 81-106
Indra 84
Inquisition 197, 200
Ipecac 173
Iraq 61
Iron 23
Iroquois (Indians) 175
Iry 13
Isis 7, 9, 10
Itch 118

—J—

Jarmo 61
Jenner, E. 213, 214
Jivaka 86
Joseph 39

—K—

Kali 81, 85
Kheme (Egypt) 2
Khufu (Cheops) 32
Kirlian photography 117
Ko Hung 122, 125-127
Knossus (Crete) 131, 132
Koch, R. 216-219
Krishna 86
Kukulcan 161

—L—

La Venta 158
Lake Titicaca 186
Lead poisoning 148
Leeching 24
Leevwenhoek, A. van 211
Legionnaires Disease 232
Leishmania braziliensis 189
Leishmania donovani 44
Leprosy 50, 80, 93, 94, 217
Li Shih-Chen 128
Lice 42, 43
Lilith 36
Linnaeus 195
Lister, J. 205, 210, 211
Loa loa 32
Locusts 45, 49

—M—

Maat 7
Macchu Picchu 192-194
Malaria 74-76, 83, 190, 191, 214
Malpighi 201

Mamma Ocllo 183
Manco Capac 183
Manson, P. 214
Mansonella ozzardi 32
Marcus Aurelius 120, 121, 148
Marduk 64, 73
Mayans 158, 159, 162
Medical instruments 15, 70, 71, 88
Medical schools (U.S.A.) 201-205
Menelaus 133
Menes (Narmer) 11
Meritaton 27
Mesopotamia 61-80
Metchnikoff 219, 220
Mexico 157
Microscope 211, 213
Minoans 4
Minos (King) 132, 133
Minotaur 132, 133
Moctezuma 157, 160, 163, 168, 172
Mohammed 149
Monte Verde (Chile) 155
Moses 41
Moslems 87, 149, 150
Moxibustion 117
Mt. Olympus 132
Mt. Parnassus 132
Mu 3, 4
Mummification 4, 39, 123-124, 187-188
Mycenae 131-134

—N—
Narmer (Menes) 11
National Institutes of Health 203
Navaho (Indians) 176
Nebuchadrezzar 35, 54, 73
Necho (Pharaoh) 156
Nefertari 10
Nefertiti 27
Nei-Ching 113-117
Nephthys 7
Nightingale, F. 205, 206
Nile River 7, 9, 10, 43
Nineveh 56, 150
Noah 37, 64
Norsemen 156
Nu Wa 108
Nun 7
Nursing 205, 206
Nut 7

—O—
Obelisk 7
Old Testament 35-39
Olmecs 157, 158
Onchocerca volvulus 32
Osiris 7, 9, 10

—P—
Panacea 135
Pandora 134
Papyri 15-17, 23
Paracelsus 197, 199
Pare 207, 208

Pasiphae 132, 133
Passover 45, 46
Pasteur, L. 215, 216
Penicillin 221
Pepi II 14
Peptic ulcer 232
Petrie, Sir Flinders 12
Peyote 173
Phaedra 132
Philip of Macedon 74
Phlebotomy 23, 24
Phoenicia 155, 156
Phoenix (bird) 7
Pinta 179
Pituitary gland 14, 27, 37
Pizzaro, F. 181-183
Plagues (Egypt) 41-46
Plato 4, 146, 149
Poppy 20
Pork 48
Pre-Olmec 158
Prometheus 133
Punt 31-33
Pyramids 32-34, 159
Pyrrha 134
Pythoness 132, 134

—Q—
Quetzalcoatl 161, 162
Quinine 190, 191
Quipus 183

—R—
Ra 7
Rabies 66, 216
Rama (India) 93
Rauwolfia serpentina 98
Red Sea 31
Reed, W. 182
Rhazes 149
Rheumatic fever 232
Rickettsia prowazeki 43
Rickettsia tsutsugamushi 125-127
Rig-Veda 82
Ringworm 215
Rome 146-149
Roundworms 77
Rudolphi 214

—S—
Salvarsan 221
Santorini (Thera) 4, 45, 132
Sarcophagus 9
Sargon 64, 65, 71
Sarsaparilla 173, 177
Sasruta Samhita 87-97, 200
Scabies 118-119
Schistosomiasis 9, 26
Schliemann 132
Scorpion 10
Scorpion King 12
Scurvy 54, 55, 181
Sekhet-n-Ankh 14
Sekhmet 8
Sennacherib 56, 71
Serpent 8, 135

Serquet (Selket) 10
Set 7, 9
Shiva 81, 85
Shu 7
Silver bullet 19, 220, 221
Sioux (Indians) 175
Smallpox 121, 122, 148, 213
Smenkhkare 27
Smith papyrus 16, 17, 200
Smith, T. 218
Solon 4
Spallanzini 213
Spell 8, 10, 50-51
Strychnine 173
Sulfa drugs 221
Sumerian deluge (flood) 67, 68
Sumerians 61, 64
Surgery 207-211, 223-228
Syphilis 19, 128, 155, 173, 179, 180, 181, 187, 192, 198, 213, 220, 221

—T—

Taglicozzi, G. 208
Tapeworm 48, 49, 214, 233
Tefnut 7
Tell-el Amarna 27
Tenochtitlan (Mexico City) 157, 160, 164-166, 172
Teotihuacan 159, 160
Tezcatlipoca 162
Thera (Santorini) 4, 45, 132
Theseus 132, 133
Thoth 4, 9, 10, 13
Thutmosis 3
Tiahuanaco 186
Tiamat 64
Tici Viracocha 183
Tobacco 173
Toltecs 157, 160, 162, 163
Tom Thumb 14
Tower of Babel 62
Toxic Shock Syndrome 232
Tracoma 22, 43
Tranquilizers 98
Transplants 11, 225, 226
Trembles 232
Trepanning 23, 144, 188
Trichinosis 48, 214

Troy 132, 133
Tsutsugamushi fever 125-127
Tuberculosis 177, 178, 217-219
Tula 157, 160
Tularemia 47
Tutankhamon 27
Typhoid fever 79, 217
Typhus fever 43, 83, 84

—U—

Ubaids 61
Ur 35, 62, 65
Usaphais 13

—V—

Vaccines 215, 216
Valdivia (Ecuador) 155
Varro 211
Vasco da Gama 181
Vedas 82
Verruga 155, 189
Vesalius, A. 200
Vishnu 86
Vitamins 20, 55

—W—

Wall of China 108
Wasson 84
Wine 8
Witch of Endor 53
Witch trials 54, 197
Wooley, L. 62
Wuchereria bancrofti 32
W. malayi 32

—X—

Xenopsylla cheopis 43, 56

—Y—

Yang and Yin 108, 116, 211
Yaws 180, 221
Yellow fever 182

—Z—

Zenograft 11
Zeus 132, 133
Ziggurat 62
Zuisudra 67, 68
Zumarraga 164